ROY J. SHEPHARD is Professor of Applied Physiology in the Department of Preventive Medicine and Biostatistics, Division of Community Health, Faculty of
Medicine, University of Toronto. He is a former president of the Canadian Association of Sports Sciences and of the American College of Sports Medicine. He
has written a number of books in applied physiology and sports medicine.

Endurance Fitness provides detailed coverage of the scientific principles on which
the general theories of physical fitness are based. It treats the subject from a
sound physiological and medical point of view, and provides a careful synthesis
of knowledge in this complex area.

This second edition has been completely rewritten, to reflect recent advances
in the field. It presents a thorough historical review as well as analyses of topics
such as the importance of cardio-respiratory fitness and techniques for its measurement, the problem of factors limiting oxygen transfer, overnutrition, obesity,
muscular development, and the influence of tobacco, drugs, and alcohol in fitness. The author discusses the role of physical activity in the prevention and
treatment of disease (particularly cardiovascular disease), and points out the economic costs both of being unfit and of promoting good health.

Dr Shephard has drawn upon his considerable experience as a member of
national and international organizations concerned with physical activity, as
director of the Fitness Research Unit at the University of Toronto and as a
teacher of graduate and undergraduate courses in Exercise Physiology.

ROY J. SHEPHARD, MD, PhD

Endurance Fitness

SECOND EDITION

UNIVERSITY OF TORONTO PRESS

Toronto and Buffalo

First edition
© University of Toronto Press 1969

Second edition
© University of Toronto Press 1977
Toronto and Buffalo

Printed in Canada

Library of Congress Cataloging in Publication Data

Shephard, Roy J

    Endurance fitness.
    Bibliography: p.
    Includes index.
    1. Physical fitness. 2. Exercise – Physiolog-
ical effect. I. Title.
    QP301.S48 1976   613.7   76-23257
    ISBN 0-8020-2250-2
    ISBN 0-8020-2251-0 pbk

This book has been published during the
Sesquicentennial year of the University of Toronto

To Muriel, Sarah, and Rachel

Contents

ix Contents

Preface to first edition

Sarah, who was seven at the time of my announcement, was not surprised when I said that I had decided to write a book. After all, she had just compressed the experiences of a lifetime into six neatly printed pages of manuscript headed 'Cats are Lovely.' However, she stipulated quite firmly that I should show her the book when it was finished later that week.

Unfortunately, I soon discovered that my chosen topic of 'endurance fitness' could neither be constrained to six pages nor committed to book form within one week. I felt that Sarah had certain advantages over me. She needed no preface. Everyone knew what a cat was, but this was by no means true of fitness. A sizable majority of girls agreed that cats were lovely, but a majority verdict in favour of fitness was less certain. Sarah even had a known and guaranteed readership – her long-suffering teacher and a few of her friends who would giggle over witticisms in a corner of the school yard; I felt intuitively that there was a place for a monograph on endurance fitness written for recent graduates in exercise physiology and the emerging discipline of physical education, but I could not test this hypothesis without first writing such a book.

The past few years have seen an amazing explosion of knowledge in many disciplines, and this is certainly true of exercise physiology. To take a very parochial example, the Fitness Research Unit in the University of Toronto has contributed over fifty papers on exercise physiology to the world literature in the last triennium. During the last year, I have edited the proceedings of one symposium on physical activity and cardiovascular health, and at least five others have appeared from different corners of the globe. In each of these symposia thirty to seventy learned authors write of fitness from disparate points of view. The controversy they have created is healthy and stimulating to the experienced research worker, but is confusing to the senior student and recent graduate, who seek a more synthesized and balanced account of the current situation.

Without being unduly immodest, I suppose that I may claim several qualifications for writing a book to meet this need. Firstly, while I think physical fitness may be beneficial to health, I am by no means certain; I would not detract from those who stand at the street corner urging people to join them in the gymnasium. They are probably right. But they are not the best men to write scientific books on fitness. Secondly, while I have considerable interest in physical education as a teacher of both graduate and undergraduate students, my primary allegiances are to physiology and medicine. I thus have no partisan urge to stake out areas of knowledge as the exclusive prerogative of a newly recognised graduate species; indeed, my personal belief is that the current complexity of knowledge demands an interdisciplinary rather than a compartmentalized approach, and I hope that this book may serve a useful purpose in breaking down a few of the artificial barriers that some seek to create. Thirdly, I have had the privilege of meeting many of the world's leading exercise physiologists over the past few years as I have worn various fitness 'hats' – chairman of the International Symposium on Physical Activity and Cardiovascular Health, director of the IBP working party on the standardization of methods for the measurement of working capacity, and rapporteur for the WHO expert committee on 'exercise tests and cardiovascular function.' Thus, although I may write with the appearance of personal expertise, my thinking has been subconsciously shaped by many great minds to which I have had the good fortune to be exposed, and to each an appropriate acknowledgement is due.

You will have gathered from my extensive use of the personal pronoun that I do not intend this book to be unnecessarily pontifical. One of the most refreshing monographs I have read in recent years is Alan C. Burton's *Biophysics of the Circulation*. Here is information presented in a pleasant and personal way. It would be impossible to approach Burton's style, but I do hope to treat the topic within the context of my personal research adventures, perhaps lightening the reader's burden by an occasional touch of humour.

It is customary to conclude a preface by enumerating the N or $N - 1$ specific individuals to whom one is indebted. My debts are so enormous, I am afraid even to contemplate their totality in print. However, I do wish to thank all who have been associated with me in the various research endeavours to be discussed, with a special word of gratitude to my very loyal secretary, Mrs. Esther Gair. I must also express my thanks to the staff of the School of Hygiene, in general, and to Dr. J.R. Brown, head of the Department of Physiological Hygiene, in particular, for unfailing support and encouragement. The generous financial support of the Directorate of Fitness and Amateur Sport, Department of National Health and Welfare, and the Ontario Heart Foundation is also gratefully acknowledged.

Toronto, September 1968   R.J.S.

Preface to second edition

Sarah is now a young lady of sixteen, and her current school assignments are much more likely to discuss the niceties of newtons than the loveliness of cats. In the years that have elapsed since the appearance of the first edition of this book, the topic of endurance fitness has shown a parallel growth and maturation. Governments are increasingly aware of the need for fitness as a means of controlling expenditures on health care. The study of 'positive health' has become the concern of a steadily expanding company of scientists. National meetings attract many hundreds of participants, not only in Canada, the United States, and Europe, but also in the distant corners of Asia and South America. Exciting discoveries are being reported with increasing frequency, and even more than in 1968 the problem seems a plethora of facts that most investigators have time neither to digest nor to read.

The ferment of new knowledge has infected every aspect of our topic. The history of man's interest in physical activity, the encyclopaedic studies of human working capacity carried out by the International Biological Programme, the random sampling of fitness in adult populations, the development of home fitness tests, the training of 'post-coronary' patients for marathon running, and the use of anabolic steroids are but a few areas where major advances have been made. Almost the entire text has been rewritten to reflect this progress. Inevitably, the length of the typescript has doubled, and the bibliography has expanded from some 360 to over 1300 items. The time has also seemed appropriate to introduce the exercise physiologist to the shocks of metrication and international standard units. It is now necessary to understand kilonewtons, kilojoules, kilopascals, and molar concentrations of gases in order to talk to our children. The transition to such terminology may even help us in discussing our problems with fellow scientists in other disciplines.

Despite extensive revision, the basic format of the original work has been retained. The aim remains to present as simply and clearly as possible current knowledge of endurance fitness, with particular reference to the health of the average sedentary city-dweller.

Toronto, April 1976   R.J.S.

ENDURANCE FITNESS

1
Introduction

THE DEFINITION OF ENDURANCE FITNESS

The definition of fitness has puzzled physiologists for several generations. When I was a student my professor felt the term so vague as to be devoid of scientific meaning, and he resolutely prohibited its use. H.E. Johnson (1946) wrote at about this time: 'Quantitative assessment of physical fitness is one of the most complex and controversial problems in applied physiology. This situation arises in part from lack of general agreement on what constitutes fitness for withstanding various types of stress, and in part from lack of agreement on what measurements allow valid comparisons to be made among different individuals exposed to the same stress.'

Twenty-one years later an expert committee of the World Health Organization wrestled with the same problem in Geneva (Shephard, 1968a). After struggling with seven successive drafts of a definition of fitness, the committee reached some measure of agreement mainly because the time available for discussion was exhausted! I may thus be accused of undue temerity in offering a definition here. However, I venture to do so, partly because it is easier to reach agreement with a committee of one, and partly because it is essential that both reader and author clarify their thoughts at the outset of this book.

The purposes for which fitness is sought legitimately include the physical, social, and psychological well-being of the human organism – in fact, the broad field of human ecology. We are dealing with man's total adaptation to his environment (Shephard, 1974f); as E.C. Davis et al. (1961) put it: 'total fitness is really a capacity for living.' Tempting as broad fields are, they do not lend themselves to concise and logical description. Social and psychological adjustments are in many respects distinctive problems, and this book will thus be concerned mainly with physical fitness. However, our initial circumscription of interest is hardly sufficient. Individuals regard physical fitness very differently, depending upon their interests, occupation, age, and sex.

Many authors have conceived physical fitness in terms of athletic perform-ance. Thus P.O. Åstrand and K. Rodahl (1970) write: 'physical performance or fitness is determined by the individual's capacity for energy output (aerobic and anaerobic processes), neuro-muscular function (muscle strength and technique) and psychological factors (e.g. his motivation and tactics).' However, the aspiring Olympic athlete seeks a standard of fitness for his chosen sport much higher than that demanded or indeed needed by the average citizen. The discipline of many hours training per day undoubtedly builds some facets of the athlete's character, but the relentless and solitary pursuit of the Olympic goal by a teenager can lead to a serious neglect of normal social and psychological development. Even the one-sided physical development of a champion weight-lifter can scarcely be re-garded as an optimizing of health. We shall have occasion to refer to the athlete at many points in this book, particularly as an example of what can be accom-plished by a combination of careful selection and rigorous training. However, our main focus will be upon the fitness needs of the ordinary sedentary citizen, metropolitan man, or 'homo sedentarius.'

From the occupational point of view, Karpovich and Sinning (1971) suggest that physical fitness is 'the degree of the ability to execute a specific physical task under specific ambient conditions.' Both the level and the type of fitness required by the individual vary with occupation. While the efficiency of a civil service clerk may be somewhat impaired by a low level of fitness, the problem is much more acute if a miner or a lumberjack is deficient in physical capacity. The latter groups often have difficulty in returning to a normal working day if their fitness has been impaired by bed-rest following industrial injury (Fried and Shep-hard, 1969, 1970). Many physically active occupations call for general endur-ance, but a painter who spends eight hours per day in decorating ceilings will benefit from a specific strengthening of his wrist muscles (I. Åstrand, 1971b) and an airline stewardess may find that retention of her job is contingent upon keeping her body weight below an arbitrary height-related target such as 55 kg.

Authors often ignore the interaction of age and fitness. Their writings seem to assume that the entire population is of university age! How does the perception of fitness change with maturation? At age 20, the male undergraduate seeks the fitness that will earn him a place on the varsity team. At age 30, the objective has altered to a fitness that will control a bulging waistline and give a greater sense of 'well-being.' At age 40, the same person may know several colleagues who have fallen prey to a myocardial infarction (the 'heart attack' of popular parlance), and he now wants a fitness that will minimize his risk of developing overt cardiovascular disease. At age 50, a new problem appears: 'working capacity' has shrunk to the point where many previously simple tasks are becoming quite formidable. Our subject now hopes simply to develop sufficient fitness to meet the demands of the office or factory, travelling, and the home without undue fatigue, leaving him some margin of energy to enjoy his leisure and cover occasional emergencies.

Man in general has a fair perception of his current fitness level as measured by the tools of the physiologist. On the other hand, there is little relationship between laboratory measurements of endurance fitness such as maximum oxygen intake (page 113) and a woman's rating of her fitness (Bailey, Shephard, et al., 1974). Bowing to the decrees of traditional western culture, a woman rates her fitness in terms of a good figure, a good posture, and a good body carriage.

No single definition of fitness could cover the needs and desires of both men and women at all ages. However, it is possible to move towards the firmer ground of traditional physiology if we make an arbitrary classification of physical fitness in terms of the period of activity that is required. In brief effort (less than one minute duration) physical effort depends upon muscle strength, coordination, agility, flexibility, reaction times, and motivation, together with the rate and extent of development of an oxygen debt in the active tissues. In activity of moderate duration (one minute to one hour), physical fitness is still influenced by almost all of these factors, but they become progressively subordinate to the ability of the body to transfer oxygen from the atmosphere to the working muscles. In protracted activity (longer than one hour) there is again a change of emphasis. Physical fitness becomes increasingly dependent on the extent and availability of the food reserves in the active tissues, and the capacity to replenish these reserves either from the diet or from depots elsewhere within the body. The capacity of the body to dissipate heat, and the establishment of an appropriate balance between the intake of water and its loss in sweat and exhaled gas, also assume increasing importance.

A substantial proportion of athletic events require fitness for brief effort (Shephard, 1976b). The marathon runner, the Eskimo hunter, and the soldier marching for 72 hours in a 'gas-mask' are interested in fitness for protracted exercise. But the great mass of ordinary citizens, if they are interested in fitness at all, will be concerned with fitness for activity of moderate duration, 'endurance fitness' as we shall call it. Endurance fitness is the main determinant of the sustained heavy work that can be performed in the factory and at home, and if we are to show a relationship between the control of obesity, the prevention of cardiovascular disease, and fitness, it will probably be through the striking of a suitable balance between the intake of food and the performance of endurance work.

We have now explored in some depth what fitness means to the subject. But what of the investigator? A valid definition of endurance fitness must take account of the latter's interests, and the tools available to him for measurement. As Karpovich and Sinning (1971) point out, all too often 'the so-called degree of fitness possessed by an individual depends on the character of the test ...' Endurance fitness is not synonymous with a large oxygen transport capacity. A full appraisal of endurance fitness should look at such features as the fat content of the body, the strength of key muscles, and the performance of the heart while under load. Nevertheless, the prime factor limiting endurance is the cardio-respiratory transport of oxygen. Information regarding this factor can be obtained by observing either physiological responses to the stress of submaximum or maximum effort, or the rate of recovery of physiological variables following exercise of standard intensity. However, if reliance is placed upon the responses to submaximum effort, the exercise procedure should be as fully learned as possible, to avoid complications from anxiety and clumsiness during performance of the test. Although it is very helpful to supplement the basic cardio-respiratory evaluation with tests of other body systems, we may note also that the person who is obese or who has weak leg muscles will score poorly on many forms of 'cardio-respiratory' appraisal. The so-called 'cardio-respiratory' item is giving an over-all index of ability to perform endurance work.

My definition of endurance fitness is thus 'the ability of a man to maintain the various processes involved in metabolic exchange as close to the resting state as is mutually possible during performance of a strenuous and fully learned task for moderate time (1-60 minutes), with a capacity to reach a higher steady rate of working than the "unfit" and to restore promptly after exercise all equilibria which are disturbed.' I acknowledge at once the debt I owe to Darling (1946) in reaching this definition. It has its faults and limitations, but to my mind it is more helpful than either the terse statement of the WHO committee ('physical fitness is the ability to perform muscular work satisfactorily,' Shephard, 1968a), or the somewhat longer verdict of the American Medical Association Committee on Exercise and Physical Fitness: 'the general capacity to adapt and respond favourably to physical effort. The degree of physical fitness depends on the individual's state of health, constitution, and present and previous physical activity' (American Medical Association, 1966).

THE PRACTICAL IMPORTANCE OF FITNESS

How important is endurance fitness to the health and happiness of mankind? There are still many scientists who maintain that the practical value of fitness – or for that matter any other topic of scientific investigation – is not a question to be discussed in polite company. The knowledge of truth is its own reward! I was once required to argue this position before a pair of crusty examiners, and if my memory of the episode is correct, I managed to marshal a reasonable number of points in favour of an esoteric approach to research. Now it is quite possible to find elegant problems for the intellect in the study of endurance fitness. To give but one example, the sequence of integrated adaptations that increase the delivery of oxygen at the onset of exercise, with the attendant questions of lengthy transmission lines and complicated feedback systems, provides a fascinating hunting ground for anyone with an interest in cybernetics (Beaver and Wasserman, 1970; H. Karlsson and Wigertz, 1971; D'Angelo and Torelli, 1971; Whipp, 1972; Vejby-Christensen and Petersen, 1973; Asmussen, 1973). The 'tightening' of the various control loops and the changes in response to a given error signal with endurance training make even more intriguing problems for those who seek intellectual stimulation through fitness research.

However, the morality of the exclusive 'pursuit of truth,' or (phrased more bluntly) the following of personal interests, is being challenged increasingly (Dubos, 1967). Expenditures on scientific research become ever smaller relative to such household necessities as nuclear weapons, cigarettes, and alcohol, but nevertheless the man in the street has a right to see something for his scientific dollar. Despite government pressures, we must admit that the current distribution of scientific talent and resources remains heavily biased in favour of the esoteric, and practical answers remain disappointingly few. This is not to plead for any extension of what is euphemistically called 'ad hoc' work – literature surveys restricted to single national journals, tables of 'normative data' based on poorly standardized methods, and batches of ill-assorted measurements literally thrown into a long-suffering computer without formulation of any discernible hypothesis. Such work is at best a caricature of science, and the fitness field has known more than its fair share of practitioners of this black art. But there is an intermediate ground between the esoteric and the ad hoc that should receive stronger support – research that answers practical questions of human health and happiness, yet preserves the rigorous scientific approach that can add to the sum of human knowledge. I would argue that the budget of the Canadian Department of National Health and Welfare, for example, remains sadly out of balance while there are annual expenditures of $2320 million on health care, yet work directed to the causation and prevention of illness is awarded a mere $124 million (Table 1). There are urgent problems of applied medical research in the areas of human life-style – the interactions of endurance fitness with physical activity, nutrition, and the use of cigarettes and other addictive drugs. What reductions in health care costs would result from a more healthful life-style? And how can a mature adult be persuaded to change the bad habits of a lifetime?

TABLE 1

Some areas of expenditure by the Canadian Department of National Health and Welfare during the fiscal years 1969/70 and 1973/74 (Lalonde, 1974)

Area of expenditure	1969/70 ($ million)	1973/74 ($ million)
Health care	1256	2320
Human biology	31	40
Environment	22	38
Life-style	12	45

Health care Expenditures under this heading include the federal contribution (50%) to provincial hospital, medical, and diagnostic costs; measures to improve the quality, supply, productivity, and distribution of health manpower and services; participation in International Health Services; provision of emergency, Indian, and northern health services; development of a prosthetic health service; and provision of a health service for federal employees.

Human biology This category of funding covers the Medical Research Council budget, but excludes aspects of human biology dealt with through national health grants and departmental laboratories.

Environment This category includes expenditures to safeguard food quality, drug quality, and environmental quality, together with health surveillance measures, including a national reference laboratory for identification of bacteria and viruses, the aviation medical service, and enforcement of international sanitary regulations.

Life-style This category embraces activities related to drug, alcohol, and tobacco abuse, fitness and recreation, nutrition, health education, and measures to control venereal diseases.

There can be little disagreement about the current inactivity of the average city dweller. The most vigorous pursuit is often the walk from the car to the elevator in the morning, and from the elevator to the car in the evening. And how the businessman complains if he cannot park right outside the entrance to his office! In traditional 'heavy' industries most of the physical work is now done by machines, and it is rare to find men who are operating at more than two or three times their basal rate of energy expenditure. In rural areas the arduous sixteen-hour day of the primitive homestead has given place to small-town life, the 'farmer' spending his eight-hour day seated in the padded comfort of an air-conditioned combined harvester. Even the hunters of the Arctic make their journeys in power boats and by snowmobile, and an ever-increasing proportion seek the sheltered pattern of western life.

Laziness is extending to ever younger ages. Primary school children remain naturally active, but from their early teens many of the current generation take much less exercise than their parents did. This is a relatively new phenomenon.

TABLE 2

Annual loss of productive years to Canadian society through deaths
occurring between the ages of 1 and 70 years (Lalonde, 1974)

Cause of death	Males	Females
Motor vehicle accidents	154,000	59,000
Ischaemic heart disease	157,000	36,000
Other accidents	136,000	43,000
Respiratory diseases	90,000	50,000
Suicide	51,000	18,000
Total (for five main causes only)	588,000	206,000

When I was attending school (during World War II) the majority of seventeen-year-old British boys could (and did) cycle quite long distances – eighty or ninety miles in six hours, six or seven hundred miles during a week's holiday. Yet now few older teenagers even own a bicycle. The long-term health effects of limited activity during the pubertal growth spurt seems a vital question posed by our present culture.

Again, what is the relationship between physical activity and cardiovascular health? Cardiovascular disease has assumed epidemic proportions in western nations. The commonest cause of death is an accident if your age lies between 1 and 44 years, some form of cardiovascular episode if you are 45 to 60, and 'cancer' if you are over 60. Looking at the years of productive life lost to Canada through deaths occurring between the ages of 1 and 70 years (Table 2), we see that ischaemic heart disease heads the list for men, accounting for 157,000 of 588,000 lost years. Unfortunately, those dying of 'heart attacks' tend to be the most productive members of the community – the managerial and executive classes in general, and the managers and executives with the most drive in particular. Ischaemic heart disease typically strikes at the most fruitful period of a man's career, and if we add to the sobering total of deaths those seriously incapacitated by non-fatal attacks, the probable economic loss from this type of illness assumes staggering proportions. There is a strong hint that lack of endurance fitness increases the risk of developing overt degenerative cardiovascular disease, but neither scientists nor those who allocate the funds for research have yet awakened fully to the health potential of exploring and exploiting this association.

And what of the spectre of automation? Ever since World War II economists have been warning us that the age of leisure and the two-day working week were just around the corner. It has been a longish corner, and you may feel the economists have miscalculated. Despite periodic recessions, in many countries the usual complaint is still that too many jobs chase too few people. However, several by-products of automation are already with us. The hard core of unemployed is rising in most countries. Many of those without work lack the personality or the intelligence to cope with modern machinery. They never will find employment, yet they deserve meaningful leisure rather than a lifetime of bleak and impoverished 'welfare.' An increasing number of companies are now adopting four- and even three-day working weeks; there is thus a need to examine the new patterns of fitness demanded by longer working days and longer weekends. There has also been a rapid growth of service industries, with an ever-increasing trend to expendable consumer goods. Irrespective of his working hours, my father never had time on his hands – there were always the family shoes to mend, the car to repair, or the vegetable garden to weed. Now, it is almost impossible to buy material to repair shoes, an annual visit to the car-dealer is essential to self-respect, and if you are sufficiently old-fashioned to prefer a house to an apartment, the vegetable garden is replaced by a neatly manicured lawn tended by a landscape gardener. The man of the house is robbed of his traditional role. How large a part can voluntary physical activity play in satisfying the search of the city-dweller for fulfilment, and in preserving his capacity to follow a simpler pattern of life if this is forced upon him by the current wastage of non-renewable resources?

Finally, let us suppose that endurance fitness has a positive effect on both immediate happiness and ultimate health. What is the most effective method of persuading someone thoroughly habituated to a life of sloth to undertake regular exercise? How much exercise should we recommend, and how often and for how long should it be performed? If the sluggard persists with his exercises, will he become a champion athlete, or will he be just an active sluggard?

These are some of the questions I propose to explore in subsequent chapters. Despite vigorous research over the past decade, there are still areas where it will be necessary to point to work that needs undertaking rather than present in tabloid form the agreed conclusions of notable authorities. However, there seems to be merit in illuminating gaps in our knowledge of endurance fitness, for if these gaps can be filled the potential improvement in the health and productivity of the world community may well repay manyfold the immediate costs of such research.

2

Development of
current concepts of fitness

In tracing the development of our current concepts of fitness, it is convenient to study first the dominant patterns of activity in successive civilizations, and then the more specific probings of enquiring minds within these civilizations.

CULTURAL PATTERNS OF ACTIVITY

Pre-history
Man, as a tool-carrying mammal, apparently emerged from other primates some 600,000 years ago. In this palaeolithic period, survival depended partly upon the natural riches of the immediate habitat, and partly upon an individual's success in hunting wild animals and birds or his industry in gathering wild fruits, nuts, and berries. Certain tropical and subtropical areas could support a man who worked only a few days per week (Lee, 1972a,b), but in other more hostile natural environments fitness was essential to life. The weakling who survived the shock of birth into a cold and cheerless world rarely reached the age of mating. This happy circumstance, which would have delighted exponents of eugenic breeding, tended to keep the human species at the peak of its genetic potential. Even where time permitted such activity the hunting and gathering society needed no specific measures to preserve its fitness. Models of such physical austerity can still be traced in the 'primitive' tribes of Africa and Oceania, and among some of the American Indians (McIntosh, 1970).

The first steps on the downward path of civilization began about 7000 B.C., when certain tribes discovered the neolithic arts of polishing stones, cultivating crops, and domesticating animals. A more settled existence became possible. Primitive bark huts were built and communities of up to 500 developed in various parts of the world. Life was still hard, but more leisure was possible. Under the leadership of the shaman or medicine man, there were ritual dancing, communal hunting, and other gamelike activities. These were valued mainly for their magico-religious significance, but were often pursued with sufficient vigour to play a useful role in maintaining the fitness of the tribe when other forms of exercise were not necessary for survival. North American Indians set great store in the game of lacrosse (Salter, 1971; Jetté, 1971). Several hundred heavily clothed participants might play for two or three days over a five to ten mile course. The French missionary Brébeuf has described how the village sorcerer would order a 'game of crosse' for a sick patient. The contests also served to prepare the tribes for war, regulated boundary disputes, and appeased the anger of the gods. Some Indian cultures associated a variety of games (archery, bowls, foot-racing, a moccasin game, and wrestling as well as lacrosse) with their funeral rites (Salter, 1972). The painter George Catlin has documented other events – canoe, horse, and foot races, a hoop and pole game, and the snowshoe dance that thanked the great spirit for the first snowfall of winter (Holbrook, 1970).

Many Eskimo sports and pastimes (Shephard, 1974d) such as whipwielding and stone-throwing games seem to have been designed not only to improve hunting skills but also to appease the spirits concerned with hunting. Simri (1969) noted a football game from northern Alaska which was supposed to contribute to good whaling conditions. If the hunt was successful, it was followed by a night of festivities, including *malukatuk* (blanket-tossing) and a lengthy drum dance. Glassford (1970) describes the winter festivities of the dark days (*kaitvitjvik*), with their emphasis on one- and two-person contests that could take place within the confined space of an igloo – arm-straightening, high-kicking (*akaratcheak*), leaping (*orsiktartut*), and drum dancing. In the spring, there were foot and dog races, a one-base ball game (*mukpaum*), and a tug of war between two teams representing the ducks and the ptarmigans. Almost all of these events apparently had both religious and fitness-developing functions.

Almost all of the other residual 'primitive' groups have vigorous physical activities with religious significance. In Meso-America there is evidence that rubber-ball games have been played in a structured court for up to 2000 years (Glassford, 1969). The Aztecs have engaged in wrestling, the Maya in the game of Thlacti, and the Samurai warriors in Jujitsu (Glassford, 1970).

A second major move towards urban life began in Mesopotamia about 4500 B.C., when one of the brighter neolithic men, perhaps watching his children playing by the river, hit upon the idea of irrigation. The combination of rich alluvial soil and the water of the Euphrates permitted the growth of much larger communities, with emergence of a ruling class living upon the industry of others. From this point in history onwards we can trace the evolution of deliberate measures to promote fitness. Initially, their use was restricted to the ruling class, but the gradual spread of leisure expanded their appeal to progressively larger segments of the population. Assyrian records show interest in hunting, swimming, and dancing (Spier, 1970). The Egyptians held contests for boxers, wrestlers, archers, jugglers, and other types of athletes (Simri, 1969; Mutimer, 1970; M.L. Howell, 1971; Ryan, 1974); their pictures suggest that women had opportunity to participate in swimming, certain ball games, archery, and (in the case of the priestesses) sacred dancing (Ziegler, 1972). Teachers in the famous medical school of Alexandria, such as Herophilus and Erasistratus, recognized the therapeutic value of moderate exercise (F. Adams, 1844).

In neighbouring Israel another use of sustained physical activity is documented – the tidings carried by a swift runner. About 1100 B.C., six hundred years before the messenger of Marathon, a 'man of Benjamin' (I Samuel 4:12) covered the 42 kilometres* from Aphek to Shiloh to notify the High Priest Eli of Israel's defeat by the Philistines (Vilnay, 1969).

Nor did other ancient civilizations neglect physical activity. The oldest Chinese historical book, the Shi-Chi, records an interest in energetic games such as *kemari* (a form of football played with a softball) and *dakyu* (a precursor of polo) throughout the legendary period prior to the second century B.C. (Sasajima, 1971). One famous emperor (Ch'ang Ti, 36–32 B.C.) was very fond of football, and when told it was too exhausting and otherwise unsuitable for his imperial majesty, he replied 'what one choses to do is never exhausting.' Dancing was apparently popular in ancient China (Ziegler, 1972). However, in many parts of the east voluntary physical activity declined with the restrictions imposed on his followers by the Gautama Buddha (563–483 B.C.).

Greek and Roman civilizations
Study of pottery and other archaeological artefacts suggests that in the Minoan civilization of Bronze Age Crete (3000–1200 B.C.) there was a substantial amount of sport – tumbling, bull-vaulting, dancing, boxing, wrestling, hunting, archery, and (at least for the soldiers) distance running and swimming. Women seem to have participated in the swimming, hunting, bull-grappling, and chariot-racing (M.L. Howell and Palmer, 1970; Boslooper, 1971; Ziegler, 1972).

The ancient Greeks set great value on the fitness of the individual, regarding it as the basis of good health and of success in war. Asclepiades (126–68 B.C.), a Bithynian physician, recommended diet, massage, walking, and running to his

---

* The distance covered by the messenger of Marathon was approximately 24 miles 1500 yards. Since the Antwerp Olympic Games (1920), the distance of Marathon races has been patterned on the 1908 contest. This was intended to be exactly 26 miles (from Windsor Castle to Wembley Stadium); however, an altered placing of the royal stand lengthened the distance to 26 miles 385 yards. (Dyson – personal communication to author)

patients (Asclepiades, 1955). Long prior to his teachings a number of the individual Greek states had organized major athletic festivals. The best known was that held at Olympia,* in honour of Zeus. We read in the eleventh Olympic Ode: 'strength and beauty are the gifts of Zeus ... natural gifts imply the duty of developing them with God's help by cost and toil' (McIntosh, 1970). Such was the importance of the Olympic festival that safe conduct was guaranteed to all contestants, irrespective of any wars that might be in progress. The origin of the Olympic celebration is obscure. One legend tells of the Phaeacian games, organized by King Alcinous for Odysseus. He pleaded tiredness and a heavy heart, but under the goading of Laodamus picked up a discus and threw it beyond the mark of the Phaeacians. Another suggestion is that the games originated as an elaborate funeral ceremony for the hero Pelops. Although the traditional date of the first contest is 776 B.C., some historians maintain that the contests extend as far back as 1300 B.C. Events were open to all men of pure Hellenic descent who had not incurred personal disgrace. Women were excluded from the official Olympic contests, and even the watching of the games by any woman except the high priestess of Hera was a capital offence. Some authors have concluded from this that while it was permissible for the young girls of Greece to run, fence, and wrestle, the properly modest Athenian woman married early, raised a large family, and was rarely heard from thereafter (Harris, 1964). However, more recent research has discovered a separate contest for women, associated with the festival of Hera (Harris, 1969).

The winners of the male games were crowned with a sacred olive wreath, one of the highest of Greek honours. Often the victors were leading figures of the day. Thus Milo, commander in chief of an army, and numbered among the Pythagoreans, won at least six Olympic contests, and is reputed to have gained twenty-six crowns at other major games. Initially, the contest was a running match, and it is tempting to read into this the implication that the Greeks prized endurance above other forms of fitness. However, sports such as chariot-racing, boxing, wrestling, and throwing the discus and javelin were featured in the Iliad and the Odyssey, both dating from about 1200 B.C. The running match of Olympia was supplemented by the *diaulos* (a double-course running event) and the *dolichos* (a 24-turn race of almost 2½ miles) in 724 B.C., but it was not until 708 B.C., with the introduction of the pentathlon (which involved a triple jump, running, throwing a copper ingot, throwing a javelin, and wrestling) that the officials at Olympia made any concession to the 'muscle men.' There were a total of 293 successive Olympiads before the final eclipse of Greek civilization. Around

---

* Olympia should not be confused with Mount Olympus, the normal 'home' of Zeus some 180 miles distant.

400 A.D., Theodosius the Great and his son sought to replace paganism by Christianity, and in 408 A.D. their decision was enforced by the burning of the temple of Zeus (McIntosh, 1970).

Natural selection of the fittest infants was given a firm helping hand in Sparta. Girls were encouraged to wrestle, run, play ball, throw the javelin, swim, and ride horseback in order that they might bear healthy children (Ziegler, 1972). Soon after birth, male children that did not meet the required standards of fitness were snatched from their mothers and thrown into the abyss. This eugenic measure seems to have been accepted even by the mothers. From early childhood, boys were drilled for military success, with the stern warning 'come back with your shield or on your shield' ringing in their ears. Philosophers such as Plato and Aristotle accepted this stern tradition, insisting that medical treatment should not be wasted on those whose condition would preclude their becoming useful members of society. The Spartan athletes were given a particularly rigorous preparation, sleeping on animal skins, eating a meagre diet, and bathing in mountain streams (Gordon, 1935). The Spartans regarded all competitive sport as a means of preparation for war, and even their dancing seemed designed to teach methods of avoiding flying missiles!

The state assumed responsibility for the education of boys between the ages of 7 and 18 in both Sparta and Athens. During the adolescent period emphasis was placed on physical rather than mental development. The dunce of Athens was a person who could neither write nor swim. Socrates is reputed to have said: 'It is disgraceful for a person to grow old in self-neglect before he knows what he would become by rendering himself well-formed and vigorous in body.' Plato (428-348 B.C.) recommended music and gymnastics to his pupils prior to their eighteenth year, and obviously he intended that their activity should be intense: 'Those (contests) which provided a training for war should be encouraged ... those which do not may be dismissed' (Plato, 1960). Aristotle (384-322 B.C.) also favoured emphasis on play, physical activities, stories, and morals to at least the fourteenth year, with physical education preceding education of the mind; however, he cautioned that the exercises should not be violent or specialized. Activities taught included leaping, running, wrestling, and wielding a weapon with grace and accuracy. The Greeks did remarkably well on this liberal regime, although I suppose that in fairness to modern educationalists it must be conceded that they had a smaller total body of knowledge to transmit than do our schools today.

The gymnasia of ancient Greece were originally quite distinct from the palestrae, where the boys of wealthy parents received their physical and mental education. The word *gymnasion* means literally a school for naked exercise. In Homeric times, the athletes seem to have worn shorts, and there are various theories as to why they were later discarded – the precedent of a winner who lost his shorts en-route to the finishing post, the less well coordinated runner who tripped over his shorts and killed himself, and the coach who attempted to alleviate heat exhaustion in his charges (Harris, 1969; Ryan, 1974). All important Greek cities boasted at least one gymnasion. Their initial function seems to have been the training of professional athletes who could compete in the public games. Competitors would spend as much as ten months at these institutions in the final year of an Olympiad preparing themselves for the new festival* (Schö-bel, 1966). Those who thought themselves ready for competition then attended Elis for a further month of intensive training under the Hellenodikai, who were also the judges for the games. Thence, those considered worthy made the final thirty-five mile journey to Olympia. There was a tendency for graduates of the palestrae to despise those attending the gymnasion. Thus Plato, himself a top-level amateur wrestler, described the professional athlete as 'but a sleepy thing and rather perilous to health ... We need a finer training for our champions ... with hard endurance training and exercise.' However, as is the way of institutions, the gymnasia were progressively upgraded. The buildings became more imposing. Dressing rooms, baths, and training quarters were added, with special areas for specific contests. The staff developed to include a physician interested in training (the *gymnastes*), a masseur (*paidotribes*), and a bath servant (*aleiptes*) (Ryan, 1974). Gradually the nature of those in charge – the *gymnasiarchs* and the *gymnastae* – changed, and instead of producing mere brawn, the gymnasia became respected institutions of learning and culture. This last phase is well illustrated by the gymnasion which has been excavated to the northwest of the Acropolis in Athens. It covered a vast area, and contained not only baths and athletic facilities but many other buildings including a number of temples. The most famous product of this system was the gymnastes Herodicus (circa 400 B.C.), himself a teacher of Hippocrates (Harris, 1966). Herodicus believed in exercise as a method of physical rehabilitation, and passed onto Hippocrates something of this belief.

The Romans seem to have regarded the final form of the gymnasion as rather effete. Ennius (239–169 B.C.) claimed that 'to strip naked among one's fellow citizens was the beginning of vice' (W.H. Bishop, 1970). The elaborate training of the athlete and the strict regulation of diet were thought to hinder preparation for active service. Thus Lucien complained: 'You will meet an army enlisted from the Greek gymnasium listless because of their palaestrae course and hardly able to bear arms.' Galen, the famous second-century physician of Pergamos,

---

* An Olympiad was a four-year interval on the calendar whose opening was celebrated by the festival of the games.

wrote: 'When athletes miss their goal, they are disgraced; when they attain it, they are not yet even above the brutes.' Again, in his 'Paraphrase of Mendotus' we read: 'Athletes live a life quite contrary to the principles of hygiene, and I regard their mode of living as a regime more favourable to illness than to health ... when they give up their profession, they fall into a condition more parlous still; as a fact, some die shortly afterwards; others live for some little time but do not arrive at old age' (Ryan, 1974). Despite these unfavourable comments, Galen wrote three works concerned with physical activity: 'On Health,' 'Whether health is the concern of medicine or gymnastics,' and 'Exercises with the small ball.' He recommended moderate therapeutic exercises for many ailments (Galen, 1951), particularly work with the small ball; the sport advocated is probably the Greek antecedent of handball, played in a walled court or *sphaeristerium*. One of Galen's pupils, the fourth-century Oribasius, commended more violent exercise, but Galen's doctrine of moderation generally prevailed.

While Fulvius Nobilior had organized a Greek athletic festival in Rome (186 B.C.), and Augustus (63 B.C.–14 A.D.) had authorized the restoration of the temple of Zeus, such gymnasia as were built in Roman cities were staffed mainly by Greeks. The Greek sophist Philostratus continued to pour scorn on athletes into the third century – the physicians overstuffed them, failed to develop endurance, and no longer enforced sufficiently rigorous training. Sports came to be thought of largely in terms of Etruscan-imported spectator events – chariot races, gladiatorial combats, and fights with wild animals – a means of buying the votes of the populace (Sawula, 1970). The Circus Maximus provided seating for 385,000! However, there were some facilities for public recreation at the *thermae*, or baths; by the fourth century A.D. there were 856 such institutions in Rome, providing facilities for simultaneous exercise by 60,000 citizens (McIntosh, 1970).

The majority of Romans valued fitness mainly in its military context, and regarded athletics as an effeminate substitute for martial training. Their attitude was essentially practical. Thus Seneca (c. 4 B.C.–65 A.D.) commended running, weight training, high and long jumping, and certain forms of dance – indeed 'any short and simple exercises which tire the body rapidly and so save time.' However, one notable exception was Quintilanius (c. 35–100 A.D.), a writer and teacher of the younger Pliny; in his 'Institutio oratoria,' he stressed the value of physical activity in the development of a graceful body. The poems of Horace (65–8 B.C.) and of Ovid (43 B.C.–18 A.D.) also suggest that wrestling and the throwing of the discus had some popularity among the wealthier young Romans. Aurelianus (fifth century A.D.) is of interest for his commendation of exercise during convalescence from surgery (Aurelianus, 1950). His techniques of rehabilitation included hydrotherapy and the use of weights and pulleys.

The Middle Ages and the Renaissance

For a time, ascetic and athletic were almost interchangeable words. Training was a method of taming the body for spiritual ends. Thus Clemens of Alexandria (c. 150-c. 215 A.D.) strongly commended games and athletics for boys and men. However, the negative aspects of asceticism – fasting and contemplation – later received greater emphasis, and in the case of the mediaeval monks became a corporate way of life. Perhaps as a reaction to the Roman debasing of sports and games, the church developed a strong opposition to athletic and recreational pursuits, and during the dark ages the only section of the European leisured class concerned with physical development was the knights. The metabolic and thermal load imposed by their protective equipment was considerable, and a high level of fitness was needed in this profession. Between military campaigns strength and endurance were preserved by frequent joustings and tournaments. The common people enjoyed occasional games of football, and despite the strictures of the church these became associated with religious festivals – Shrovetide, weddings, and baptisms. As in more primitive societies, the games often had a somewhat pagan mystical significance; thus the Good Friday football game at Wreyland was intended to ensure a substantial potato crop. Edward III prohibited football in London, because it was taking his citizens away from the more practical sport of archery. Occasionally even the clergy succumbed to the temptations of the football field, and in the Diocese of Oxford it was ruled (1584) that any minister or deacon convicted of playing football was to be banished and reported to his bishop.

An important medical writer of the mediaeval period was the Arabian philosopher Avicenna (980–1037). He stated (Kruger, 1962): 'Among physical exercises there are some moderate ones; it is to them that one ought to devote himself. They ... are factors of good nutrition for adults and of happy growth for the young. Unmoderated exercise is an overload ... and causes the body to age before its time ... preserve a happy medium ... exercise your limbs ... until you succeed in panting.' Another notable thinker of this era was the Jewish physician Maimonides (more properly Rabbi Moses ben Maimon, 1135-1204). He lived in a suburb of Cairo, and rose to become the doctor of Saladin. His writings attest to a strong belief in a healthful life-style: 'A person should ... walk prior to the meal until his body begins to be warmed ... Anyone who lives a sedentary life and does not exercise ... even if he eats good foods and takes care of himself according to proper medical principles – all his days will be painful ones and his strength shall wane' (Ryan, 1974).

With the Renaissance and the Reformation, it again became respectable for Europeans to mention the body and even to think of preserving it in a functional sense. Historians distinguish three categories of reformers: the verbal realists, who desired a strong body for the help it could give the mind in its search for piety; the social realists, who saw physical education as part of the development of an integrated personality; and the sense realists, who desired physical fitness for its contributions to health and thus to learning (Van Dalen and Bennett, 1971). Luther (1483-1546) is a good example of the first category. He wrote approvingly of the recreative and moral value of physical exercises such as fencing and wrestling, and expressed the hope that such pastimes would become possible for the world at large. In England, Henry VIII set a vigorous personal example in his younger days, laying down bowling alleys at Whitehall, building tennis courts at Hampton, and wrestling with the King of France. During his reign running, wrestling, leaping, casting the bar, and football were widely practised by the general population (McIntosh, 1963). This enthusiasm for vigorous games continued throughout the Elizabethan period and on to the time of the Stuarts. In 1618 we find James I promulgating his 'Declaration on Lawful Sport.' This allowed the 'meaner sort' 'who labour hard all the week' to practise 'lawful recreations' (archery, leaping, vaulting, and dancing) upon Sundays 'after Evening Prayers ended.' The liberal attitude ended with the Commonwealth, and the Puritans quickly moved from attacking sport on Sundays to condemning all sport for sport's sake. John Bunyan (1628-1688) gives a vivid description of his wickedness: 'I shook the sermon out of my mind and to my old custom of sports and gaming I returned with great delight.' Nevertheless, fitness remained welcome if it offered the prospect of service to God and man. Thus John Milton (1608-1674), in his essay 'Of Education,' recommended that boys should devote three and a half hours of each day to physical exercise, mainly military-type drill.

Several Renaissance physicians deserve brief notice. In Italy, Mercuriale (1530-1608) published six popular books on the art of gymnastics; he distinguished preventive and therapeutic exercise, and warned of the dangers of strenuous military training and athletics. In France, Paré (1510-1590) became concerned at the condition of his patients following surgery for gunshot wounds, and suggested that treatment of fractures should be followed by specific exercise of the limbs. At Montpellier University, Joubert (1529-1583) advocated daily exercise, and introduced therapeutic gymnastics into the regular medical curriculum. Duchesne (1546-1609) prescribed swimming and gymnastics to promote 'the strengthening of the heart and joints, the opening of the pores of the skin, and the stronger circulation of the blood in the lungs by strenuous breathing.' In Spain, Mendez meanwhile was writing 'The easiest way of all to preserve health ... is to exercise well.'

The Renaissance brought about dramatic changes in the patterns of education. At the Mantuan court the Italian da Feltre (1378-1446) treated his scholars with individually prescribed physical exercise as well as mental training. The more traditional Dutch teacher Erasmus (1446-1536) found no place for sport in his educational thinking, and his attitude is reflected in schools, such as St Paul's, founded under his guidance. However, England had its share of schoolmasters with 'advanced' ideas, notably Mulcaster (c.1530-1611), the first headmaster of the Merchant Taylors' school in London, and John Locke (1632-1704), inspirer of the 'age of enlightenment.' Locke was greatly concerned about the effeteness of the aristocracy and advocated riding as 'one of the best exercises for health which is to be had in those places of ease and luxury.' In Czechoslovakia, Comenius (1592-1670) was bold enough to suggest that as the soul was nourished by books, so the body was nourished by movement. On this basis, he proposed that students be given thirty minutes of exercise for every hour of study. He also commended light exercise to pregnant women, in order that they might produce vigorous offspring. As with so many ardent reformers, Comenius seems to have had a fiery temperament. He had the misfortune to be on the wrong side in the Thirty Years War and spent most of his life in exile. In 1642 he was invited to Sweden to promote a national system of education, but was unable to accommodate his views as a Moravian bishop to the wishes of the Lutheran hierarchy. One is left with the impression of an energetic man with valuable ideas that were not adopted because he allowed his substantial powers to be dissipated in numerous rather meaningless disputes and conflicts of personality.

National emphases
The subsequent course of physical education followed divergent paths, reflecting differences in national personality. In France, the early humanist Michel de Montaigne (1533-92) had written: 'It is not enough to toughen (man's) spirit, his muscles also must be toughened.' The Age of Reason developed under Rousseau (1712-78). He reacted against interference by church and state, preaching a naturalism in education, with a strong emphasis on health and the unity of mind and body. Games and sports had a therapeutic value, taking from man 'all the dangerous inclinations that spring from idleness.'

The British placed an emphasis on sports and organized games within the 'public school' tradition. Interest spread steadily from the upper to the developing middle class. The latter engaged vigorously in such pursuits as association football, hockey, tennis, rowing, cycling, cricket, and track and field. There were also many long-distance walks; thus in the year 1808 a Captain Barclay Allardice accepted a thousand guinea wager to cover 1000 miles in 1000 hours (McIntosh, 1963). He finished his walk two stone lighter, but otherwise apparently in good fettle.

In Germany, gymnastics developed as a political tool. This emphasis is generally traced to another stormy petrel, Johann Basedow (1723-90). Born in Hamburg, Basedow was a disciple of Rousseau, and is widely credited with the reform of the Prussian educational system. After summary dismissal from academies in Denmark and Altona, he remained in Dessau (northern Germany) long enough to establish a *philanthropinum*, or model school. This operated on a rather drastic ten-hour schedule, five hours being allocated for studies, three hours for recreation, and two hours for manual labour. Basedow's knowledge of physical education came from his brief acquaintance with the Knights' Academy in Soroe (Denmark), and in Dessau he attempted to adapt the pleasures of riding, dancing, and ball-games to the baroque taste (Wildt, 1971). Nevertheless, the avowed objective of philanthropism was an education based on human nature rather than on the privileged life of the nobility. The concept that both general education and physical instruction should be made available to the poorest of children was enthusiastically endorsed by Pestalozzi (1746-1827) and others of the Froebel school in Switzerland. The trend from knightly exercises to gymnastics progressed under the influence of Simon (1776), Dutoit (1778), and Johann Guts-Muths (1759-1839), who wrote a number of books on gymnastics and games; his program embraced running, jumping, lifting, carrying, climbing, dancing, and balancing, in addition to the more traditional items of vaulting, fencing, shooting, and military drill. Spiess (1810-58) originally taught at Froebel's school in Switzerland, but later moved to Germany, taking with him a keen interest in gymnastics.

The person commonly blamed for the political element in German gymnastics is Friedrich Jahn. He was born at Lanz in 1778, and spent much of his youth brooding over Napoleon's humiliation of the German nation. Current historians doubt the originality of his methods of physical education (Wildt, 1971), since the gymnastic exercises he used were very similar to those of Guts-Muth. Jahn is remembered rather because he sought to restore national morale by a program of outdoor gymnastics. Through his efforts, the year 1811 saw the first *Turnverein*, or outdoor gymnasium, established in Berlin. The young gymnasts regarded themselves as a guild, pledged to the emancipation of the Fatherland, and because of the political overtones of the movement, outdoor gymnastics were banned in Prussia and other German states from 1820 to 1842. As might have been anticipated by the legislators, exercise continued behind closed doors, with an emphasis on those movement patterns that were possible in a confined space. One of Jahn's pupils, Carl Voelker, opened a *Turnplatz* near Regent's Park in London; we read of facilities for exercises on horizontal and parallel bars, rope and ladder climbing, and pole-vaulting. In 1848, Jahn's followers sided against the monarchists, and many found it prudent to depart for the United States and Canada. A German-speaking colony was established in Cincinnati, complete with its *Turngemeinde*, and the latter continued to have both physical and political functions ('the strengthening of democracy and the im-provement of cultural opportunities through physical and mental development'). Through men such as Beck, Follen, and Lieber, the *Turngemeinde* played an im-portant role in the shaping of physical education within the school system of a number of U.S. states (Barney, 1972; Ziegler, 1972).

Mass gymnastics also became popular in Bohemia, and the Bohemian gymnas-tic society (Sokol) established its first gymnasium in Prague in 1862. During the latter part of the nineteenth century, increasing reaction against the industriali-zation and urbanization of central Europe was reflected in the 'open air move-ment' – an attempt to get exercises out of the gymnasium and back into the open air. The birth of the third Reich gave a sinister militaristic emphasis to acti-vities of this class. Hitler wrote: 'Education by a national state must aim primar-ily not at the stuffing with mere knowledge, but at building bodies which are physically healthy to the core' (Berridge, 1974).

The Swedes and the Danes developed an interest in physical education follow-ing the Napoleonic defeats. However, whereas Germans of this era conceived gymnastics as a political tool, the Swedes saw exercise more as an instrument of pedagogy. In contrast to the German emphasis upon muscle-building through apparatus work, the Swedes favoured free exercises, seeking to perfect the rhythm of movement in their pupils. The first advocate of free exercises was pro-bably Salzmann (1744–1811), but they became popular through the work of Per Henrik Ling (1776–1839). He originally taught fencing at Lund, in eastern Swe-den, but in 1813 became principal of the renowned Royal Central Gymnastic Institute in Stockholm. There, he elaborated a system of gymnastics with four objectives (pedagogical, medical, military, and aesthetic); of these, the thera-peutic component (movement cure, or Swedish massage) is best known. For a time the demand for exponents of his system outstripped the graduation of trained therapists, and this stimulated the development of machines that would provide active, assisted, and resisted exercise and massage. The aesthetic beauty of Scandinavian gymnastic teams has also gained worldwide recognition.

Neighbouring Denmark had a keen interest in organizing physical education for the general population through such pioneers as Nachtegall (1777–1847) and Niels Bukh. It was the first nation to introduce compulsory physical education into its schools.

The earliest plea for physical education in Canadian schools was made by Egerton Ryerson in 1846. He had just returned from a tour of Germany, Switzer-land, the United Kingdom, and the United States, and had been greatly impressed by the ideas of men such as Pestalozzi, Ling, and Guts-Muth. He proposed that in winter pupils should participate in gymnastics, calisthenics, and work with dumb-bells and Indian clubs, while in the summer months there should be walking, skipping, dancing, and lawn bowling. Enthusiasm for games and sports was initially channelled into the private school sector, and in 1860 the *Journal of Education for Upper Canada* wrote of the 'social necessity' of more uniform recreational opportunities if 'the children and youth of our Canadian cities are to grow up with half the proper quantity of bone and muscle and with but a fractional part of the elasticity of spirit which, of right, belongs to them' (Lindsay, 1970). The year 1862 saw the first normal school equipped with a gymnasium for the training of teachers, and in 1865 a bounty of $50 was offered to schools introducing 'drill and gymnastics' into their curriculum. The terminology reflects the early source of instructors, usually retired army sergeants. The subject was made compulsory in 1892, the elements of drill, calisthenics, and gymnastics being preserved with a view to developing discipline. At this time, military readiness was considered a necessary corollary of a long border with a powerful and unpredictable neighbour. The McGill University calendar of 1900 noted: 'the gymnasium is fully equipped in accordance with the regulations of the Swedish system.' In Catholic Quebec, Henri Scott led a wave of enthusiasm for Swedish drill, but in the Maritimes and in Ontario the military emphasis continued under the provisions of the Strathcoma Trust 'for the encouragement of physical and military training in the public schools of Canada' (MacDiarmid, 1970).

After World War I, there was an increasing reaction against 'the issuing of commands in a parrot-like fashion without any understanding of the motives underlying the commands that are given.' Dr Lamb of McGill University led the movement from drill to fitness (Cosentino, 1970; Eaton, 1970), stressing a principle stated but perhaps previously ignored ('physical training at school should form the groundwork of healthy exercise and recreation in later life.' [H.M. Stationery Office, 1919]). Greater emphasis was placed upon learning by doing, and upon activities that were natural, spontaneous, and enjoyable; education through the physical began to supersede education of the physical (T.D. Wood and Cassidy, 1927). In Canada, as in other industrialized countries, mechanization and automation led to a rapid growth of leisure time for adults. A great contrast was seen between the early exploits of the homesteader, the miner, or the voyageur and current demands of metropolitan life. But a few years earlier, Mackenzie had described the workload at Grand Portage thus: 'Voyageurs, hired from the St. Lawrence villages for one to three years, would set off with two packages of ninety pounds each and return with two others of the same weight, in the course of six hours, being a distance of eighteen miles over hills and mountains' (Schellberg, 1970). However, with the new affluence of the developing nation, lack of regular activity was no longer just a problem of the ruling class, but was spreading to the humblest of citizens. For a while, some desire to emulate the pioneers persisted. Even after World War II, one American encyclopaedia (Menke, 1947) wrote: 'no country in the world is more devoted to sport than Canada.' However, as Canadians became accustomed to life in cities, interest in the outdoors and the physical waned. In common with most other industrial nations Canada now shows only a limited social acceptance of voluntary activity by the adult. It remains permissible for teenagers to preserve some of their fitness through modern forms of tribal dancing, but the adult who indulges half-heartedly in calisthenics at the local YMCA is regarded at best with a tolerant smile. Perhaps part of the problem lies with the educational system, for despite Lamb's advice it has all too frequently placed an emphasis on team games and star performers. If the youngsters, irrespective of skill, were taught activities they could enjoy as adults, they might be more inclined to persist with them.

The role of government

Low levels of national fitness have been of serious concern to the military in both world wars, substantial batches of otherwise acceptable 'cannon-fodder' being rejected simply on the basis of poor physical development. In the United States, President Eisenhower and his advisors were apparently greatly shocked by the proportion of U.S. children who failed the Kraus-Weber performance test battery in 1956. More recently, governments have become frightened by the spiralling costs of national health services, and in Canada both the prime minister and the minister of health have had frequent occasion to quote cost/benefit analyses of the likely results of an increase of physical activity (Chapter 12). Government concern in the U.S.A. found practical expression through the formation of the President's Council on Physical Fitness. In Canada, the National Physical Fitness Act was enacted in 1943. A National Council on Physical Fitness was given a budget of $250,000 to promote fitness on the basis of matching provincial funds. The council urged every university to institute a physical fitness program for all students, and recommended an annual month of canoeing for children aged five to fourteen. Neither of these suggestions was taken very seriously, and although some of the promised money was used to develop recreational programs and improve fitness in schools, the Act was repealed in 1954. Nevertheless, some Canadian provinces continued to expand recreational services, contingent upon the formation of local boards of citizens prepared to share in the developmental work (McFarland, 1970).

In 1959 His Royal Highness, the Duke of Edinburgh became the first lay president of the Canadian Medical Association, and in his inaugural address he spoke with characteristic bluntness of the poor physical condition of Canadian youth. His words were noted and widely distributed via a Royal Bank newsletter, which carried an article, 'In search of physical fitness,' that pointed the finger squarely at existing school programs of physical education. The resultant furor spread to Parliament, and in 1961 Bill C-131, 'an act to encourage fitness and amateur sport,' received royal assent. A Directorate of Fitness and Amateur Sport was established with an initial operating budget of $5 million per year. Some $500,000 of this total was earmarked for research. A reorganization of the directorate began in 1969, and in 1971 separate sport and recreation divisions were created, the latter giving increased emphasis to participation and development of personal fitness. Shortly afterwards, a Crown corporation ('Participaction') was formed, modelled after the German *Trimm* program; it has sponsored various forms of advertisement (radio, television, and bus displays) and mass media campaigns to increase the physical activity of the general populace. A national conference on fitness was convened by the federal government in 1973, and recommendations of this conference (such as the development of a home fitness test) are currently being implemented.

Development of professional organizations
The present century has seen a useful blending of divergent national traditions through such groups as the Fédération Internationale de Gymnastique and the International Council on Physical Health, Education and Recreation. However, the current basis of most training methods remains a combination of cultural heritage and the inspired hunches of coaches. Serious study of physical activity is in its infancy, and the new knowledge is only now being translated into improved practical programs for the development of fitness, Ernst Jokl (1971) made an exhaustive tabulation of textbook contents and university curricula, seeking an answer to the question: 'What is Sports Medicine?' Unfortunately, no consensus was possible, since views differed markedly in different parts of the world. In Eastern Europe, sports medicine early attained the status of a respected specialist certification for physicians. The Fédération Internationale de Médicine Sportive held its founding meeting at St Moritz in 1928. It has remained European-based, and has sustained a physician-oriented concept of sports medicine. In theory, the forty participating national federations of sports medicine require medical qualification on the part of their members. In most recent years, the Fédération has sponsored a two-week postgraduate course in sports medicine. The principal subjects have been sports injuries and their surgical treatment, and the course has often been arranged in conjunction with regional contests such as the Mediterranean games. Every fourth year, the Fédération has also sponsored a World Congress of Sports Medicine; the 1974 conference was in Melbourne, and the 1978 conference is set for São Paolo, Brazil.

The American Association of Health, Physical Education and Recreation dates back to 1885. In recent years it has served a professional rather than a scientific function. The dominant U.S. research group of the past decade has been the American College of Sports Medicine. Founded by less than a dozen enthusiasts in the early 1950s, the membership has grown to about 3300, drawn rather equally from physicians, exercise physiologists, and physical educators. The quarterly house journal *Medicine and Science in Sports* and the annual scientific meetings have shown a strong bias towards exercise physiology and biochemistry, with only occasional contributions relating to sports injuries, exercise cardiology, biomechanics, sociology, and psychology. Understandably, practising physicians have felt somewhat isolated from discussions of increasingly fundamental research, and at least a proportion of sports doctors in the U.S. have found an alternative forum in that section of the American Medical Association devoted to athletic injuries.

In Canada, the professional history is even more complex. The Canadian Physical Education Association was formed in 1933. Despite all the problems of the depression, 86 members travelled to the first annual meeting of the association. The group was reconstituted as the Canadian Association of Health, Physical Education and Recreation in 1946, to accommodate the recreational interests supported by the National Fitness Act (Devenney, 1974). A peak membership of 1300 was reached in 1961. Shortly afterwards, the need to marry the expertise of the physical educator and the physician was recognized, and in 1965 a joint subcommittee of the Canadian Medical Association and the Canadian Association of Physical Health Education and Recreation was established under the chairmanship of Dr Sam Landa, to deal with problems relating to sports medicine and national fitness (Merriman, 1967). Perhaps originally a marriage of convenience, the value of the union was soon recognized, and in 1967 conjugal activity led to the birth of a sturdy infant, the Canadian Association of Sports Sciences. Naturally, much thought was given to the naming of the child. It could well have been called the Canadian Association of Sports Medicine, but in view of the increasing importance of such disciplines as sociology and psychology, the more broadly based title of Sports Sciences was finally chosen. CASS has grown vigorously since its inception, and it has played the major role in initiating the 2000-registrant International Congress of Physical Activity Sciences that accompanied the Montreal Olympic games.

A second strand in the Canadian tradition has been the Grey Cup symposium; for a number of years, this has brought together surgeons, coaches, and trainers with an interest in football and other team sports. A one-day meeting is held each year, immediately preceding the Grey Cup game.

A third force has been the medical committee of the Canadian Olympic Association. This body has traditionally assumed responsibility for medical coverage of the Canadian Olympic team. It commenced preparations for the Mexico City Olympics with a small research study in the fall of 1965. Unfortunately, our Canadian athletes fared rather badly in Mexico City, and somewhat unfairly this was blamed upon poor medical coverage. Both the Canadian Olympic Association (which apparently lacked the necessary funds to send more medical support) and the Canadian Association of Sports Sciences (which was just holding its first annual meeting!) shared in this ill-deserved criticism.

The Canadian federal government reacted in a predictable manner, appointing a 'task-force.' Through an unfortunate clash of personalities, the report of the task force (Queen's Printer, Ottawa, 1969) chose to ignore existing structures, and added to the confusion by persuading the Canadian Medical Association to father a second child, the Canadian Academy of Sports Medicine. Membership of this group is restricted to physicians. Its prime responsibilities have been seen as (i) providing top-level medical coverage for Canadian athletes, and (ii) the development of an increasing cadre of physicians with an interest in sports medicine (through the formation of specialist sections in national and provincial medical associations). In the meantime, other specialist groups have emerged, with particular interests in motor learning, sociology, psychology, and history of sport, while a declinine Canadian Association of Physical Health, Education and Recreation has begun an agonizing reappraisal of its identity.

The last few years have thus seen an alarming fragmentation among those interested in the phenomena of human physical activity. To a point, this has fostered growth, but the information obtained has often been narrow in outlook, and poorly integrated into the over-all framework of developing knowledge. In the future, a number of the more specialized societies may persist, but it seems likely that many will meet together periodically under some type of federated structure such as that adopted at the International Congress of Physical Activity Sciences in 1976.

International athletic competitions
Our survey of cultural patterns would not be complete without brief mention of the resurgence of international athletic competitions. Britain led the way by establishing athletics on a national basis in 1866. The Amateur Athletic Association of Canada was also founded as early as 1883. The Olympic games were revived in 1896, largely through the enthusiasm of Baron de Coubertin. The number of participants has increased steadily throughout the present century (Table 3). A Canadian Amateur Athletic Union was formed in 1904, and its Olympic

TABLE 3

Growth of participation in the Olympic Games*

Location	Date	Sports	Events	Participants M	F	Nations
Athens	1896	9	43	311	–	13
Paris	1900	17	80	1319	11	22
St Louis	1904	14	84	617	8	12
Athens	1906	11	76	877	7	20
London	1908	24	104	1999	36	22
Stockholm	1912	14	105	2490	57	28
Antwerp	1920	22	155	2543	64	29
Paris	1924	18	136	2956	136	44
Amsterdam	1928	15	120	2724	290	46
Los Angeles	1932	15	124	1281	127	37
Berlin	1936	20	141	3738	328	49
London	1948	18	146	3714	385	59
Helsinki	1952	17	145	4407	518	69
Melbourne	1956	17	145	2813	371	67
(incl. Stockholm)	(1956)	(26)	(149)	(3486)	(371)	(69)
Rome	1960	17	146	4738	610	84
Tokyo	1964	19	160	4457	683	93
Mexico	1968	18	176	4750	781	112
Munich	1972	21	198	6077	1070	122
Montreal	1976					

* Figures vary somewhat from one authority to another. The data are based largely on Kamper (1972), and do not include participation in the Winter Olympic Games (commenced in 1924).

subcommittee submitted the first entries to the St Louis games. Dramatic successes were attained in 1908 and 1912; however, a formal Canadian Olympic Association was not constituted until 1937.

Women were first admitted informally to the Olympic contest of 1900. Official participation dates from 1928 (Shephard, 1976c), and such has been the rate of development of records for both sexes that current female performances now threaten the best efforts of the male in previous generations.

The influence of superb competitive feats upon the general level of world fitness is problematical. Ordinary citizens who take twenty or thirty minutes to cover a mile may react negatively to the Bannisters and Zatopeks of this world. It can also be argued that the Olympics have become one more weapon in the struggle between rival ideologies. Certainly true amateurs such as the majority of Canadian competitors are at a strong disadvantage relative to 'state amateurs' and 'scholarly' athletes. A reasonable national pride in victory has become sub-servient to hard political goals. Competitors from some quarters scarcely dare to lose! To the extent that government interest in a scientific approach to fitness is kindled by the contests, their influence undoubtedly remains good. However, for the countries hosting the Olympic extravaganza, it is arguable that the money spent on vast arenas could have been distributed more usefully among a much larger number of simpler local facilities.

THE DEVELOPMENT OF FITNESS AS A SCIENTIFIC CONCEPT

The ancient world

It is difficult to separate early developments in the area of fitness from the gen-eral growth of scientific knowledge. Our historical survey must thus trace the origins of medicine and of science. The first civilization known to have had an interest in health was that of Egypt; the medical attainments of the Egyptians reached a peak about 3000 B.C., with careful descriptions of the signs of illness and suggestions of appropriate medication by such physician statesmen as Imho-tep.

Moses is thought to have studied both medicine and hygiene at the Egyptian temple school of Os, and much of his concern with public health can presumably be traced to this fact. He gained a distaste for quackery and magic, and sought to avoid this in Israel by insisting that God was the sole physician. In our present context, it is interesting that he appreciated the value of a day of rest after six days of hard physical labour.

The early Chinese civilization developed elaborate rituals for pulse-taking. Arteries were palpated at up to six sites, using each of three fingers, and applying strong, medium, and weak pressure three times with each finger. The whole exer-cise, which sounds almost like a statistically designed experiment, could occupy a physician for up to three hours. The objective was to detect an imbalance of Yang (the male principle, active, light, and represented by the heavens) and Yin (the female principle, passive, dark, and represented by the earth). Importance, both physiological and philosophical, was also attached to proper breathing; this transmuted the inspired air into an essence vital to life.

Similar views developed in ancient Greece. In Homeric times, medicine had been entrusted to very practical army surgeons, but in succeeding centuries a group of shrewd practitioners emerged from the temples of Aesculapius, bring-ing to their task of healing the accumulated wisdom of Egypt, Babylon, Phoe-necia, and other eastern powers. Thales of Miletos ($\sim$640-548 B.C.) conceived an all-pervading first principle of water as essential to life. Anaximenes ($\sim$570-

525? B.C.) held a similar view, although his first principle was the pneuma, or air. Heraclitus of Ephesos (550–475 B.C.) in turn suggested that fire was the dominant principle. For the mathematician Pythagoras of Samos (580–489 B.C.), numbers were the origin and essence of all things. The human body was ordered according to rigid musico-mathematical rules, and a sick man was essentially out of harmony with himself. The physician had but to tune him up, and he would be as fit as a fiddle. Pythagoras founded a sect that believed in a strict and health-ful life-style; its rules included celibacy, a rigid diet, and the absence of laughter. A pupil, Alcmaeon of Croton, put forward the idea that health depended on the balance of a number of opposing qualities (wet/dry, cold/warm, acid/sweet, and so on). A second pupil of Pythagoras, Empedocles of Agrigente (∿495–435 B.C.), suggested that four was a particularly potent number, and proposed that all mat-ter was composed of four basic elements (air, fire, water, and earth). These were bonded by love and separated by strife. Both the rhythmic motion of the pneuma into the body and the ebb and flow of the blood as a carrier of innate heat were essential to health.

Hippocrates (∿460–377 B.C.) was a noted physician of this period. He was born on the island of Cos, and probably commenced work as an apprentice to his father, who was a physician at the local health resort. Ptolemy commissioned an over-zealous collection of his writings, the Corpus Hippocraticum; the total of more than fifty volumes gives a good picture of the thinking of his school of medicine. Several aphorisms are of interest in the context of fitness:

Exercise strengthens and inactivity wastes.
Weariness without cause indicates disease.
To eat heartily after a long illness without putting on flesh is a bad portent.

Hippocrates himself seems to have had a fairly simple view of the nature of life. In his treatise 'On Diet' he spoke of living organisms as consisting simply of fire and water. His son-in-law Polybus, also a physician, was probably responsible for final elaboration of the theory that health (*eucrasis*) was contingent upon an appropriate balance of four humours (Figure 1): blood (a combination of fire and water), phlegm (a combination of earth and water), yellow bile (a combination of fire and air), and black bile (a combination of fire and earth). Practical application of the theory is well indicated by the medical history of a patient named Silenius. He had eaten some cheese before bedtime and awoke with painful indigestion. It transpired that he had spent a strenuous day in the gymnasium, and the Hippocratic physician deduced that he was tired and over-heated when he ate the cheese. A surplus of fire had thus upset his humoral bal-ance. The patient was advised to avoid strenuous exercise, or alternatively to

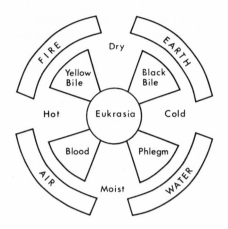

Figure 1 The theory of four body humours, as proposed by Polybus. Health (Eukrasia) was contingent upon an appropriate balance of yellow bile, black bile, blood, and phlegm within the individual.

cool off before eating. Shades of the doctrine of Polybus linger still in the well-adjusted personality, and in sanguine, phlegmatic, choleric, and melancholic temperaments.

Aristotle (384–322 B.C.) recognized clearly the animal nature of man. However, an emphasis on logical thinking rather than upon observation kept him from much progress in physiology. He regarded the heart as a blood-producing organ, and (through the alternate contraction and expansion of its fibres) as the source of all movement. The pulse wave, cardiac contractions, and even the respiratory movements had their origin in the heat produced by the formation of blood, the essential function of the lungs being to cool the overheated fluid emerging from the heart. The brain, in contrast, was a cold and insensitive organ, where the heat of ascending fluids was tempered sufficiently to form the mucous secretions of the nose.

Epicurus (342–270 B.C.) was another noteworthy figure of the Greek period. He held that the body was full of atoms and pores, and good health prevailed while the atoms were kept on the move.

At this time, Alexandria had developed as a major citadel of Hellenistic learning. The 'Museum' served as a combined University, research laboratory, and hall of residence. Here, Praxagoras (350–300 B.C.) made post-mortem examinations of animal blood vessels. He concluded that since the arteries were empty of blood, they must serve as channels to conduct air, or 'vital spirit.' He also revived the ancient Chinese concept that certain types of pulse had medical significance. Herophilus (∿300 B.C.) made many dissections of human cadavers, and possibly carried out some vivisections of criminals. He drew a clear distinction between arteries and veins, and is remembered also for use of a water-clock to obtain accurate estimates of pulse rate. His rival Erasistratus (∿304 B.C.) used this technique to diagnose the ailment of prince Antiochus. He noted a dramatic speeding of the pulse in the presence of the voluptuous queen, the prince's step-mother. The prescription was an early divorce for the queen, and according to the story the prince's ailment was soon resolved. Although of the Alexandrian school, Erasistratus spent much of his life in Chios. He described the valvular action of the heart correctly, and thus came very close to an understanding of the circulation. Nevertheless, he accepted the dogma of Praxagoras that since the arteries were empty, they must be serving as channels to conduct to the tissues air or vital spirit (*pneuma zotikon*) necessary to the vegetative aspects of life. The veins were conducting blood to the heart and peripheral tissues as needed for nutrition and growth. The left ventricle was separating off a distinct species of spirit, the *pneuma psychikon*, and delivering this to the head. In later years, he suggested further that this psychic pneuma or animal spirit was conveyed to the muscles via the nerves, and that the resultant swelling of the muscle belly shortened its fibres, built up a tension, and led to movement of the body part.

The Romans were content to leave medical science, like other forms of manual labour, to immigrant Greeks, slaves, and freedmen. The low opinion of the medical profession is illustrated by Pliny the Elder (23-79 A.D.). In his 'Natural History,' he wrote: 'It is at the expense of our perils that they learn ... they experiment by putting us to death ...' (Bettmann, 1956). Nevertheless, the stature of Greek physicians was increased by a decree of Caesar (46 B.C.) granting Roman citizenship to Greek doctors practising in Rome. Asclepiades ($\sim$124-40 B.C.) rose to become physician to both Cicero and Mark Anthony. He subscribed to the atomic theory of Democritus and the Epicureans – health depended on maintaining a normal relationship between the body pores and their contents, with the humours playing only a secondary role.

Galen (130-199 A.D.) was also of Greek origin. He travelled widely among the medical schools of the world before settling as team physician to the group of gladiators owned by the ruler of Pergamon. Unlike most physicians of the period, he gained a sound knowledge of anatomy by dissecting a wide variety of species, including a hippopotamus, an elephant, and a drowned man. In terms of physiology, he further elaborated the humoral theory (Figure 2). Food was conveyed by special ducts from the intestines to the liver, where it was transformed into nutritive spirits. The vital heat of the liver converted food into blood, and excessive particles passed to the gall-bladder and spleen as yellow and black bile respectively. The blood carried nutritive spirits to other tissues through an ebb and flow motion in the veins. A part also passed along the vena cava to the right ventricle; here, it penetrated pores in the cardiac septum to reach the left side of the heart. In the left ventricle, the blood was warmed by the innate heat of the heart and mixed with the pneuma to form the vital spirits necessary to life. Vivi-

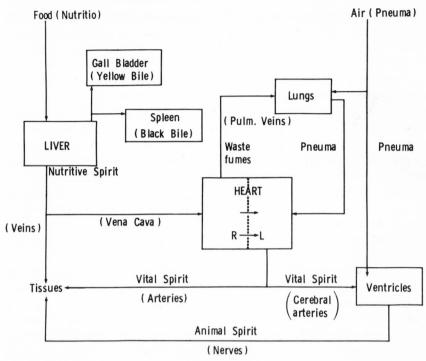

Figure 2 Galen's concepts of human physiology.

section convinced Galen that the arteries were normally filled with blood. Cardiac systole served to distribute vital spirit via the arteries, and allowed the ascent of excessive vapours and waste fumes back through the pulmonary veins. Respiration was necessary to cool the fire in the left ventricle. Part of the arterial blood penetrated the cribriform plate, to enter the brain. Here, the vital spirits were mixed with further supplies of pneuma inhaled via the nostrils and converted to animal spirits, stored in the lateral ventricles. After distribution by the nerves, animal spirit was responsible for sensation and could also call the voluntary muscles of the body into action. While Galen added much to anatomical knowledge, he followed the tradition of Aristotle in placing a teleological explanation on what he saw (De Usu Partum Corporis Humani); thus his physiology is essentially an elaboration of what was known at the time of Plato.

Nevertheless, his views were held in great reverence. More than 1300 years later (1559), the College of Physicians in London formally asked a Dr John Geynes to retract a suggestion that the works of Galen contained errors. In our day, when every hypothesis is tested by searching experiment, it seems incredible that the readily disproved views of Galen could hold sway for so long. Part of the problem lay in the absence of analytical and experimental tradition, and part in the repressive attitude of the authorities of the day (the Christian, Jewish, and Muslim religions). While the existing knowledge of Greece and Rome was stored in monastic vaults, medicine became regarded as a Godless science; all that was necessary for health and healing was a sound belief in the one true God. Thus Gregory of Tours threatened to class as a heretic anyone seen visiting the local physician. The body, also, was regarded as sacred, and stern prohibitions of dissection did not help to improve poor anatomical knowledge. Added to these problems were the dogmatism and teleology of classical scholars, and a too ready acceptance of their teachings by mediaeval pupils. Like Alice, professors and students were required to repeat things until they seemed to be true. Even today, we can learn the danger of reiterating ill-proven concepts until we believe them ourselves and force them upon our pupils.

The Renaissance
Enlightenment came from the east. The Arabic followers of Mohammed respected, preserved, and studied the traditions of their conquered neighbours, and through a band of displaced Nestorian Christians at Jondishapur, in Persia, they gained a wide knowledge of classical Hippocratic and Galenic medicine. Unfortunately, the stern proscriptions of Allah kept them not only from dissecting human flesh, dead or alive, but also from drawing it! Nevertheless, it was an Arabic physician of Damascus (Ibn Nafis, 1210–82) who was the first person to question the teachings of Galen. He rejected the idea that blood passed through pores in the ventricular septum, and suggested that the functions of the lungs included cooling and aeration of the blood, with removal of 'fuliginous vapours.' Damascus was not regarded as a major teaching institution at this time, and it is not certain how far these heretical views filtered back to the leading medical schools of Italy. Possibly some word of the new concepts may have been brought back by the crusaders.

By the fifteenth and sixteenth centuries the absolute authority of the church was weakening, and scientific humanism gained a foothold in Italy. Factors leading to the changed intellectual climate included the separation of theological and philosophical faculties at many European universities during the twelfth and thirteenth centuries, the emergence of a wealthy urban middle-class, and such inventions as the compass and the printing press which greatly extended the bounds of man's curiosity. In Bologna, professors such as da Varignana again began to dissect the human body. At first their objective was merely to illustrate the points made by classical scholars, but gradually discrepancies came to light. Leonardo da Vinci (1452–1519) made many dissections, including a series of sketches illustrating the function of the semi-lunar valves of the heart. He suggested that friction of the blood against the rough walls of the heart generated the heat needed for the formation of vital spirit. He pointed out that since the isolated lungs could be kept inflated, there could hardly be a direct connection between the blood vessels and the bronchi. Only the freshness and cooling action of the inspired air could be transmitted in the depths of the lungs. Leonardo planned to publish a systematic textbook of anatomy, but unfortunately was kept from a realization of this project by the premature death of his collaborator. Thus his daring ideas had little impact on the course of physiology.

Another early critic of the established order was the Spanish physician and theologian Servetus (1511-53). He seriously questioned not only religious doctrines such as the Trinity, but also the scientific 'facts' endorsed by the church. In his 'Christianismi Restitutio,' Servetus gave a clear account of the change in colour of the blood during its passage through the lungs. However, the book was mainly a criticism of current theology, and it brought upon its author the combined wrath of the Roman church and of Calvin. Servetus was arrested while attending church in Geneva, and was burnt at the stake with a copy of his work in his hands. He certainly published his findings in an 'obscure journal,' and as with Ibn Nafis, it is uncertain how widely known the scientific views of Servetus were in his own day. Even in our generation, if a scientist were to describe his choicest discoveries in a theological journal such as the *Oecumenical Review* or the *Critical Quarterly*, there is a good chance that his work would be overlooked.

Several of the Paduan school helped in the overthrow of Galen. Vesalius (1514-64), a Flemish physician, became professor of anatomy in Padua, and carried out careful personal dissections of the human cadaver. He began to appreciate the limitations of the information Galen had drawn from animal dissections, and went so far as to cast discreet doubt on the existence of pores in the ventricular septum of the heart. Despite the caution of his criticism, he was branded by his former teacher Sylvius as an 'ignorant, slanderous liar, inexperienced in all things, ungrateful and godless, a monster of ignorance.' An assistant of Vesalius, Columbus (1516-59) went on to give a good description of the mitral valves in his 'De re anatomica,' and apparently independently of Servetus he repeated the description of the aeration of the blood. Evidently the time was ripe for such a discovery. During the years 1545-48 Columbus stressed to his pupils the absence of pores in the intraventricular septum and the presence of blood in the 'artery-like vein.' Since Servetus did not make the fatal mistake of sending his manuscript to Calvin until 1546, Columbus can perhaps claim equal priority with him in the rediscovery of the pulmonary circulation. However, the persistent strength of Galenic ideas is seen in the Paduan's warning about the temperature in the left ventricle, where the heat is 'Intolerable to the exploring hand.'

Another Paduan anatomist, Hieronymus Fabricus (1537-1619), devoted a long treatise to a description of the venous valves, but ended by concluding that their purpose was to delay the flow of blood to the periphery, thus averting a catastrophic flooding of the extremities. Caesalpino (1519-1603), professor of botany and physiology in Pisa, corrected this error when he observed that veins became swollen on the distal side of a ligature; this phenomenon could only be explained if the blood was flowing towards the heart!

Final proof of the circulation of the blood was provided by William Harvey (1578-1657). Born at Folkestone in England, he studied under Fabricus in 1600-02 before returning to Britain as physician to Charles I. A series of painstaking dissections revealed many anomalies in current concepts of circulatory function. If the functions of the two ventricles were so different, why did they have an almost identical structure? How did the pulmonary vein succeed in carrying air in one direction and fuliginous vapours and blood in the opposite direction without intolerable confusion? If it did function in this manner, why was there never any sign of air or vapour within the vessel? During systole, the heart did not absorb blood as Vesalius had proposed, it became hard and expelled about half an ounce of blood. Over the course of the day, it would expel many times the blood manufacturing capacity of the liver. Harvey went on to bleed animals such as the sheep, and estimated the total blood volume fairly accurately. From these measurements, he reasoned that the entire blood volume must be pumped by the heart in a matter of minutes; the blood seen in the great vessels was therefore the same blood, circulating again and again. There was within the body a microcosm of that perfect circular motion seen in the course of the planets. His classical monograph 'De motu cordis' (Harvey, 1628) altered the whole course of physiology, yet it was no more than 70 pages in length. Here is a lesson in brevity for us all.

Later knowledge of the circulation

Harvey had boldly affirmed that he could find no connection between the arterial and venous systems, and he apparently assumed that blood oozed through the walls of the smaller arteries into the veins. He also continued to accept the traditional view that the heart recharged the blood with heat and vital spirit.

His first misconception was soon corrected by a new generation, armed with microscopes. Hand lenses had first appeared about 1280, but initially they only permitted a magnification of about ten orders. The improved glass technology of the Renaissance allowed scientists not only to study the distant planets, but by an inversion of their telescopes to begin a search for the 'atoms' of Democritus.

Malpighi (1628-94) was born in Bologna, but after a period of teaching in that city he moved to Pisa, where he came in contact with Borelli and began microscopic investigations. Close examination of a frog lung showed that it was not solid, as had been supposed, but contained a network of vesicles, crossed by small and tortuous blood vessels. The latter were populated by tiny reddish globules with a definite outline; although he mistook the globules for fat, he stated categorically that the blood was not a mixture of four humours, but consisted of white serum and red atoms.

Malpighi's primitive description of the capillaries and red cells was amplified over the next few years by another famous histologist, Antonj van Leeuwenhoek (1632-1723). The latter built over 410 microscopes, some with a magnifying power of 270, and provided much-needed histological background such as the striated appearance of skeletal muscle and the netlike arrangement of cardiac muscle.

Attention was next focused on the mechanics of the circulation. Borelli (1608-79) was a professor of mathematics at Pisa and Messina who began a systematic application of Galilean mechanics to the problems of human motion, interesting himself not only in external movement but also in the internal movement of fluids and particles. He wrote papers on the flight of birds, on swimming, and on the mechanics of the limbs. He further proposed designs for a submarine and a SCUBA underwater breathing set. He held that swelling of the cardiac muscle caused expulsion of blood at systole, and by comparing the mechanism to a winepress made some ingenious (if erroneous) calculations of the force exerted by the heart at each beat. By placing a thermometer within the contracting heart, he showed that the temperature of this organ was no greater than that of other body parts. Lastly, he realized the role of the elastic arterial wall in translating the pulsatile action of the heart into a smooth flow of blood to the tissues, although he concluded wrongly that the muscle of the arterial wall played an active role in helping the peripheral flow of blood.

In Denmark, a goldsmith's son named Niels Stensen (1648-86) developed a rigid mechanical and geometric view of muscular contraction. He examined the heart closely, and concluded it was not the source of body heat and vital spirit, but simply a muscle.

A keen experimentalist of this period was the Reverend Stephen Hales (1677-1761), the somewhat unusual vicar of Teddington. He succeeded in introducing a tube into the femoral artery of a horse with the aid of no other anaesthetics than could be found in his cellar, and reported that the blood rose to a height of 8 foot 3 inches above the heart, varying with the heart beat and with respiration. In contrast, blood in a venous tube rose to little more than a foot. Making full use of the creature, Hales later·filled the heart with wax, thereby estimating the volume of the cardiac chambers and gaining some insight into the cardiac output. He drew attention to the fact that the globules described by Malpighi and van Leeuwenhoek were only slightly smaller than the capillaries; in consequence, the circulation of the blood was greatly slowed by friction encountered in its passage through the tissues.

Theoretical application of the blood pressure concept was soon made by the Dutch physician and mathematician Bernouilli (1700-82). He multiplied a revised estimate of stroke volume (1½ ounces) by the required lifting force and obtained an acceptable figure for the resting cardiac output. Measurements of the cardiac force and the length of the resultant impulse also enabled him to correct Borelli's estimates of the cardiac work-load.

Clinical application of Hales's work was much slower, coming finally with refinement of the sphygmomanometer cuff by Riva-Rocci (1863-1937) and the description of a stethoscopic procedure for the indirect measurement of blood pressure by Nicolai Korotkoff in 1905.

Knowledge of the regulation of cardiac activity began with the demonstration by Ernst Weber (1795-1878) and his brother Eduard (1806-71) of the inhibitory function of the vagus nerve. Marey (1830-1904) showed that the action of the heart could be depressed by a rise of blood pressure, and Bezold (1836-68) described the sympathetic accelerator nerves to the heart, while Czermak (1828-73) slowed the heart by pressure in the neck. Thus were laid the foundations for studies of the action of adrenaline (by Cannon, 1871-1945), of acetylcholine (by Loewi, 1873-1961), of the pressor-receptor reflexes (by Hering and Heymans, commencing in 1924), and autoregulation of the circulation (Pavlov, 1849-1936).

Carl Ludwig (1816-95) was a dominant figure of this epoch. Succeeding Weber at Leipzig, he attracted over 200 students to the institute, many of whom subsequently achieved international recognition. However, in contrast to some of his European colleagues, Ludwig was so modest that his name rarely appeared on the work he had inspired and directed. He insisted throughout on a physical rather than a vital approach to the explanation of physiological phenomena, and perhaps for this reason gave much time to the perfection of objective measuring devices such as the kymographion (for recording blood pressure and respiration rate) and the stromuhr (for measuring blood flow). Another significant contribution was the initiation of work on isolated organs. This concept was followed up in the famous heart-lung preparations of Ernest Starling, and led to descriptions of the 'Law of the Heart' and the Bainbridge reflex.

Otto Franck (1865-1944) spent some time with Ludwig, and inherited his passion for the application of physical and mathematical principles to the circulation. He developed capsules that were capable of recording impeccable pulse curves, and used this technology to give accurate descriptions of distension, isometric, and isotonic contraction curves for the heart muscle. Application of wave theory also enabled him to estimate cardiac stroke volume from the amplitude of the pulse wave and the elasticity of the great vessels.

A simple polygraph for clinical recordings of the pulse wave at the wrist was devised by MacKenzie (1853-1925). He distinguished three types of irregularity of the pulse: the 'youthful' type found in healthy young subjects (corresponding to our sinus arrhythmia), the 'adult' type seen during anxiety or exertion (corresponding to our ventricular extrasystoles), and the 'dangerous type,' with a completely irregular rhythm (corresponding to auricular fibrillation). However, the diagnostic promise of the polygraph was soon eclipsed by the discoveries of a Dutch scientist, Willem Einthoven (1860-1927). Such was the intellect of this investigator that he was appointed professor at Utrecht even before his graduation. However, he adopted an extremely cautious approach to publication, locking his reports in a drawer for one year, and only submitting them to a journal if they agreed in detail with his subsequent researches. He described the electrical changes occurring in cardiac muscle, set these in a theoretical framework (the Einthoven triangle of limb leads), and in 1906 evolved a delicate string galvanometer that would record the electrocardiogram. Sir Thomas Lewis (1881-1945) carried out much further research on irregularities of cardiac rhythm, using a combination of the string galvanometer and a plethysmograph.

There were various attempts to make clinical measurements of cardiac output in the early part of the twentieth century. We have already noted the pulse-wave analysis that was developing in Germany. In Denmark, Lindhard (1870-1947) used the newly designed spirometer and bicycle ergometer of his colleague August Krogh (1874-1949) and deduced the exercise cardiac output from the absorption of nitrous oxide by the lungs. Grollmann applied similar concepts to the absorption of acetylene in the early 1930s. However, both techniques were soon overshadowed by a more direct approach. This chapter of cardiac history began with a Dr Forsmann, the young surgeon to a small hospital at Eberswalde in Germany. One day in 1929, while his colleagues were busy eating their lunch, he introduced a slender flexible tube into the right side of his heart via an arm vein. To complete this feat, he found it necessary to carry out radiographic screening of himself, viewing the fluoroscope in the wall mirror. Then, when the tube was securely in place, he marched briskly upstairs and demanded an x-ray plate of his chest from the astonished radiographer. His motivation seems to have been to evolve a method of injecting drugs directly into the heart, but the technique has since been exploited by others, notably Cournand and Richards, for the direct measurement of cardiac output. There are laboratories where this procedure has been applied to normal subjects during exercise, but such relatively drastic intervention is undesirable for research purposes.

Later knowledge of respiration

For many years, the nature of respired gas remained something of a mystery. The first to disrupt the Galenic concepts of matter was Paracelsus (1493–1541). He was both an alchemist and a lecturer in medicine at Basel. In a blanket rejection of tradition, he literally burned the works of Galen, and taking Arabic astrological concepts of 'mercury' (volatility) and 'sulphur' (combustibility), he added a residue ('salt') to form the 'tria prima,' the three basic elements of which he believed man was made. Because of his dalliance with eastern mystical ideas and the search for the transmutation of metals, he has been regarded by many historians as a quack. However, by insisting that vital phenomena had a chemical basis, he laid the foundations of modern biochemistry. He rejected the idea that the heart was the source of vital heat, postulating that this came rather from digestion, and he suggested that rather than exerting a cooling action, the pulse and the respiration served to distribute heat around the body.

Van Helmont (1577–1644) was in some respects the successor to Paracelsus, seeking a comprehensive chemical explanation of both health and disease. However, he rejected the tria prima, and maintained that there were only two basic elements, 'air' and 'water.' Although this was not in itself a great advance, Van Helmont also appreciated that 'air' differed in its quality from time to time. 'Gas' was not the same thing as steam. Again, 'air' produced by adding acid to limestone or by fermentation of malt contained a 'gas sylvestre' with a wild, chaotic quality that extinguished a naked flame. No doubt fascinated by his studies of malt and grapes, Van Helmont concluded that the body contained a sequence of ferments, decomposing food in the intestines, turning chyle into blood, and changing the colour of the blood within the lungs as vital spirit was introduced.

Boyle (1627–91) and his pupil Hooke (1635–1703) appreciated the need for careful observations rather than wild speculation, and thus conducted some of the first human experiments. A decompression chamber was built in their laboratory, and they discovered that a flame was extinguished and various unfortunate creatures such as a lark, a sparrow, and a mouse died when a vacuum was created. Hooke himself then ventured inside a larger version of the chamber. Fortunately, the inefficiency of his pump was such that the only noticeable effect was a pain in his ears. Hooke next showed that the primary function of respiration was not to pump blood through the pulmonary circulation, but to provide a fresh air supply to the lungs. He succeeded in keeping a dog alive by blowing air into the lungs with a bellows and allowing it to escape through pinholes at the lung surface. The animal even survived for brief periods without movement of the bellows, although if the 'menstruum' from the atmosphere was denied too long the dog convulsed and died. Hooke's experiments were continued and extended by his younger colleague Lower (1631–91). The latter used the technique of artificial ventilation to establish categorically that the change in colour of the blood occurred in the lungs. If dark blood was injected into the pulmonary artery, it emerged from the vein a brighter red, the transformation being contingent upon a continuation of ventilation. A similar change of colour could be observed in the upper layers of blood obtained at letting; the process was related in some way to an exposure of the blood to air.

The last of this remarkable group of English physiological chemists was Mayow (1643–79). He found that the survival time of animals enclosed in a small glass vessel was halved if a lighted candle was also present. This he attributed to the combustion of 'nitro-aereal particles.' By a happy accident, his bell jar was inverted over water, and he was thus able to observe a decrease in gas volume accompanying both combustion and respiration. We now realize that this reflects a metabolic gas exchange ratio* of less than unity and differences in the relative water solubilities of oxygen and carbon dioxide. However, Mayow suggested that the nitro-aereal particles had been used up by the candle and by various forms of tissue fermentation, the latter giving rise to body heat. Breathing served merely to facilitate contact between air and blood, allowing a transfer of the nitro-aereal particles from the atmosphere to the blood stream. The increased breathing of exercise reflected primarily the greater effervescence occurring in the muscles, and the consequent increased demand for the nitro-aereal particles.

These sound discoveries were soon forgotten with the advent of the 'phlogiston' theory of Stahl (1660–1734). Stahl held that combustible materials contained phlogiston, which could turn into fire on heating. Flames died out in closed bell-jars because the air became saturated with phlogiston. This ill-founded theory influenced many great minds over the next hundred years. Even Joseph Priestley (1733–1804) in England and Carl Scheele (1742–86) in Sweden, who each independently rediscovered oxygen, managed to constrain their findings within the bounds of the phlogiston tradition. Air supported life and fire because it was partly 'dephlostigated'; 'pure' air derived from heating mercuric oxide supported life and fire better because it was completely dephlostigated. If a candle was burned to extinction within a closed vessel, living plants could progressively dephlostigate the air to the point where it would again support combustion.

In the meantime, the work of Van Helmont on 'gas sylvestre' was repeated and extended by Joseph Black (1728–99). He described a 'fixed air' that was produced by burning charcoal, by the fermentation of beer, and by respiration. It could be detected by the white deposit that formed when it was passed into limewater, and in one dramatic demonstration of human carbon dioxide produc-

---

* See Glossary.

tion, Black introduced a dish of limewater into the roof ventilator of an over-crowded chapel.

It was left to Antoine Lavoisier (1743-94), a French tax-collector and later inspector of powder and saltpetre works, to demolish the phlogiston theory. Lavoisier stressed an observation apparently known to Stahl, that when metals such as mercury were burned they gained rather than lost weight. He showed further that the resultant oxides could be reconverted to pure metal and combustible air with a loss of weight. Again, when living organisms respired there was a disappearance of 'eminently respirable air' (he first used the term *oxygène* in 1777) from a closed vessel, with a corresponding production of 'aeriform calcic acid' (carbon dioxide). Combustion and respiration were, in fact, analogous processes, and during respiration there was a slow combustion of carbon in the lungs. In collaboration with Seguin, Lavoisier went on to study the oxygen cost of effort, and they found that the performance of 9195 foot-pounds of work increased the oxygen consumption of the body by 200 per cent. Unfortunately, not long afterwards a revolutionary tribunal decided 'nous n'avons plus besoin des savants,' and a guillotine halted a brilliant career.

The concept that combustion occurred in the lungs was soon disputed. A French colleague, Jean Hassenfratz (1755-1827), pointed out that since the lungs were no hotter than other tissues, it was more logical to assume that combustion occurred throughout the organism. At Pavia, the Italian naturalist Lazarro Spallanzini (1729-99) demonstrated that lowly animals without lungs still used oxygen. Furthermore, excised skin and muscle continued to absorb oxygen and give off carbon dioxide for a considerable time after removal from the body. Support for the theory of tissue respiration came from Heinrich Magnus (1802-70); he developed an improved mercury pump for the analysis of blood gases, and observed that the arterial blood contained more oxygen and less carbon dioxide than the venous blood. In 1835, Becquerel and Breschet succeeded in introducing a thermocouple into the arm muscles, and noted that the recorded temperature rose by at least $1°C$ during violent exercise, and in 1848 Helmholz demonstrated a similar rise of temperature during contraction of an isolated muscle. Finally, Claude Bernard (1813-78) amplified work from Liebig's laboratory, showing that although the temperature of the active muscles was higher than that of the blood entering them, the blood on the left side of the heart was cooler than that on the right. It was thus impossible that any substantial heat production occurred in the lungs.

It was important for the progress of knowledge to establish that the law of the conservation of energy applied to man, that energy could be neither created nor destroyed within the body. The first steps towards proof of this hypothesis were taken by Santorio Santorio (1561-1636), professor at Venice and later at

Padua. He compared the weight of his ingested food and excreta for more than thirty years, and commonly ate and slept in a weighing chair; usually, he lost about 1¼ kg over the course of the day, attributable to insensible perspiration. Audry (1658-1742) gave tacit acceptance to the principle in prescribing increased exercise for those of his patients that needed to lose weight. However, in the early nineteenth century people as well educated as Charles Dickens seriously discussed the possibility that people could meet their death by spontaneous combustion. Disproof of such ideas needed accurate measurements of energy expenditure during rest and work. Von Regnault (1810-78) perfected a closed-circuit metabolism apparatus, and obtained figures for the oxygen consumption and carbon dioxide production of animals as diverse as dogs and silkworms. He found that the smaller the animal, the greater the oxygen consumption per unit of body weight. In this same period, Helmholz used his sensitive thermomultiplier to show the relationships between muscular work and the production of heat. Voit (1831-1909) obtained a very substantial research grant (8000 guilders, about $3600) in order to carry out similar studies on man (1861). He built a chamber large enough to accommodate either a bed or a bicycle ergometer, and found that the protein requirements of his subjects were determined largely by body mass rather than the intensity of their daily activity. He thus rejected Liebig's view that protein was the principal fuel for muscular work; fat and carbohydrate provided interchangeable sources of energy during activity. Voit used his apparatus to make accurate measurements of body heat production; he also determined the energy contents of food and excreta with some precision, and was able to demonstrate convincingly that the principle of the conservation of matter applied in man. However, the first figures for the efficiency of human effort were probably obtained by Robert Von Mayer (1814-78), a German country doctor; he estimated that only about a fifth of the energy of foodstuffs was converted to mechanical energy, the remainder being dissipated as heat. Max Rubner (1854-1932) was one of Voit's most distinguished pupils; he further established the principles of direct and indirect calorimetry, and set energy equivalents for the principal forms of food. Two other well-known students were Atwater (1844-1907) and Benedict (1870-1957); they carried Voit's interest in human metabolism and studies of energy balance back to the United States. Other notable contributors to exercise biochemistry include Meyerhof (1884-1951) and A.V. Hill, each of whom studied lactic acid and oxygen debt, and Lohmann, who described energy storage in the adenosine triphosphate molecule.

Understanding of the characteristics of haemoglobin began with Lothar Meyer, who appreciated that oxygen was carried in the blood not only as a simple physical solution, but also as a loose and unstable compound from which it was readily freed. Reichert (1811-84) was the first to describe haemoglobin;

shortly afterwards Hoppe-Seyler (1825-95) succeeded in obtaining a crystalline preparation and reported its characteristic absorption spectrum. The importance of haemoglobin to human activity was emphasized by Sir Joseph Barcroft (1872-1947). In the first volume of his classical monographs on 'The respiratory function of the blood,' he pointed out that in the absence of the red blood pigment man would have been forced either to restrict his activity to that of the lobster or reduce his body size to that of a fly (J. Barcroft, 1914). In Copenhagen, Bohr (1855-1911) contributed much to an understanding of the oxygen-carrying capacity of the blood, including the description of widely accepted blood gas dissociation curves. His students Hasselbach (1874-1962) and Krogh (1874-1949) continued this interest, giving us respectively a series of blood gas nomograms and a microtonometric method for the accurate determination of blood gas tensions.

The inspiratory volume of the chest was measured by Borelli in 1680, but the first large-scale survey of lung volumes was published by John Hutchinson in 1846. An improved form of spirometer was used to measure the vital capacity of 2130 subjects ranging from 'paupers' to 'gentlemen,' and including artisans, servicemen, pugilists, and wrestlers. Borelli appreciated the existence of a residual gas volume that persisted after a complete exhalation, but it was not until the early nineteenth century that Humphrey Davy used hydrogen as a 'tracer' gas to estimate the residual volume of the lungs. Spirometry was further advanced by Krogh in Denmark and Benedict in the United States. Open circuit methods of measuring gas exchange were developed by Douglas and Haldane in England, while in Germany Zuntz reduced a respirometer to the size where it could be carried on the back of a worker or a mountaineer.

Other respiratory concepts important to oxygen exchange are the dead space of the airways, first discovered by Zuntz (1847-1920), and diffusion across the pulmonary membrane. For many years, Haldane and his associates held that the transfer of oxygen from the alveolar gas to the pulmonary capillaries was assisted by some active secretory process, but with improved techniques for the measurement of gas tensions in the alveoli and in the blood August Krogh (1874-1949) finally proved that diffusion was based on known physical principles.

Later knowledge of muscle and nerve
This topic we shall treat quite briefly. However, it is at least important to dispel the idea that muscle contractions are the result of a swelling produced by passage of a mysterious fluid down the nerves!

Cardano (1501-76), an Italian physician and mathematician, first conceived the idea that muscle movement could be explained from a mechanical standpoint. This approach was greatly developed by the physical scientist Borelli

(1608-79), who believed that all the phenomena of life and death had their basis in the newly discovered laws of physics. He suggested that muscular forces were dissipated by such factors as unfavourable leverage, air resistance, and water resistance. His studies of locomotion were particularly thorough, and his views predominated until the classical studies of the Weber brothers in 1834. Nevertheless, Borelli clung to the traditional explanation of muscular contraction itself: agitation within the brain produced a flow of spirits along the nerves, filling and enlarging the porosities within the muscles and causing their turgescence.

The idea of muscle swelling during movement was questioned almost immediately. Francis Glisson (1597-1677) used a plethysmograph to show that muscles contracted rather than expanded during activity. He went on to suggest that all viable tissue was 'irritable' and could react to stimuli. This concept was expanded by Albrecht von Haller (1708-77), who stressed the inherent irritability of muscle – an ability to contract in response to any suitable stimulus, independently of the nervous system. The nerves, also, could call a muscle into action independently of the will, but the basis of the contraction was then the 'extrinsic nerve force' which he distinguished from the 'inherent muscle force.'

Luigi Galvani (1737-98) was the first of a long series of eminent students of the 'frog jerk'; he found that contraction of the frog's muscles could be induced by application of metal such as a scalpel blade to either the muscle itself or the sciatic nerve. He concluded that movement of a muscle was due to a combination between its external negative charge and positive electricity passing down the nerve. From this time the theory of animal electricity rather than spirits began to dominate discussions of muscle action, through authors such as Emil DuBois Raymond (1818-96).

An Edinburgh surgeon (Robert Whytt, 1714-66) established that reflex actions were mediated via the spinal cord. Subsequently, Hughlings Jackson (1835-1911) and Sir Charles Sherrington (1857-1952) each made major contributions to our understanding of patterns of organization within the central nervous system.

Angelo Mosso (1848-1910) invented the ergograph, thereby allowing quantification of muscle contractions. The string galvanometer was first adapted to the recording of muscle action potentials by Piper (1912), and the use of the technique was popularized by Adrian (1925). Subsequent developments have paralleled the growth in knowledge of electricity, membrane structure, and protein chemistry; although fascinating topics, they fall outside the scope of this book.

Specific interest in endurance fitness
We have noted already a number of clinicians who believed in the therapeutic value of exercise. Ramazzini (1633-1714), in a classical textbook of occupational

medicine, commented on the prophylactic value of increased activity; sedentary workers needed regular exercise to avoid poor health. Stahl (1660-1734) also wrote of the preventive value of exercise. Nevertheless, general scientific interest in endurance fitness is quite a recent development.

Several probable reasons may be advanced for this state of affairs. Until recently physicians had inadequate remedies for major acute diseases. While a few hours of infection by the pneumococcus promised death to many patients, it would have been unrealistic to devote major consideration to the more remote hazards of habitual inactivity. Further, while Ramazzini wrote about sedentary workers, in his day lack of endurance fitness was a rare phenomenon, at least as far as the ordinary working man was concerned. The nineteenth-century miner who toiled for 14 hours a day had many ailments, but he was not worried by lack of fitness! Lastly, the sports sciences have until recently been the Cinderellas of the universities. Although some European schools boast a fairly long tradition of sports medicine (Ryan, 1974; Shephard, 1974g), it is only during the last two or three decades that there has been a determined effort to establish physical education and its occasional pseudonyms (kinesiology, kinanthropology, movement studies) as worthy areas for graduate work in North America. Master's and doctoral dissertations are now being presented in many schools of physical and health education; although the topics are subdivided among such areas of study as work physiology, biomechanics, sociology and psychology of sports, motor learning, and the history and philosophy of sport, a substantial proportion have relevance to fitness research.

The natural scientist first examined fitness in the context of its survival value. Darwin (1809-82), who had just read the 'Essay on the principle of population' joined the ideas of Malthus with his own observations to write *On the Origin of Species by Means of Natural Selection, or the Preservation of Favoured Races in the Struggle for Life* (1859). However, the well-worn phrase 'survival of the fittest' was coined by Herbert Spencer. Spencer originally held the Lamarckian view that abilities acquired by an animal were inherited by its offspring, but later he became converted to the Darwinian concept of evolution. The International Biological Programme has shown great interest in applying such principles to questions of adaptation and survival in the twentieth century, comparing the sedentary city dweller with the primitive tribesman in terms of such variables as working capacity (Shephard, 1976e). In order to influence the course of natural selection, an adverse environment (be it an extreme of heat, cold, or altitude, the energy demands of hunting or territorial defence, the competition for a mate, or debilitating disease) must demand a high level of fitness for successful adaptation of the individual; it must also exert any selective effect (such as an increase of illness or death rate) before the reproductive period has passed. Thus death from atherosclerotic disease at the age of 55 or 60 – even if attributable to a lack of personal fitness – would have little influence upon the survival prospects of any offspring.

The first serious attempts to assess the effects of lack of fitness on the life expectancy of 'civilized' populations were based on comparisons of mortality statistics for athletes and non-athletes. J.E. Morgan (1873) compared the age at death of 294 oarsmen who had rowed for Oxford or Cambridge with the life expectancies of the 'average' Englishman of insurance statistics. His objective was to refute the prevalent view that competitive oarsmen did not survive beyond the age of fifty, and he noted that far from showing early deaths, the oarsmen had an average advantage of two years longevity relative to the statistical norm. A similar study of Harvard oarsmen (Meylan, 1904) showed an advantage of 2.9 years over average U.S. citizens. Indeed, if allowance was made for the high incidence of accidental deaths in the athletes, the advantage was extended to 5.1 years. Although these studies served the immediate purpose of disproving the early demise of the competitive athlete, they took no account of the privileged life of the nineteenth-century university graduate. It was both unfair and unrealistic to compare him with the 'average' man (P.H.S. Hartley and Llewellyn, 1939). More recent investigations (Dublin, 1932; Rook, 1954; Montoye et al., 1956, 1957) have drawn control groups from the same college. The ex-athletes then fare no better than average graduates and live about two years less than the top honour students. This is hardly surprising, for Montoye et al. present figures showing that by the age of 45 the ex-athlete has gained as much weight and is less active than his 'sedentary' classmate; he is also drinking and smoking more than his sedentary counterpart. Evidently, the typical athlete finds some difficulty in abandoning the life of heavy eating and general merry-making previously associated with his athletic feats. The cross-country skiers of Finland seem to be an exception to this indictment. The majority of this group continue participating in ski-events through to old age. Karvonen (1959) showed that successful competitors from the period 1889 to 1930 had a seven-year advantage of life expectancy relative to unselected Finnish men.

Interest in the quantitative assessment of fitness was greatly stimulated by the need for objective grading of troops and aircrew during World War I. Undernutrition of the poorer segments of the population was still an appreciable problem at that time, and in a book entitled *The Assessment of Physical Fitness* Dreyer (1920) drew up extensive tables showing expected relationships between weight and body build. He also believed that a useful assessment of fitness could be obtained from the relationship of vital capacity to body weight, trunk height, and chest circumference, and he published tables of expected values for subjects with three grades of fitness (A, B, and C). Although Dreyer undoubtedly demonstrated differences of vital capacity between sportsmen and sedentary individuals of similar body dimensions, it now seems probable that he was testing the strength of the chest muscles rather than cardio-respiratory fitness. A large vital capacity has value in some sports such as swimming, but the measurement is no longer seriously advocated as a routine assessment of fitness. Two other respiratory tests were popular with the service physicians of World War I. One was the measurement of breath-holding time. This was routine in the British Royal Air Force until 1939, and a monograph from a German laboratory of Aviation Medicine discussed 'Die apnoische Pause' as recently as 1962 (Kallfelz, 1962). Breath-holding continues to have importance for some specific athletic and military situations, but confidence in the measurement as a test of fitness has waned since it was shown that the duration of apnoea could be doubled if subjects were faced by a clock with a second hand moving at a half the correct speed! The second air force respiratory test was a development of the breath-holding procedure; subjects were required to maintain a column of mercury at a height of 40 mm for a minimum of 45 seconds (Flack, 1920). As with breath-holding per se, results were found to depend very much on the motivation of the subject and his ability to withstand unpleasant sensations arising from the sustained positive pressure within the chest.

The first to make dynamic measurement of ventilatory capacity was Hermansen (1933). He studied the *Atemgrenzwert*, the maximum volume that a subject could breathe in 30 seconds. As the maximum breathing capacity, and latterly as the maximum voluntary ventilation, the test has enjoyed considerable clinical popularity. When the ventilation of a sendentary individual is more than 50 per cent of his maximum voluntary ventilation, he feels short of breath. To the extent that shortness of breath limits the exertion of many subjects (Shephard, 1974b), the concept of a respiratory reserve (Cournand and Richards, 1941) has some validity as one measure of cardio-respiratory fitness; however, the calculation of respiratory reserve has limited usefulness. The maximum voluntary ventilation depends greatly on the motivation of the subject, and there is little doubt that endurance athletes can push their ventilation to a greater proportion of maximum voluntary ventilation than a sedentary subject would tolerate.

The first observations on fitness and circulatory function are probably those of Harvey (1628). He noted that powerful, muscular men had stronger, thicker, denser, and more fibrous hearts than their weaker brethren. Interest in heart size and activity was revived with a report by Bergmann (1884) that domesticated animals had smaller hearts relative to body weight than the corresponding wild species. In the same period, Mosso used his ergograph to study exercising muscle and formulated the hypothesis that muscular efficiency depended on circulatory factors. Hirsch (1899), Linzbach, and Reindell further documented the association between heart weight and a well-developed musculature in men, while Külbs (1912) demonstrated that, after caging, the heart weight of the wild rabbit declined to the level of the tame animal. With the development of radiography, it became possible to show similar differences of heart size between active and inactive men during life (Schieffer, 1907). Herxheimer (1929) found that long-distance runners and cyclists had relatively larger hearts than weight-lifters and participants in short-distance events, while Steinhaus et al. (1932) applied the radiographic technique to puppies, observing that those exercised regularly developed larger hearts than their litter-mates. The procedure has more recently been refined to include lateral as well as postero-anterior radiographs of the chest (Blumchen et al., 1966; Reindell et al., 1966; Roskamm & Reindell, 1972), and it is still quite popular, particularly in Germany. The main weaknesses of the current method are: (1) development of the cardiac musculature is not distinguished from the development of fat or fibrous tissue and (2) any increase of tissue mass is not readily distinguished from an increase in the cardiac blood volume. Such difficulties are largely overcome if the heart volume is considered in conjunction with other measures of fitness, such as the working capacity and the total blood volume (Holmgren et al., 1964).

Following the refinement of the sphygmomanometer by Riva-Rocci, attention was directed to the blood pressure as a possible measure of fitness. Barringer (1917) described the rise of blood pressure that followed sixty seconds of vigorous work with dumb-bells, and considered this a measure of the reserve power of the heart. Bock (1928) suggested that more importance should be attached to the rise of systolic pressure during work. A second approach was to examine circulatory adaptations to changes of posture. The English physiologist Leonard Hill (1895) noted that the capacity of the visceral vessels was sufficient to contain the entire blood volume, and he postulated that as a person became fatigued the regulating autonomic nerves failed to bring about the necessary constriction of the visceral vessels on shifting from a lying to a standing position. The tests of Crampton (1905) and Schneider (1920) each presuppose that, when a fit individual moves from the supine to the upright position, the systolic blood pressure remains unchanged or rises slightly without a large increase of heart rate. However, Schneider admitted that the correlation between the postural change of blood pressure and other simple indices of fitness such as the resting pulse rate was poor. Scott (1924) provided further evidence that training improved tolerance of shifts to a vertical posture. It has since been widely accepted that one cause of poor physical performance is an inadequate control of venous reservoirs (the syndrome of 'vaso-regulatory asthenia,' Holmgren, 1967a), a problem that can be remedied through an appropriate exercise program. Wyman (1913) suggested that strenuous training produced some reduction of resting systolic blood pressure, and the Barach index - (systolic + diastolic pressure) X pulse rate/100 - incorporates this concept (Barach, 1914). On the other hand, Damez et al. (1926) reported that pulse pressures were greater in athletic than in non-athletic girls. The situation was clarified somewhat by German studies of the pulse wave, initiated by Otto Franck and carried forward by Wezler and Böger (1937); it was shown that, other factors being equal, the size of the pulse pressure was a reflection of stroke volume and thus of endurance fitness. The physical fitness laboratory of the University of Illinois, directed by Thomas Cureton, was greatly attracted to the possibilities of the indirectly recorded pulse pressure and its derivatives as a fitness test (Cureton, 1945; Franks, 1969). Critics of their work were quick to point out that the other factors contributing to the observed 'heartometer' pulse (elasticity of the great vessels, peripheral resistance, mean systemic blood pressure, and transmission of the pulse wave through overlying tissues) were so seldom equal that the information yielded by this approach was necessarily of limited value. Nevertheless, both the cardiac stroke volume and the timing of the various phases of the cardiac cycle have become of considerable interest in assessing the prognosis for patients with ischaemic heart disease, and with the development of more sensitive electromechanical transducers suitable for positioning over the carotid arteries, pulse wave analysis is currently enjoying a phase of renewed popularity.

The electrocardiogram has been the subject of exhaustive scrutiny since its introduction by Einthoven. A study of 260 competitors at the Amsterdam Olympic Games suggested that the two main features of the 'fit' individual were a long P-Q interval and a large T wave (Hoogerwerf, 1929). Neither measurement has proved of great practical value. The long P-Q interval is difficult to dissociate from the slow heart rate of the athlete, and many factors other than endurance fitness influence the recorded voltage of the electrocardiogram. Of more significance was Master's observation (1929) that depression of the ST segment immediately following vigorous exercise was associated with the risk of a subsequent heart attack (Master, 1969). His proposals for the use of loads adjusted for age, sex, and weight have only recently been superseded in exercise electrocardiography.

It has been known since the work of Lindhard (1915) that training is associated with an increase in the stroke volume of the heart. Some authors have also suggested that there is an increase in resting cardiac output with training. However, according to current views the latter differs relatively little, either between the athlete and the non-athlete, or between the trained and the untrained individual. For this reason, an increase of stroke volume with training is reflected in a slowing of resting heart rate, and laborious estimations of resting stroke volume are hardly justified in assessing fitness. In Lindhard's classical paper, the cyclist showed a progressive decrease of his resting pulse rate over the course of training. Unfortunately, readings are often unstable, particularly in a nervous athlete, and for this reason the resting heart rate has not been widely used as an index of fitness. Now that monitoring devices such as portable tape-recorders allow measurements to be made during sleep, heart rate determinations may have more practical value.

Lindhard (1915) and Grollman (1929, 1931) both tested cardiac output during submaximum effort, and Grollman noted a considerable scatter of results for a given oxygen intake. He suggested that the rate of muscular movements, and thus changes of venous return to the heart, was responsible for the variations of cardiac output at a specific loading. He further speculated that training would give better coordination, greater economy of movements, and a lesser venous return for a given intensity of work. During the last few years improvements in both Grollman's acetylene rebreathing technique (Simmons, 1969) and carbon dioxide rebreathing methods (Defares, 1956; Jones et al., 1967) have permitted rapid and repeated measurements of cardiac output during maximum exercise. It has been established that training increases not only the resting but also the exercise stroke volume. However, the strong negative correlation between heart rate and stroke volume has persisted during work, and it thus remains uncertain how much new information such sophisticated observations contribute to much simpler measurements of heart rate and oxygen consumption at graded work loads.

Perhaps because of difficulties in counting the pulse during exercise, many early tests were based on pulse recovery measurements, following running on the spot (15 seconds at 180 paces/minute, Foster, 1914), or stepping (Hunt and Pembrey, 1921; Tuttle, 1931; Brouha, 1943). Rapid restoration of the pulse rate following exercise is certainly a feature of the fit individual; indeed, on the basis of Hunt and Pembrey's investigation, the British Medical Research Council concluded that the recovery curve gave the best simple indication of general physiological condition. During the first 10–15 seconds of recovery, the pulse rate corresponds closely with values recorded in the final seconds of effort (Cotton and Dill, 1935: Bailey, Shephard, and Mirwald 1976). However, subsequent events are influenced by many extraneous factors, and if readings are taken 30–60 seconds after vigorous effort only about two-thirds of the 'information content' is related to the pulse rate during exercise (Ryhming, 1954; Shephard, 1967g; Millahn and Helke, 1968; McArdle et al., 1969). Complicating influences include: (a) the extent of the reflex increase in heart rate during exercise, (b) the heat load imposed by the exercise and body build (obesity), (c) pooling of blood in the legs following exercise, and (d) the extent and rate of repayment of any oxygen debt. One example of the difficulties of interpretation is provided by Knehr et al. (1942);

they reported that recovery curves were unchanged in subjects who increased their maximum oxygen intake over six months of training. Presumably, a larger oxygen debt was accumulated after training, and this accounted for the lack of change in the recovery curve.

Another approach adopted by those with limited equipment has been to describe the performance of the individual. Initially, this was done in the field. Thus Sargent (1921) proposed an index of muscular strength based on the product of weight and vertical jump height, divided by stature; others suggested various forms of endurance run. In the laboratory, the duration of effort on the step, bicycle, or treadmill was timed (as in the Harvard step-test [Brouha, 1943], and the all-out-treadmill run [Cureton, 1945]), or the loading of a bicycle ergometer was increased at minute intervals until exhaustion was reached. Tests of this type examine the second characteristic of endurance fitness – a high level of maximum performance. It is possible to show a dramatic improvement of performance following training. However, it is less certain how far the gains in performance reflect physiological adaptations to chronic exercise, and how far they indicate that the subject is becoming accustomed to the unpleasant sensations that accompany maximum exercise. In physiological terms, a small gain of maximum oxygen intake can turn an exhausting, 'supramaximal' effort into an easily tolerated submaximum run. Furthermore, the end-point is influenced largely by the motivation of the subject, unless an objective terminal criterion (such as reaching a pulse rate of 180/minute [Balke, 1954]) is adopted.

A more satisfactory method of examining maximum performance is to increase the work load in a stepwise manner until a plateau of oxygen intake is reached, and to report this physiological limit. The first to make extensive measurements of maximum oxygen intake was S. Robinson (1938); his work was repeated and extended by the Åstrands (P.O., 1952; I., 1960) and by Mitchell et al. (1958). If a true plateau of oxygen consumption is achieved, there can be little question regarding this criterion of endurance fitness. However, some subjects fail to reach a plateau, and a study of heart rates and blood lactate levels suggests that in such instances the explanation is poor motivation. Maximum tests are also not without risk for older subjects (McDonough and Bruce, 1969; Rochmis and Blackburn, 1971; Shephard, 1974k), and are clearly contraindicated in many cardiac disorders. For these reasons, interest has also focused on the first characteristic of endurance fitness – a lesser increase of variables such as heart rate during submaximum exercise. Some authors have reported their data with minimal interpolation, for instance the physical working capacity at a pulse rate of 170 beats/minute (Sjöstrand, 1947; Wahlund, 1948) or the heart rate at an oxygen consumption of 1.5 litres/minute (Cotes, 1966). This approach has the advantage of simplicity, but ignores the important difficulty of variations in maximum heart rate with age (Asmussen and Molbech, 1959; Lester et al., 1968). Others have attempted to extrapolate the heart rate/oxygen consumption line to a predicted maximum oxygen intake (P.O. Åstrand and Ryhming, 1954; Maritz et al., 1961; Margaria, Aghemo, and Rovelli, 1965). This approach involves the assumptions of a linear heart rate/oxygen consumption relationship and a similar maximum heart rate in all populations at a given age. Nevertheless, it has proved a very useful tool for field studies.

At one point there was considerable interest in the prediction of performance from body build. This concept has the great merit that little co-operation is required from the subject, other than the removal of most of his clothing. Hippocrates had originally distinguished two physical types – the long and thin man with the 'phthisic' habitus, and the short, thickset, muscular man with the 'apoplectic' habitus. Halle (1797) distinguished the fat *type digestif*, the strong *type musculaire*, and the large-headed *type cerebrale*. More recently Kretschmer and Enke (1936) contrasted the round and compact body form of the 'pyknic' build with the muscular 'athletic' individual and the long, thin leptosome. Sheldon et al. (1940) described fat 'endomorphs,' muscular 'mesomorphs,' and thin 'ectomorphs.' Fitness laboratories put much effort into Sheldon somatotyping and its later elaboration by Lindsay and Heath-Carter, but it is now widely accepted that if body form is worthy of attention, it is best described by parametric variables such as the weight of lean tissue, the standing height, and the percentage of body fat. Predictions of maximum oxygen intake from such measurements are still sometimes made (Davies, 1972a; Shephard, Weese, and Merriman, 1971).

In the past, the main emphasis of fitness assessment has seemed to be directed towards divergence, with the development of an ever-increasing number of tests and criteria. However, there have been sporadic attempts at synthesis, based on the statistical techniques of principal component and factor analysis. Thus McCurdy and Larson (1939) analysed 26 possible test items and advocated the use of a combination of five tests (sitting diastolic pressure, breath-holding time after exercise, increase of pulse rate after exercise, standing pulse pressure, and vital capacity). More recently, Cureton and his colleagues have reported many principal component analyses (Cureton, 1945; Franks, 1969; Franks and Cureton, 1969). In general, the results have been disappointing. 'Factors' have been extracted, but owing to the heterogeneity of the original data, their practical meaning has been obscure. The present author's adventures in this field, using both principal component (Shephard and Callaway, 1966) and sequential multiple regression analysis (Shephard and McClure, 1965), have served to emphasize that a large part of the interpretable variance in endurance fitness data can be ascribed to the heart rate response to submaximal exercise. Currently, a new approach is being tried. Instead of taking the favourite test of every research worker, and attempting to combine it mathematically into an omnibus expression for fitness, a serious attempt is being made to reach international agreement on a few simple basic tests of endurance fitness (Shephard, 1968a; Shephard, Allen, et al., 1968b,c; Weiner and Lourie, 1969; Larson, 1974). These focus on relatively unrelated (orthogonal) determinants of human performance and typically include an assessment of oxygen transport (the directly measured maximum oxygen intake or its prediction from heart rate and oxygen consumption during submaximal exercise), body composition (weight relative to height, skinfold thicknesses, body fat), muscle strength (knee extension, back extension, handgrip), and the electrocardiographic response to standard effort. Substantial advances in our understanding of endurance fitness seem likely as this standard protocol is applied to a variety of populations and experimental problems.

Many early fitness programs conceived training in terms of the development of prodigious strength. Morpugo (1897), a pathologist from Siena, reported a 55 per cent increase in the girth of the sartorius muscle when he trained dogs by running in an exercise wheel; this reflected a growth (hypertrophy) of existing fibres rather than an increase in the total fibre population (hyperplasia). Petow and Sibert (1925) went on to show that the extent of hypertrophy depended on the intensity rather than the duration of training. Thus was laid the groundwork for the researches of Germans such as Hettinger (1961), Müller, and Rohmert, who sought the development of muscle strength through as little as six seconds of exercise per day (Steinhaus, 1963).

Early work on endurance training centred around the Harvard Fatigue Laboratory. This was conceived by Henderson, and opened in a building attached to the Harvard School of Business Administration in 1927. Henderson saw that the role of the laboratory would encompass both physiology and sociology (Dill, 1967); 'The physiological pattern of the individual is an important factor in determining fitness for work, just as it is in determining excellence as a sprinter or as a football player. It also explains the kind of changes that work produces in a worker. Further, it probably determines some of the diseases that a man suffers and it can hardly fail to modify the course and result of all his diseases.' Interest was first directed to fatigue, and it was soon shown that tiredness sprang not from a single 'fatigue toxin,' but had many facets including an accumulation of lactic acid in the muscles, a build-up of lymph in the legs, and loss of salt by sweating. The first treadmill was borrowed from the Carnegie Nutrition laboratory in Boston. Apparently it did not stand up to the regular demands of the Fatigue Laboratory, for we read of a much more rigid machine being built by a conveyor belt company and fitted with a four-speed regulator taken from a streetcar. The influence of the Fatigue Laboratory can be surmised from a partial list of the investigators who worked there. Among many leaders of exercise physiology may be noted Bruce Dill, Talbott, Forbes, the Consolazio brothers, Sid Robinson, Lucien Brouha, Hugo Chiodi, Rudolfo Margaria, Howu Christensen, Erling Asmussen, and Marius Nielsen. A typical longitudinal training experiment is that reported by Knehr, Dill, and Neufeld (1942). Fourteen relatively sedentary students participated in a six-month training program to the limits imposed by their initial physique. Both body weight and maximum oxygen intake increased slightly during the experiment, but other more important variables contributing to a greater final performance on the treadmill were gains in mechanical efficiency and a higher tolerance of intramuscular lactate.

Tait McKenzie (1909, 1916) was an early advocate of endurance training for the cardiac patient. He spent much of World War I at a military hospital in Aldershot, and quickly found the value of graduated physical training in counteracting the several kinds of cardio-respiratory inefficiency variously described as 'soldier's heart,' 'neuro-circulatory asthenia,' and 'disorderly action of the heart.' Of 220 hospitalized cases, 64 were returned to full duty, 117 to light duty, and 39 were discharged from the services. During World War II, Howard Rusk (1943) and his associates began a program of physical reconditioning for men of the U.S. Army Air Force with rheumatic heart disease. Use of a simple step test as a guide to exercise prescription enabled the time to initiation of active treatment to be cut from 77 to 16 days, without deterioration in the long-term experience of the patients (Karpovich et al., 1946). More recently, physicians such as Gottheiner and Hellerstein have pioneered the use of similar treatment for patients recovering from myocardial infarction, to the point where such people can compete in marathon races (Kavanagh, Shephard, and Pandit, 1974).

Limitations of space preclude discussion of many other fascinating historical facets of endurance fitness. The interested reader is referred to other excellent sources of detailed information, including McKenzie (1909), Fulton (1930), Steinhaus (1933), Cureton (1945), Bettmann (1956), Steinhaus (1961), Husain (1962), McIntosh (1963), Perkins (1964), Fishman and Richards (1964), Harris (1964, 1966), Leake (1964), Munro (1965), Dill (1967), Ryan (1968), Howell and Howell (1969), Cox (1970), Boylan (1971), Gerber (1972), Rothschuh (1973), and Ryan (1974).

3
Physiological determinants
of endurance fitness

In this chapter we shall discuss the various physiological determinants of human performance in relation to the duration of activity (Keul, 1973). After a brief review of the 'oxygen debt,' we shall analyse in more detail factors contributing to the steady transfer of oxygen from the air to the working tissues, and arguments will be advanced sustaining the centrality of this oxygen transfer process as a determinant of activity lasting from one to sixty minutes.

THE FACTORS LIMITING HUMAN PERFORMANCE

The immediate basis of human movement (Figure 3) is the coupling of energy stored in certain high-energy phosphate bonds (adenosine triphosphate, ATP; creatine phosphate, CP) to the contractile proteins of skeletal muscle (actin and myosin). However, the total energy stored in such phosphate bonds is extremely small, about 7 millimoles of ATP and 18 millimoles of CP per kilogram of muscle (Bergstrom, 1967; Hultman et al., 1967). The total weight of muscle in an average man is about 28 kg, and if 20 kg is involved in endurance effort, the total potentially available phosphagen (ATP + CP) is 500 mmol. Some 11 kcal of energy, about 46 kilojoules (kj), are yielded for every mole of ATP that is broken down to adenosine diphosphate (ADP), but because energy is used in such reactions as the pumping of calcium ions through the muscle's sarcoplasmic reticulum, no more than 40-50% of the liberated energy can be applied to the bonding of actin and myosin (Banister, 1971). Very rapid sprints are further limited because the breakdown of ATP occurs faster than the potential rate of resynthesis by CP (Figure 3). Thus a runner may stop from exhaustion while his CP stores remain relatively intact (Margaria, di Prampero, et al., 1971). But even if ATP and CP stores are both used to the full, the potential performance of external work by phosphagen breakdown is no more than 2-3 kcal (8.4-12.6 kJ), and the body can readily exhaust this store within a few seconds. Sustained physical activity thus demands the replenishment of phosphate bonds. In the presence of oxygen, energy is made available through a breakdown of foodstuffs to carbon dioxide and water. If oxygen is not available, the reaction is halted at the lactate/pyruvate stage.

As activity continues, there must be an equilibration of income and expenditure for all accounts within the muscle cell (Figure 4). No one has yet succeeded in living on credit indefinitely! Theoretically, an overdraft could develop with respect to the delivery of normal fuels (carbohydrate and fat) or the removal of waste products (lactic acid, formed from carbohydrate in the absence of oxygen, carbon dioxide formed from carbohydrate and fat in the presence of oxygen, and heat due to inefficiencies in the conversion of chemical energy to mechanical work). However, within the time frame chosen for our discussion of endurance fitness (one minute to one hour), the principal bottleneck is the ability of the body to transfer oxygen from the atmosphere to sites of biochemical activity within the working tissues.

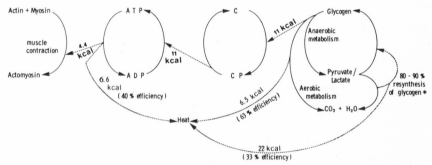

Figure 3 Sequence of chemical reactions involved in the contraction of muscle. The cycle is illustrated for the breakdown of one gram-molecule of adenosine triphosphate (ATP). Under aerobic conditions the efficiency is approximately 40 x 63/100, or 25%. Under anaerobic conditions, subsequent repayment of the oxygen debt and resynthesis of a portion of the glycogen yield an ultimate efficiency of approximately 40 x 33/100, or 13%.

* Recent studies have shown that the resynthesis of intramuscular glycogen is not complete for 24 hours or more after vigorous aerobic exertion (Hultman, 1971). However, this does not necessarily invalidate the traditional view of 80-90% resynthesis during repayment of the oxygen debt, since limiting concentrations of intramuscular and blood lactate are reached with the anaerobic breakdown of only a small percentage of muscle glycogen stores. Even if resynthesis proceeds more slowly than the disappearance of blood lactate, the net effect on the energy balance of the body will be as illustrated.

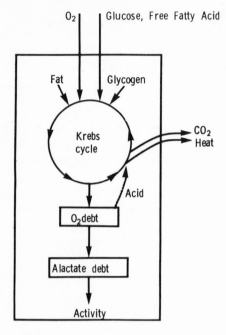

O$_2$ Glucose, Free Fatty Acid

Fat Glycogen

Krebs cycle

CO$_2$
Heat

Acid

O$_2$ debt

Alactate debt

Activity

Figure 4 Potential factors limiting endurance performance. In theory, activity could be restricted by the input of oxygen and foodstuffs to the Krebs cycle, or by the build-up of heat, carbon dioxide, and acid waste products. However, in practice, the factor limiting activity of 1 to 60 minutes' duration is usually the steady transport of oxygen from the atmosphere to the working tissues.

Consider first the food reserves. The muscles contain some 400 g of glycogen and the liver a further 100 g (Hultman, 1971; Saltin and Karlsson, 1973). Assuming this to be exhausted within 60 minutes, it would provide fuel for an energy expenditure of almost 32 kcal min^{-1} (134 kJ min^{-1}). The corresponding oxygen consumption would lie between 6.2 and 6.3 l min^{-1}, a figure encountered only in endurance athletes. Plainly the endurance effort of the ordinary sedentary person could not be limited by intramuscular food reserves or the delivery of metabolites via the blood stream except on rare occasions when near maximum effort was sustained for several hours.

Now let us look at waste products. Here the answer is less clear-cut. During brief and very intense muscle contractions that impede local muscle blood flow, the accumulation of the waste products of metabolism can create so acidic an intracellular environment that certain key enzymes cease to function (Figure 5). Various authors have noted an inhibition of phosphofructokinase (Trivedi and Danforth, 1966), a failure of phosphorylase activation (Danforth, 1965), and an alteration of the Michaelis constant of phosphofructokinase (Hofer and Pette, 1968), all of these changes slowing the rate of combustion of glycogen. However, the root of the problem is a failure of oxygen delivery to the active muscle fibres, with a consequent switching to alternative (anaerobic) methods of energy release

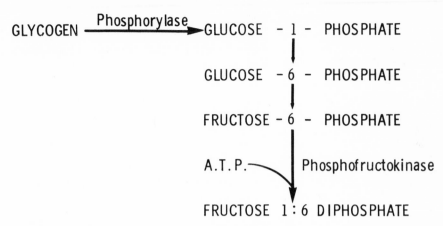

Figure 5 The enzymes phosphorylase and phosphofructokinase, essential to the breakdown of glycogen, are inhibited by the accumulation of acid metabolites within the muscle fibres.

and a build-up of lactic acid within the working tissues. With some types of more sustained rhythmic activity, performance may again be limited, at least partially, by increasing intramuscular concentrations of lactic acid. This reflects both a poor delivery of oxygen to the most active tissues and a slow diffusion of lactate from the muscle fibres into the blood stream.* However, if the activity is distributed over the majority of the large muscles of the body, lactate build-up is a less significant problem than oxygen delivery per se. Carbon dioxide transport becomes limiting only under unusual circumstances – underwater exercise and certain forms of chronic respiratory disease. When under water, ventilation is hampered by an increase in the density of respired gas, and the circulatory transport of carbon dioxide is often further impeded by the increased partial pressure of oxygen in the respired mixture.

Body heat accumulates in sustained exercise. We have noted already that the efficiency of energy transfer from ATP to actin and myosin is no better than 40-50%. Further energy is wasted in the resynthesis of ATP, so that the maximum production of useful work is about 25% of the energy content of glycogen under aerobic conditions and about 13% under anaerobic conditions (Figure 3). The remaining energy from the metabolized food appears as heat. Even under temperate conditions the rectal temperature of marathon runners may reach 40-41°C (Pugh et al., 1967; Wyndham and Strydom, 1972; Kavanagh and Shep-

---

* Theoretically, lactic acid could also accumulate because of a deficiency of enzyme systems converting pyruvate to CO_2 and water (Kaijser, 1970).

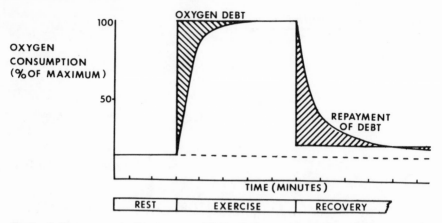

Figure 6 The concept of an 'oxygen debt' and the problem of its estimation owing to an incomplete return to the initial resting conditions after exercise. Some authors (for example, F.I. Katch et al., 1972) have adjusted the area of the repayment curve to allow for the cost of increased ventilation following activity.

hard, 1975c). However, unless the climate is extreme or the clothing inappropriate, neither the rise of body temperature nor the depletion of fluid and mineral reserves seems likely to impede the first hour of activity.

By a simple process of elimination, we can thus see that the usual factor limiting activity of 1 to 60 minutes duration is the maximum oxygen intake of the body.

The role of the oxygen debt

When considering the tolerance of fairly short periods of activity (1-10 min), it is necessary to note not only the 'cash flow' of oxygen, but also the rotating charge account, or oxygen debt (A.V. Hill et al., 1924-5). The latter reflects the various obligations incurred during vigorous activity – not only the partial breakdown of glucose and glycogen to lactic acid, but also an 'alactate debt' corresponding to the depletion of body oxygen stores and the breakdown of high-energy phosphate compounds (de Coster, 1971; di Prampero, 1971).

Measurement of the oxygen debt is difficult. If it is incurred in the early phases of work, one possibility is to look at the accumulated deficit of oxygen consumption before the individual reaches a steady state where oxygen delivery equals usage (Figure 6). However, if a man is performing maximum work to exhaustion in perhaps 10 minutes, a true steady state is never reached – the debt continues to grow until work becomes impossible, and there is then no basis for calculating the accumulated deficit. The alternative is to examine the status of the subject during the recovery period. It is not too practical to estimate intramuscular concentrations of lactate, but blood lactate determinations are commonly made on specimens collected from the heated finger tip, the heated earlobe, or (less satisfactorily) the arm veins (Mohme-Lundholm et al., 1965; Barker and Summerson, 1941; Shephard, Allen, et al., 1968b). Blood lactate analyses are time-consuming and not particularly accurate except in experienced hands. Furthermore, problems arise from the excretion of lactate in sweat and urine and a non-uniform distribution of lactic acid in body water (Alpert and Root, 1954), while the alactate debt (possibly as much as 40% of the total oxygen debt) is necessarily ignored. Another possibility is to continue measuring oxygen consumption from the end of exercise until the initial resting readings are regained. It is then assumed that the total excess oxygen consumption of the recovery period corresponds with the repayment of an accumulated oxygen debt. The traditional chemistry of the process has been that a portion of the lactate (10% [Margaria, 1967a,b; di Prampero, 1971], or 20% [Hill et al., 1924–5]) is broken down to carbon dioxide and water, providing the necessary energy for the resynthesis of the remainder to glycogen. One immediate apparent fallacy in the repayment calculation is that, as oxygen again becomes available, some of the accumulated lactate replaces other carbohydrate as a normal metabolic fuel, both within the active tissues and elsewhere in the body; this has the effect of reducing the apparent debt. Other factors operate in the opposite sense (Stainsby and Barclay, 1970). A persistent increase of ventilation, pulse rate, and tissue temperature (Brooks et al., 1971) all increase oxygen consumption during the recovery period. Energy needed to restore intracellular levels of sodium, potassium, and calcium ions, a depletion of carbohydrate stores, and the liberation of adrenal secretions all further conspire to prevent a return to the initial oxygen consumption within a reasonable time. Measurements of excess oxygen consumption during the recovery period thus become rather arbitrary and unsatisfactory (Figure 6). Different authors quote debt repayments ranging from 5 to 20 litres, with repayments usually exceeding the initial debt (de Coster, 1971; Katch et al., 1972). Taking into account the likely magnitudes of errors and alternative methods of validating estimates (Table 4), I favour the 'low' values suggested by Margaria and his associates (Margaria, 1967a,b; di Prampero, 1971), with total debts ranging from about 5 litres in a sedentary young man to about 8 litres in a wellmuscled athlete.

The debt can be accumulated in as short a time as 30 seconds if the body is engaged in maximum activity; equally, repayment begins as soon as the continuing energy expenditure falls appreciably below the maximum oxygen intake. The

TABLE 4

Maximum likely value of oxygen debt in moderately athletic young man*

Component of debt	Tissue weight	Concentration	Contribution to debt
Depletion of oxygen stores			
Venous blood	4 kg	-100 ml $l.^{-1}$	400 ml oxygen
Myoglobin	20 kg	-10 ml $l.^{-1}$	80 ml oxygen
Body fluids	38 kg	-0.5 ml $l.^{-1}$	19 ml oxygen
Phosphagen	20 kg	25 mmol kg^{-1}	500 mmol = 1.65 $l.O_2$
Lactic acid			
Muscle	20 kg	44 mmol $l.^{-1}$	
Blood	5 kg	11 mmol $l.^{-1}$	
Combustion of lactic acid, 10% of formation			9.4 mol = 6.00 $l.O_2$
Total			8.149 $l.O_2$

*   The calculation is based on the limiting assumptions of total depletion of phosphagen in active muscles, with an intramuscular lactate concentration of 44 mmol kg^{-1} and a blood lactate of 11 mmol kg^{-1}. The calculations of Margaria (1967a) have previously assumed 20 rather than 25 mmol kg^{-1} of phosphagen and a limiting lactate concentration of 16.5 mmol $l.^{-1}$ uniformly distributed throughout the body water.

practical importance of the debt can be seen when it is considered in relation to the normal cash flow – a steady oxygen intake of perhaps 5 litres per minute (5 l. min^{-1} STPD†) in an average young athlete, 3 l. min^{-1} in a sedentary young man, and 1.5-2.0 l. min^{-1} in an older person. If a subject performs maximum exercise for one minute, 50–70% of his energy expenditure will be based on credit (Figure 7). If the exercise is continued for five minutes, credit still accounts for at least 20% of the total, but at one hour credit has dropped to less than 2%.

Irrespective of the duration of activity, there is some initial depletion of phosphagen and accumulation of lactic acid, since time is needed to adjust muscle blood flow to the demands of exercise. In an athletic contest, this involuntary debt may be reinforced by early efforts while 'jockeying for position.' However, as with most charge accounts, if the oxygen debt is not repaid promptly there are unpleasant sequelae. The accumulation of unoxidized metabolites such as

† See Glossary for a discussion of symbols and abbreviations.

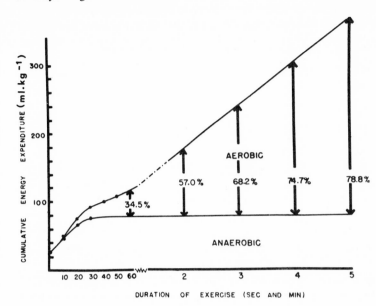

Figure 7 The relationship between the duration of exhausting activity and the proportion of the energy expenditure attributable to steady oxygen transport (from Shephard [1970e], by permission of the *Journal of Sports Medicine and Physical Fitness*).

lactic acid leads to discomfort and weakness in the active muscles and it also causes excessive ventilatory efforts. The wise distance competitor thus learns to slow his pace to a point where the early accumulation of lactic acid is oxidized, and he defers renewal of the debt until a final 30-second sprint (A.V. Hill, 1925).

From the foregoing it might seem that a complete description of endurance fitness should include an estimate of oxygen debt. Margaria (1966) proposed a field test for anaerobic power based on the maximum rate of ascent of a short flight of stairs, and this laboratory recently timed the endurance of an anaerobic treadmill run (Niinimaa et al., 1974). However, measurements of oxygen debt are still relatively uncommon. Apart from the difficulties of measurement, the oxygen debt is important mainly to athletes. It is rare for ordinary citizens even to approach their maximum oxygen intake in normal daily activity, and it is difficult to arouse their enthusiasm for measurement of an unused mechanism. In addition, it is uncertain how much 'new' information can be gained from studies of oxygen debt. Although there is evidence that the maximum tolerated debt is greater in trained than in untrained individuals, and that tolerance can be increased by training (Knehr et al., 1942; Helbing and Nowacki, 1966; Haskell,

1966), the increase of debt is commonly paralleled by an increase of maximum oxygen intake. If subjects differing widely in fitness are taken to exhaustion, they reach surprisingly similar terminal blood concentrations of lactate (about 100 mg 100 ml^{-1} of blood, 11 mmol l.$^{-1}$). Thus the larger oxygen debt of the trained athlete may reflect mainly a larger pool of blood and lean tissue in which unoxidized metabolites can accumulate.

INDIVIDUAL COMPONENTS OF THE OXYGEN TRANSFER PROCESS
AND THEIR INTERRELATIONSHIPS

The sequence of processes involved in the transfer of oxygen from the atmosphere to the working tissues is shown diagrammatically in Figure 8.

1. *Ventilation.* The bellows action of the chest brings an almost continuous stream of air to the alveolar interface within the lungs. However, not all of the observed external ventilation is 'gainfully employed.' Some of the respired volume is 'wasted' in ventilating the dead space of the airways, where no gas exchange can occur, and only alveolar ventilation helps forward the process of oxygen intake. Also a part of the total intake of oxygen is used by the muscles of the chest and heart, and oxygen consumed in this way is not available to the muscles engaged in external physical activity.

2. *Pulmonary gas exchange.* The interface between alveolar gas and pulmonary capillary blood next imposes some resistance to oxygen transfer. The ease of gas exchange across this interface is commonly characterized as the 'pulmonary diffusing capacity.'

3. *Blood transport.* The third stage of oxygen transfer is from the capillaries of the lung to the capillaries of the tissues via the blood stream. Here, the rate of transport is controlled by the haemoglobin level and the cardiac output, although as with ventilation a fraction of the cardiac output is 'wasted'; within the chest, there are shunts that by-pass ventilated areas of the lung, while within the tissues part of the cardiac output is directed to organs other than skeletal muscle.

4. *Tissue gas exchange.* Lastly, a long sequence of events is concerned in the movement of oxygen from the tissue capillaries to the metabolically active sites within individual cells; for convenience, these will be considered jointly as the 'tissue diffusing capacity.'

Which of these several transfer processes limits oxygen intake and thus human performance? In seeking an answer to this question, it is helpful first to develop a mathematical equation corresponding to Figure 8, and then to study the relative magnitude of the various terms in the equation. Hatch and Cook (1955) suggested that individual elements of the transfer process could be treated as conductances. In electrical terms, a conductance is the reciprocal of a resistance. If

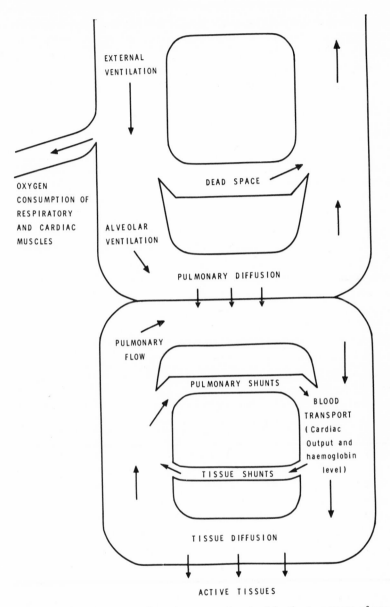

Figure 8 The sequence of conductances involved in the transport of oxygen from the atmosphere to the working tissues (from Shephard [1968b], by courtesy of *Ontario Medical Review*).

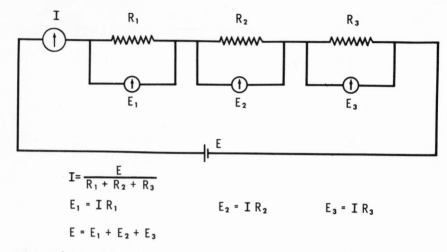

$$I = \frac{E}{R_1 + R_2 + R_3}$$

$$E_1 = I\,R_1 \qquad\qquad E_2 = I\,R_2 \qquad\qquad E_3 = I\,R_3$$

$$E = E_1 + E_2 + E_3$$

Figure 9 To illustrate the behaviour of three conductances arranged in series. The total potential E, or the corresponding pressure, distributes itself over the three elements in proportion to their individual resistances (or the reciprocal of the individual conductances).

resistance is represented by R, potential difference by E, and current flow by I, then from Ohm's law

(1) $R = E/I$

and

(2) $1/R = I/E$.

Thus conductance expresses the current flow through an element per unit of potential difference. Now let us suppose that we have three conductances, $1/R_1$, $1/R_2$, and $1/R_3$, arranged in series (Figure 9). If a current I is passed through the system, a potential difference $E = I(R_1 + R_2 + R_3)$ is developed, and this distributes itself between the three elements in proportion to their resistances, or in other words to the reciprocal of their conductances.

We must now leave the simple world of physics for the more complex problem of man. In man, oxygen intake can be regarded as the equivalent of current flow, and oxygen partial pressure or oxygen concentration gradient as the equivalent of potential difference. Oxygen uptake ($\dot{V}_{O_2}$) can thus be represented by an over-all conductance G and an appropriate gradient of oxygen concentration from the atmosphere (C_{I,O_2}) to the tissues (C_{t,O_2}). Rearranging equation (2), we have

(3) $I = (1/R)E$

and, by analogy,

(4) $\dot{V}_{O_2} = \dot{G}(C_{I,O_2} - C_{t,O_2})$.

The units for $\dot{G}$ are l. min^{-1} STPD, and those for C_{I,O_2} and C_{t,O_2} are ml l.$^{-1}$; thus, $\dot{V}_{O_2}$ is expressed in ml min^{-1} STPD. Similar equations can be written for the individual elements involved in oxygen transfer. Thus, alveolar ventilation ($\dot{V}_A$) can be regarded as a conductance, with a corresponding gradient of oxygen concentration from the atmosphere (C_{I,O_2}) to alveolar gas (C_{A,O_2}):

(5) $\dot{V}_{O_2} = \dot{V}_A (C_{I,O_2} - C_{A,O_2})$.

For example, if $\dot{V}_A$ is 80 l. min^{-1}, C_I is 209 ml l.$^{-1}$, and C_A is 160 ml l.$^{-1}$,

$$\dot{V}_{O_2} = 80(209 - 160) = 3920 \text{ ml min}^{-1} \text{ STPD.}$$

In the same way blood transport can be regarded as the product of two conductance terms, $\dot{Q}$ (the cardiac output), and λ (the solubility coefficient for oxygen, an expression of both the haemoglobin content of a unit volume of blood and the manner in which this haemoglobin reacts with oxygen). Again there is an appropriate gradient of oxygen concentration, from arterial blood (C_{a,O_2}) to mixed venous blood ($C_{\bar{v},O_2}$):

(6) $\dot{V}_{O_2} = \lambda\dot{Q}(C_{a,O_2} - C_{\bar{v},O_2})$.

A little more difficulty is presented by the terms relating to pulmonary and tissue diffusion. At first sight, the remaining gradients of concentration (from alveolar gas to arterial blood, $C_{A,O_2} - C_{a,O_2}$, and from mixed venous blood to tissue gas, $C_{\bar{v},O_2} - C_{t,O_2}$, respectively) seem incorrect. Pulmonary diffusing capacity ($\alpha\dot{D}_L$) is normally related to a gradient of oxygen concentration extending from alveolar gas to 'mean pulmonary capillary' blood ($C_{\overline{p.c.},O_2}$) rather than to arterial blood:

(7) $\dot{V}_{O_2} = \alpha\dot{D}_L(C_{A,O_2} - C_{\overline{p.c.},O_2})$,

while tissue diffusion $\alpha\dot{D}_t$ is normally related to the gradient from the mean tissue capillary oxygen concentration ($C_{\overline{t.c.},O_2}$) to the tissues (C_{t,O_2}):

(8) $\dot{V}_{O_2} = \alpha\dot{D}_t(C_{\overline{t.c.},O_2} - C_{t,O_2})$.

An explanation of this anomaly is suggested by further examination of Figure 8. We are not dealing with a simple series arrangement of conductances. Transfer of gas at both pulmonary and tissue capillaries depends upon the interaction of blood flow and diffusion. However, it is possible to treat gas exchange as a simple series system if we create two new conductances expressing these interactions (Beeckmans and Shephard, 1967; Shephard, 1972c). For the lungs the conductance becomes $(1 - B)/B.\lambda\dot{Q}$, so that we may write

(9) $\dot{V}_{O_2} = (1 - B)/B.\lambda\dot{Q}(C_{A,O_2} - C_{a,O_2})$,

while for the tissues the corresponding conductance is $(1 - K)/K.\lambda\dot{Q}$, and we may write

(10) $\dot{V}_{O_2} = (1 - K)/K.\lambda\dot{Q}(C_{\bar{v},O_2} - C_{t,O_2})$.

The derivation of the constants B and K is beyond the scope of this book, but we may note that the two terms include integrals describing the shape of the oxygen dissociation curve, with $B = \exp(-\dot{D}_L / \int\lambda\dot{Q})$ and $K = \exp(-\dot{D}_t / \int\lambda\dot{Q})$. We have now succeeded in partitioning the over-all conductance $\dot{G}$ of equation (4) into four series elements: alveolar ventilation (equation 5), the interaction between pulmonary blood flow and diffusion (equation 9), blood transport (equation 6), and the interaction between tissue blood flow and diffusion (equation 10). It follows from Figure 9 that the reciprocal of the over-all conductance is equal to the sum of the reciprocals of the individual elements:

(11) $\dfrac{1}{\dot{G}} = \dfrac{1}{\dot{V}_A} + \left(\dfrac{B}{1 - B}\right)\dfrac{1}{\lambda\dot{Q}} + \dfrac{1}{\lambda\dot{Q}} + \left(\dfrac{K}{1 - K}\right)\dfrac{1}{\lambda\dot{Q}}$.

There are a number of rather obvious limitations to this simplified mathematical representation of the cardio-respiratory system (Shephard, 1971a).

1. The lungs are represented by a simple chamber, uniformly and continuously ventilated and perfused, whereas we know that in practice it is a complex organ, that the distribution of ventilation and blood flow are far from uniform, and that both ventilation and blood flow tend to be discontinuous cyclical processes (Lacquet et al., 1967; Graeser et al., 1969). The effective values of alveolar ventilation and blood transport applicable to equation (11) are thus determined in part by the spatial and temporal matching of ventilation and blood flow within the lungs.

2. The lung diffusion term $\alpha\dot{D}_L$ reflects not only the ease with which oxygen diffuses across the alveolar and capillary membranes of the lungs, but also the volume of blood in the pulmonary capillaries and the rate of reaction between oxygen and haemoglobin. Similar considerations apply to the tissue diffusion term $\alpha\dot{D}_t$.

3. Neither $\alpha\dot{D}_L$ nor $\alpha\dot{D}_t$ is completely independent of cardiac output. An increase of cardiac output may distend existing capillaries, or it may open up new vessels. In either case, there will be an increase in both the effective surface available for diffusion and in the capillary blood volume, and this will be reflected in larger values for both $\alpha\dot{D}_L$ and $\alpha\dot{D}_t$.

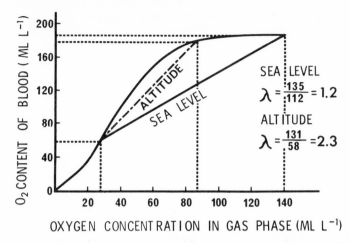

Figure 10 Illustration of the method of calculating the solubility of oxygen in a unit volume of blood (λ). The average slope between arterial (a) and venous (v) points is used. Note that at high altitude the increase in λ is not always as marked as the oxygen dissociation curve might suggest, since with the decrease in atmospheric pressure a given oxygen tension gradient is equivalent to a larger concentration gradient (ml l.$^{-1}$).

4. The tissues are assumed to behave as a single homogenous 'oxygen sink,' with an equivalent diffusing capacity $\alpha\dot{D}_t$ and terminal oxygen concentration C_{t,O_2}. In fact, a substantial part of the blood flow during maximal exertion is directed to tissues other than muscle, particularly the skin, and terminal oxygen concentrations are very different for the several components of the circulation (Shephard, 1968e).

5. The properties of the red cell pigment are such that the average value of the solubility term λ increases with a decrease in the oxygen concentration of alveolar gas (Figure 10). Thus there is an increase in λ as the blood passes from the arterial to the venous side of the circulation, and the second and fourth terms of equation (11) require an integral of λ based on the changes occurring in the capillaries. A nomogram has been devised that provides approximate integrals suitable for these calculations (Shephard, 1971a).

6. There is no guarantee that the largest over-all conductance is optimal in terms of the performance of external work. If large values of alveolar ventilation or cardiac output are achieved at the expense of a gross increase in the work of the respiratory and cardiac musculature, it is possible that the oxygen remaining for the performance of 'useful' work may be less than during more modest respiratory and cardiac efforts.

Despite these various important limitations, the conductance equation (11) provides a convenient framework for summarizing the interrelationships of the various factors limiting oxygen transfer (Piiper et al., 1971; Shephard, 1971a), and at least in children there is good agreement between the observed maximum oxygen intake and values predicted from the equation (Shephard, 1969c). We shall now look at the magnitude of some of the individual conductances.

EFFECTIVE ALVEOLAR VENTILATION $\dot{V}_A$

External ventilation

Ventilation is not usually regarded as the main factor limiting endurance fitness, since the maximum exercise ventilation (MEV) is less than the maximum voluntary ventilation (MVV) induced when a subject is asked to hyperventilate at rest. S. Robinson (1938) found an average MEV of 118 l. min^{-1} BTPS in healthy young men, and values as high as 160 l. min^{-1} BTPS have been reported in champion national athletes (Saltin and Åstrand, 1967). If the MVV is measured at optimum respiratory rates, using low-resistance apparatus that does not impede ventilation, figures of 160-200 l. min^{-1} BTPS are found in ordinary young men (Needham et al., 1954; Shephard, 1957; Ghiringhelli et al., 1957; Bartlett et al., 1958; Dittmer and Grebe, 1958; Altman and Dittmer, 1971) and values of 220-240 l. min^{-1} are encountered in athletes.

This does not necessarily prove that there is a large margin of ventilatory power during sustained exercise. The full MVV of the young adult is not realized at respiratory rates of less than 90 breaths per minute (Shephard, 1957), whereas it is uncommon to find a respiratory rate of more than 40 to 50 breaths per minute during maximum exercise. In addition, when the MVV is measured at rest, subjects are not normally asked to hyperventilate for more than 15 seconds. However, if subjects are encouraged to increase their respiratory rate to 100 breaths per minute, they can sustain 75-80% of their MVV throughout 15 minutes of exercise (Shephard, 1967h), and 70-75% of MVV can be developed for 4 minutes under resting conditions (Freedman, 1970). Furthermore, the main factor limiting greater ventilatory effort is not physiological but psychological, a reaction to the unpleasant sensations of vigorous chest movement (Schmidt and Comroe, 1944; Shephard, 1974i), since, with more forceful encouragement, subjects can push themselves to 100% of the resting MVV, even in the 15th minute of exercise.

The MVV falls with age, being 20-25% less in the sixth decade of life (Needham et al., 1954; Gilson and Hugh-Jones, 1955); it is also 20-25% less in the female at any given age (Dittmer and Grebe, 1958; Altman and Dittmer, 1971). However, it seems probable that the MEV is proportionately reduced in the aged

(S. Robinson, 1938) and in the female (I. Åstrand, 1960), so that throughout life the margin between the MEV and the MVV is maintained.

Some authors, such as Ishiko (1967), have found a fair correlation between vital capacity and the endurance of top athletes (Shephard, 1972a); in Ishiko's study of Japanese national competitors, vital capacity had a correlation of $r = -0.34$ with times for the 5000-metre run and $r = -0.71$ for rowing times. It is also known that training can induce substantial increases in maximal inspiratory and expiratory pressures (Delhez et al., 1967-68). Cureton (1936) and G.R. Cumming (1971) have argued that much, if not all, of the demonstrated correlation reflects a mutual dependence of performance and vital capacity upon body size. After allowance for standing height, Cumming (1971) found no correlation between athletic performance and vital capacity or maximal mid expiratory flow rate; nevertheless, the MVV remained related to performance of the 100-yard run, hurdling, the shot put, and the decathlon, possibly reflecting the dependence of MVV scores upon motivation, coordination, muscle strength, and speed. Swedish studies provide further evidence that training may augment lung volumes. Ekblom (1969a) trained a small group of 11-year-old boys for 32 months; over this period, gains of vital capacity in control subjects were as predicted from increases in stature, but the increase of vital capacity in the experimental subjects exceeded height predictions. Similarly, the vital capacity of 29 girl swimmers increased more than would have been predicted from size changes between the ages of 13 and 16 years, the largest increments of lung volumes being seen in the girls who trained the hardest (Engström et al., 1971).

Despite such increases of static and dynamic lung volumes with endurance training, recent studies confirm that ventilation does not normally limit exercise (Hyatt, 1972). During a forced expiration (Figure 11), there is a critical transpulmonary pressure (P_{max}) at any given lung volume (Macklem and Mead, 1967; Olaffson and Hyatt, 1969; Van de Woestijne and Zapletal, 1970; Yamabayashi et al., 1970); further increase of expiratory effort leads to a dissipation of pressure in compression of the airways without any increase of expiratory air flow. Plots of pressure/volume loops during exhausting exercise (Hyatt, 1972) show that P_{max} values are never reached during physical activity, at least in healthy young adults. Further, the flows attained during maximum exercise average only 63% of those recorded during a forced expiration and 40% of those seen in a forced inspiration (Pierce et al., 1968).

Alveolar ventilation
At rest, some 30% of external ventilation is 'wasted' in the dead space. The major component (130-160 ml in a young man) is attributable to the 'anatomical dead space' of the conducting airways, but a sizable minor component (30-40 ml) is

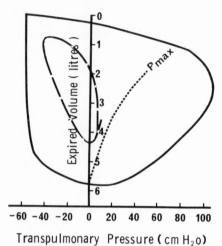

Transpulmonary Pressure (cm H₂O)

Figure 11 The relationship between transpulmonary pressure and respiratory flow. The outer solid loop shows a maximal expiration succeeded by a maximal inspiration, while the smaller interrupted loop indicates the findings during exhausting exercise. At no point during expiration does the latter loop exceed the limiting pressure (P_{max}) at which expiratory effort is 'wasted' through increasing compression of the airways. (Based on data of Olafsson and Hyatt, 1969)

'alveolar dead space,' reflecting temporal and spatial mismatching of ventilation and blood flow within the lungs (Shephard, 1959; Lacquet et al., 1967; Graeser et al., 1969; Kinne and Seagrave, 1974).

The size of the dead space during exercise is more controversial. Most observers have found some increase. Perhaps the most widely quoted study is that of Asmussen and Nielsen (1955a); unfortunately, only four subjects were used in their experiment, and no details were given of either the respiratory rate or the intensity of effort relative to the aerobic power of the individuals concerned. Some authors (Enghoff, 1938; Rossier and Bühlmann, 1955; and de Coster et al., 1958) have reported that the ratio of alveolar to external ventilation ($\dot{V}_A/\dot{V}_E$) remains about 0.7 as at rest, while others (Asmussen and Nielsen, 1955a; Jones et al., 1966) have found that $\dot{V}_A$ approximates more closely to $\dot{V}_E$ as respiration is increased. All of the observations cited were at respiratory rates chosen by the subjects – sometimes unspecified, but probably in the range 25–50 breaths per minute. Observations from the author's laboratory (Shephard and Bar-Or, 1970) suggest that an optimum $\dot{V}_A/\dot{V}_E$ ratio is reached at a respiratory rate of about 32 breaths per minute, but even at the high respiratory rates where maximum ventilatory effort can be developed (50–100 breaths min⁻¹), the ratio $\dot{V}_A/\dot{V}_E$ is no poorer than 0.70–0.75 in the adult and approaches 0.80 in the child.

The matching of ventilation and blood flow within the lungs (Cuomo et al., 1973) is improved by moderate exercise (Bryan et al., 1964; Bake et al., 1968), so that the 'alveolar dead space' may actually be smaller than at rest. During vigorous effort, most of the dead space of up to 500 ml is due, not to the large conducting airways, but rather to the brief time allowed for a mixing of gas between the terminal air passages and alveolar gas (Roos et al., 1955; Shephard, 1956; Beeckmans and Shephard, 1971). Although somewhat ignored when first proposed, the concept of such a 'stratified inhomogeneity' has now gained widespread acceptance in explaining the slow mixing of aerosols in the lung (Altshuler, 1961; G. Cumming et al., 1966; Muir, 1967), differences in the rate of mixing for gases of differing density (Arnott et al., 1968; Magnussen & Scheid, 1974), and the behaviour of various computer simulations of gas mixing within the bronchial tree (Stibitz, 1969; LaForce and Lewis, 1970; Beeckmans and Shephard, 1971; Cumming et al., 1971; Paiva and Paiva-Veretennicoff, 1972; Paiva, 1973; Stibitz, 1973; L.G. Baker et al., 1974). All of the models contain many uncertainties, ranging from the basic anatomy of the bronchial tree (a simple dichotomous model as proposed by Weibel [1963] or an asymmetric system as proposed by Horsfield et al. [1971]) to difficulties in making allowance for the simultaneous bulk movement of gases and diffusion (W.W. Wagner et al., 1969; Cumming et al., 1971). At the end of inspiration, the extent of stratified inhomogeneity is less than would be predicted by many of the models (Beeckmans and Shephard, 1971; L.G. Baker et al., 1974), and it seems that as gas passes through the bronchial tree its mixing is aided by some combination of local turbulence at airway bifurcations, convection, and axial streaming (L.R. Johnson and Van Liew, 1974; Engel et al., 1973). Nevertheless, little of the air that is inspired initially reaches the alveoli proper (Figure 12). Fortunately, much of it is contained in the atria and alveolar ducts, and is thus within a few millimetres of the main alveolar gas volume. During the remaining one to five seconds of a typical breathing cycle, the inspired gas mixes with alveolar gas by a process of diffusion, equilibration being helped forward by the massaging action of the heart beat ('cardiogenic oscillation') and physical movement of the bronchi. The interface between mixed and inspired gas gradually retreats up the bronchial tree, leaving a progressively diminishing effective dead space within the airway (Figure 12).

From the viewpoint of the conductance equation, we may accept that young healthy men can realize 75–80% of their maximum voluntary ventilation during sustained exercise. The external ventilation thus reaches 110–160 l. min^{-1} in a sedentary subject, and somewhat more in an athlete. Furthermore, some 75% of this respired volume normally mixes with the alveolar gas, giving a maximum alveolar ventilation of 85–120 l. min^{-1} BTPS, or 65–100 l. min^{-1} STPD.*

---

* Oxygen uptake has traditionally been expressed as litres per minute of dry gas, measured under standard conditions of temperature and pressure (STPD). Accordingly, all elements of the conductance equation are expressed at STPD, rather than at body temperature and pressure, saturated with water vapour (BTPS).

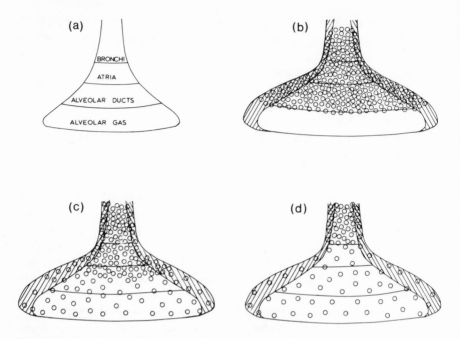

Figure 12 Simple conical model of a single-chamber lung, to illustrate the
concept of 'stratified inhomogeneity' of respired gas: (a) *At the end of
expiration.* (b) *At the end of inspiration.* Expansion of the constituent parts
is shown by diagonal shading. The fresh air, shown by open circles, has penetrated to the atria and alveolar ducts by bulk movement, supplemented by the
effects of local turbulence, convective mixing, and axial streaming. (c) *After a
short post-inspiratory pause.* The fresh air has mixed with alveolar gas and
through a mixture of diffusion and physical massage by the heart, the interface with fresh air has been displaced backwards towards the atria. (d) *After a
longer post-inspiratory pause.* Mixed gas now fills both the atria and the alveolar
ducts, and the effective dead space corresponds simply with the dimensions of
the bronchial tree.

We may note that the sensation of dyspnoea (shortness of breath) develops
when the exercise ventilation is more than 50% of the MVV. Although athletes
talk much about breathlessness and 'second wind' (Shephard, 1974b), dyspnoea
does not normally limit their performance. In contrast, a poorly motivated seden-

tary individual often fails to realize the potential of his cardio-respiratory system because of this symptom. Indeed, shortness of breath can be the main complaint of the unfit person who is forced to exercise, and in an older individual with some chronic obstructive lung disease a vicious cycle may develop, lack of fitness causing dyspnoea, with reduction of habitual activity, further loss of fitness, and worsening dyspnoea (Bass et al., 1970; Nicholas et al., 1970; Mertens et al., 1976).

THE OXYGEN COST OF BREATHING

While a healthy young subject remains at rest, the oxygen used in breathing is quite small, probably less than 10 ml min^{-1} (Otis, 1964). However, costs increase disproportionately with an increase of ventilation. There are several reasons for this. Turbulent airflow develops in an increasing proportion of the bronchial tree; a larger proportion of energy is diverted to movement of the liver and other heavy abdominal viscera; the efficiency of the respiratory pump is decreased as inspirations become larger and accessory muscles not normally concerned with ventilation are brought into play; and finally, the chest movements may become so rapid that the optimum speed of muscle contraction is passed.

If ventilation is plotted against the added cost of further respiratory effort ($\partial \dot{V}_{O_2 (R)}/\partial \dot{V}$), it is possible to envisage a subject reaching the point where this cost (Figure 13) becomes equal to the total additional oxygen introduced into the body by the extra ventilation ($\partial \dot{V}_{O_2}/\partial \dot{V}$). Increase of ventilation beyond this critical point is not only uneconomical, but actually restricts the oxygen supply to the muscles performing 'useful' external work.

At one time most attention was focused on the progressive increase of respiratory costs during vigorous effort; in near maximum exercise, $\partial \dot{V}_{O_2 (R)}/\partial \dot{V}$ rises to 4-5 ml of oxygen per litre of ventilation, four or five times the resting figure (Shephard, 1966e). However, if there is excessive ventilation during exercise, a larger problem arises from the rapid decline of $\partial \dot{V}_{O_2}/\partial \dot{V}$ (Figure 13). During maximum effort, $\partial \dot{V}_{O_2}/\partial \dot{V}$ is normally 30-40 ml per litre of ventilation, but if the subject hyperventilates, this quotient rapidly drops to less than 5 ml per litre of additional ventilation. This happens because blood leaving the lungs is normally almost completely saturated with oxygen; little additional uptake of oxygen is achieved by a further increase of ventilation, unless there is a matching increase in the maximum cardiac output.

In sedentary young men the critical point where $\partial \dot{V}_{O_2 (R)}/\partial \dot{V}$ equals $\partial \dot{V}_{O_2}/\partial \dot{V}$ is reached at a ventilation of about 130 l.min^{-1}. If the same were true of ath-

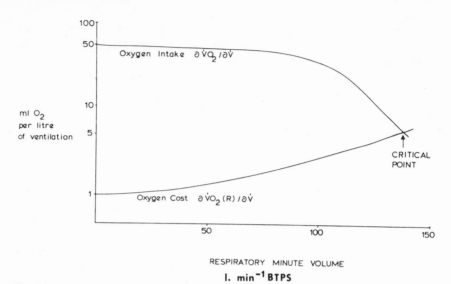

Figure 13 The relationship of respiratory minute volume to (a) the oxygen cost of added respiratory effort ($\partial \dot{V}_{O_2}/\partial \dot{V}$) and (b) the added oxygen intake resulting from the increased respiratory effort ($\partial \dot{V}_{O_2}/\partial \dot{V}$). Note the critical point beyond which the oxygen consumed by the respiratory muscles per litre of added ventilation exceeds the oxygen intake achieved thereby.

letes, the oxygen cost of breathing (or perhaps more correctly, the oxygen intake achieved by breathing) could be an important factor limiting their endurance performance. However, the maximum cardiac output of the athlete is substantially greater than that of the sedentary individual, and thus the drop of oxygen intake per unit of ventilation does not occur until a larger respiratory minute volume is reached; indeed, it is recognized that in maximum exercise the athlete has a lower ventilatory equivalent (and thus a higher reciprocal, the oxygen intake per unit of ventilation) than a sedentary subject. On the other hand, the critical point is readily exceeded in older subjects whose airways are blocked by chronic obstructive lung disease (Levison and Cherniak, 1968); for this reason, such individuals may well be forced to cease exercise before their hearts have been fully taxed.

In young normal subjects even the imposition of a substantial external resistance has little effect upon the oxygen cost of effort or the work that can be performed (Shephard, 1962; Deroanne et al., 1968; Flook and Kelman, 1973; Demedts and Anthonisen, 1973). However, this shows man's capacity to adapt rather than the unimportance of the work of breathing when airflow resistance is increased. Among the adaptive mechanisms open to the healthy young person are (1) the adoption of a slower, deeper, and more efficient pattern of respiration, with a reduction of the respired minute volume, (2) some increase of alveolar carbon dioxide pressures, with dilatation of the bronchi and a reduction of internal airflow resistance, and (3) an increase in the mean thoracic gas volume during breathing, with consequent mechanical expansion of the airways.

PULMONARY DIFFUSING CAPACITY

The idea that pulmonary diffusing capacity ($\dot{D}_L$) might be an important determinant of endurance fitness dates from reports that the resting diffusing capacity is higher in athletes than in non-athletes (Bates et al., 1955; Bannister et al., 1960; Newman et al., 1962), with swimmers showing a particularly large diffusing capacity (Mostyn et al., 1963). Some of the very high figures quoted for subjects with slow breathing patterns are artefacts arising from an inadequate sampling of alveolar gas (T.W. Anderson and Shephard, 1968a); however, the breathing pattern cannot explain high single-breath estimates of $\dot{D}_L$ (Bannister et al., 1960), and if due allowance is made for technical problems in steady-state estimates of $\dot{D}_L$, the results still seem somewhat greater in athletes than in non-athletes (T.W. Anderson and Shephard, 1968b). Furthermore, although physical training does not alter $\dot{D}_L$ at a given submaximal oxygen consumption (Anderson and Shephard, 1968b; Hanson, 1969), it does increase maximum oxygen intake and thus leads to a small increment of maximum diffusing capacity (Anderson and Shephard, 1968b). Although training produces some increase of maximum diffusing capacity, this does not prove the importance of the latter as a determinant of endurance fitness. Indeed, the increment of $\dot{D}_L$ may reflect no more than a close association between diffusing capacity and cardiac output (Holmgren, 1965; K.L. Andersen and Magel, 1970).

The level of exercise at which subjects reach their maximum pulmonary diffusing capacity has been the subject of some controversy. Holmgren (1965) accepted the belief of some earlier authors that a plateau of diffusing capacity was reached at a relatively low heart rate (120 min^{-1}), and more recently Scherrer and Bitterli (1970) have reiterated this finding with respect to oxygen diffusing capacity. Most measurements by the carbon monoxide method have failed to show a plateau of diffusing capacity (T.W. Anderson and Shephard, 1968c; di Prampero et al., 1969; Pirnay, Fassotte, et al., 1969; Lawson, 1970; Jebavy and Widimsky, 1973). In some individuals, possibly those who are less well trained, the slope of the $\dot{D}_L$/heart rate line does become less steep between heart rates of

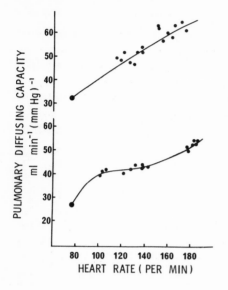

Figure 14 The relationship between heart rate and pulmonary diffusing capacity for carbon monoxide. In one of two healthy subjects the slope is less steep at heart rates of 120–155 min^{-1}, but it remains significantly greater than zero at all levels of exercise (data of T.W. Anderson and Shephard, 1968c).

120 and 155 per minute (Anderson and Shephard, 1968c; K.L. Andersen and Magel, 1970), but the slope remains significantly greater than zero and increases again at the highest work loads (Figure 14). Thus, the only maximum of $\dot{D}_L$ is that which occurs at the maximum oxygen intake.

For technical reasons, pulmonary diffusing capacity is usually measured in terms of carbon monoxide rather than oxygen transfer. We have found the maximum $\dot{D}_{L,CO}$ to be 40-50 ml min^{-1} mm Hg^{-1} (300-375 ml min^{-1} kPa^{-1}) in sedentary young men; it is 50-70 ml min^{-1} mm Hg^{-1} (375-525 ml min^{-1} kPa^{-1}) in the moderately athletic, and decreases slowly over the span of adult life (Cotes, 1965; Anderson and Shephard, 1968c; Pasquis et al., 1973). Values for the maximum $\dot{D}_{L,CO}$ of the female are still urgently required. Oxygen is transferred somewhat more easily than carbon monoxide, the maximum $\dot{D}_{L,O_2}$ being 1.23 times the maximum $\dot{D}_{L,CO}$. For the purpose of the conductance equation, it is also necessary to express diffusing capacity as the volume of gas transferred per unit of concentration gradient (ml l.$^{-1}$) rather than the transfer per unit of partial pressure (mm Hg or kPa). Accordingly, a correction factor α is applied, such that $\alpha = (\pi - 47)/1000$, where π is the barometric pressure measured in mm Hg and 47 is the corresponding vapour pressure of water within the body. The maximum value of $\alpha\dot{D}_{L,O_2}$ for a sedentary young man is thus about 35-43 l. min^{-1}.

The last figure is much smaller than would be expected from the anatomical surface area of the lung. The theoretical conductance of such a membrane is readily determined. Fick's law of diffusion for an infinite plane surface states that

(12) $\dot{D}_M = AD'\lambda\,.60/1000h$ (l. min^{-1}),

where $\dot{D}_M$ is the diffusing capacity, A is the area (cm^2), D$'$ is the diffusion co-efficient of the gas in a watery medium (cm^2 sec^{-1}), λ is the coefficient of partition of the gas between air and fluid, and h is the mean thickness of the membrane (cm). Anatomical dimensions required for this calculation have been given by Weibel (1963, 1970, 1973) and Scrimshire et al. (1973). Details of the anatomical assumptions can be disputed, particularly the pattern of bronchial branching and the use of a two-dimensional model to represent a three-dimensional structure (Hansen and Ampaya, 1974), but nevertheless the calculations reveal an interesting disparity between observed and theoretical values for $\dot{D}_M$. The area A is about 80×10^4 cm^2, and the harmonic mean thickness of the tissue layers h is about 0.55×10^{-4} cm. According to Weibel (1970), there are no fundamental differences of structures among the various terrestrial mammals, although there remains a need to verify the preliminary estimates of tissue thickness in man, using further samples of post-mortem material (Weibel, 1973). Assuming that such studies confirm that the thickness of the membrane is as in other species, the calculated value of $\dot{D}_M$ would be 450–500 l. min^{-1}, much in excess of the highest observed experimental value.

Part of the difference between theoretical and experimental figures is due to the time taken for oxygen and carbon monoxide to react with the haemoglobin of the red cells. The delay caused by this relatively slow reaction is equivalent to the introduction of an additional series conductance between alveolar gas and the blood stream. The resistance that is imposed varies inversely with the rate of reaction (θ) and with the volume of blood in the pulmonary capillaries (Q_c, often written as V_c). Thus if $\dot{D}_M$ is the diffusing capacity of the membrane proper, we may write

(13) $\dfrac{1}{\dot{D}_L} = \dfrac{1}{\dot{D}_M} + \dfrac{1}{\theta Q_c}$

The reaction constant θ is about 0.6–0.7 for carbon monoxide, and close to unity for oxygen (Forster, 1964). Anatomists such as Weibel (1963, 1970, 1973) and Miyamoto (1972) have found a capillary blood volume of 100–200 ml. Measurements of Q_c by physiological methods based on gas transfer have generally yielded substantially smaller values (Johnson et al., 1960). Given normal forward perfusion and restriction of the measured volume to blood vessels engaged in gas exchange (the capillaries and arterioles and venules smaller than 40 μ), it seems unlikely that Q_c exceeds 200–250 ml even during vigorous exercise. Thus, we may set an upper limit of 200 ml O_2 min^{-1} mm Hg^{-1} (143 l.min^{-1}) to the conductance θQ_c. Putting this value into equation (13), and taking $\dot{D}_L$ as 40 l. min^{-1}, we find that $\dot{D}_M$ is about 50 l. min^{-1}, around a tenth of the figure estimated from equation (12). The probable reason for the large remaining discrepancy between anatomical and physiological figures for $\dot{D}_M$ is that under normal conditions the lung capillaries cover only a small part of the membrane. The effective surface area is thus much smaller than the anatomical area. This view gains credence from the substantial increase of $\dot{D}_M$ during exercise (Mostyn et al., 1963; Anderson and Shephard, 1968c); it is difficult to conceive of much enlargement or thinning of the membrane during exercise, but it is easy to visualize an increase of $\dot{D}_M$ arising from a more complete covering of the alveolar surface by capillary blood vessels. Recent calculations of 'capillary loading' based on estimates of capillary surface and volume (Weibel, 1973) support this interpretation of the exercise response. We may conclude that, while the alveolar and capillary membranes would pose a negligible barrier to oxygen transfer if they were coextensive, in normal life a measurable resistance is found because parts of the alveolar surface are not related to perfused capillaries and vice-versa.

In view of difficulties in measuring the pulmonary diffusing capacity accurately, it is useful to consider other evidence regarding the equilibration of alveolar gas and pulmonary capillary blood. Staub and Schultz (1968) traced the path of individual capillaries in various small mammals, and found that a typical vessel coursed over five to seven alveoli, a total length of about 600 μ separating small arterioles from small venules. Under resting conditions, the transit time of the red cells through this system (and thus the opportunity for gas equilibration) ranged from 0.35 to 1.7 seconds, with an average of 0.8 second. Calculations suggested that this period was adequate to allow both diffusion of oxygen across the pulmonary membrane and the subsequent reaction between haemoglobin and oxygen. Miyamoto and Moll (1971) found a similar capillary path length; according to their calculations, if the alveolar oxygen pressure was 100 mm Hg (13.2 kPa) and red cells kept to the axis of the capillaries, as much as 0.5 second might be required to allow diffusion of oxygen through the lung membrane and peripheral plasma film to the centre of the red cell. Other authors (P.D. Wagner and West, 1972; Hlastala, 1972; E.P. Hill et al., 1973) quote figures of a similar order. Such slow equilibration could compromise gas transfer during severe exercise, when the average capillary transit time is apparently reduced to 0.3 second or less (Roughton, 1945; Fishman, 1963; Frech et al., 1968). However, the calculations of authors such as Miyamoto and Moll (1971) do not take account of the facilitation of diffusion by rotation of the red cells, their occasional displacement from the axial stream, and a possible movement of haemoglobin and cytochrome molecules within the erythrocytes (Kreuzer, 1970; Hill et al., 1973); these various processes could speed capillary equilibration appreciably.

The size of the oxygen concentration gradient from alveolar gas to pulmonary capillary or arterial blood provides further evidence on the resistance to oxygen uptake at the lung surface. From the technical point of view the most convenient gradient to measure is that used in the conductance equation (9), from alveolar gas to arterial blood $(C_{A,O_2} - C_{a,O_2})$. The size of this gradient reflects not only the incompleteness of equilibration across the lung membrane, but also any mis-matching of ventilation and perfusion within the lungs and the amount of blood by-passing the lungs in venous-arterial shunts. Despite the composite nature of the gradient, it remains remarkably small. Vigorous exercise typically gives rise to an increase of both C_{A,O_2} and C_{a,O_2}, with some widening of the alveolar-arterial difference (Holmgren and McIlroy, 1964; Hartung et al., 1966; di Pram-pero et al., 1969; Whipp and Wasserman, 1969; Vale, 1970; Rosenhamer et al., 1971; Doll, 1973). One early study (Linderholm, 1959) set the alveolar-arterial gradient at 16-20 mm Hg (2.1-2.7 kPa) in moderate work, and 50 mm Hg (6.7 kPa) in maximum effort; however, errors can arise from the effect of rising body temperatures upon the recorded oxygen pressures in arterial blood (Holmgren and McIlroy, 1964), and recent estimates show the gradient as increasing from about 10 mm Hg (1.3 kPa) at rest to 20 mm Hg (2.6 kPa) in exhausting effort. Riley (1974) summarizes the position by commenting that if there is a gradient, it arises from the shunting of venous blood rather than incomplete equilibration across the pulmonary membrane.

In any event, the oxygen-carrying properties of the blood are such that even the alveolar-arterial gradient of 50 mm Hg, as suggested by Linderholm (1959), would have relatively little influence upon oxygen transport. The solubility fac-tor λ of equation (11) increases from around 1.2 to about 2.3 as the oxygen content of arterial blood falls from 97 to 90% of saturation (Figure 10). However, any further decrease of arterial oxygen concentration brings a subject onto the steep part of his oxygen carriage curve, and oxygen transport is then markedly impeded by the falling oxygen content of arterial blood. Shepard (1958) has cal-culated the pulmonary diffusing capacity needed to keep the arterial oxygen saturation above the critical figure of 90%. If the maximum oxygen intake is 4 l. min^{-1}, a $\dot{D}_{L,O_2}$ of 60 ml min^{-1} $(mm\ Hg)^{-1}$ (455 ml min^{-1} kPa^{-1}, or 43 l. min^{-1}) is required, and if the maximum oxygen intake is 6 l. min^{-1}, $\dot{D}_{L,O_2}$ must rise to 100 ml min^{-1} $(mm\ Hg)^{-1}$ (758 ml min^{-1} kPa^{-1}, or 71 l. min^{-1}). These theoretical figures are of the same order as the observed maximum $\dot{D}_L$, emphasizing that although there is little physiological advantage to be gained from an increase of diffusing capacity (Johnson, 1967), a decrease can have serious repercussions on oxygen transport.

EFFECTIVE CARDIAC OUTPUT

General considerations
The maximum cardiac output $\dot{Q}$ attained during exercise depends on the working capacity of the cardiac muscle, the tolerance of a rising systemic blood pressure,

the peripheral resistance encountered in the muscles and elsewhere, the total blood volume, and the venous return to the heart. The effectiveness of a given cardiac output in meeting the oxygen needs of active tissues is influenced by the fraction of pulmonary arterial flow that perfuses underventilated alveoli or by-passes the lungs. Account must also be taken of blood flow distributed to the skin and internal organs rather than muscle. Finally, as with respiration, cardiac output has a theoretical upper limit, beyond which the consumption of oxygen by the heart muscle would make excessive inroads upon the over-all oxygen intake.

Working capacity of the heart muscle
Under resting conditions, some 20% of the oxygen consumption of the heart muscle is attributable to its basal metabolism, and a further 1% is accounted for by the cost of activating the tissue; only a small component (some 3%) is used in pumping blood around the arterial system, the main expense being the development (and to a lesser extent the maintenance) of tension within the ventricular walls (Sonnenblick et al., 1968; Jorgensen, 1972). The work performed thus depends largely on the determinants of ventricular tension (intraventricular pressure, the square of the ventricular radius, and the inverse of wall thickness), on the number of times the tension is developed per minute (heart rate), and the efficiency of conversion of chemical energy into mechanical tension (proportional to the reciprocal of contractility). During exercise, the contractility of the heart muscle is increased by the rise of heart rate itself and to a greater extent by the associated augmentation of β-adrenergic discharge. The stroke volume also increases with physical activity, but even in maximum endurance effort the external work associated with the pumping of blood around the circulation accounts for no more than 10–15% of cardiac metabolism (Burton, 1965; Shephard, 1968e). Internal tension work remains the major component, and the energy expenditure of the heart thus depends greatly upon the systemic blood pressure.

Rhythmic exercise of the large muscles of the body gives rise to some increase of systolic pressure, particularly if the activity is prolonged, but there is little change of diastolic pressure (Mellerowicz, 1962; P.O. Åstrand, Ekblom, et al., 1965; Hanson et al., 1968). Larger increments of the systolic reading are seen in older subjects (Reindell et al., 1960; Hanson et al., 1968) and in conditions where there is difficulty in perfusing the active muscles (use of small or weak muscles [Åstrand et al., 1965; Bevegard et al., 1966], particularly movements of the arms above the head [I. Åstrand, 1971b]). Sustained isometric contractions at more than 15% of maximum voluntary force lead to major increases in both systolic and diastolic readings, with corresponding augmentation in the work of the heart (Lind and McNicol, 1967).

Oxygen lack in the heart muscle is shown by the symptom of 'angina' and by the laboratory evidence of a depression in the ST segment of the electrocardiogram with a transition from lactate metabolism to lactate excretion in the coronary venous blood (Blomqvist, 1974). Normal healthy young subjects do not develop cardiac oxygen lack during endurance effort. However, as many as a third of 60-year-old men present the characteristic electrocardiogram of ischaemia during maximum effort (Cumming, 1972). In some elderly subjects the heart rate fails to increase to the anticipated maximum value during exercise (Powles et al., 1974); in others, the onset of angina, alarming electrocardiographic changes, and evidence of failing ventricular function such as a gallop rhythm or a falling systemic blood pressure lead to a 'symptom limitation' of maximum effort (Kasser and Bruce, 1969; Sheffield, 1974).

Maximum heart rate
Heart rates as high as 250-300 min^{-1} may be encountered during short bursts of very intense activity (Christensen and Höberg, 1950), but in sustained maximum exercise the heart rate of young men and women is a little under 200 (P.O. Åstrand and Ryhming, 1954). The maximum heart rate is sometimes lower in athletes than in sedentary subjects (Saltin and Åstrand, 1967; Lester et al., 1968). There is also a negative correlation between the maximum heart rate of an individual and his aerobic power (Davies, 1967), and some types of training reduce maximum heart rate by 5-10 beats min^{-1}. In our experience, athletes develop maxima comparable to sedentary individuals when the form of the test activity differs from that of their sport (for instance, swimmers tested on a treadmill [Shephard, Godin, and Campbell 1973]); however, low values are encountered when test and athletic activities are similar (for instance, runners tested on a treadmill). The maximum heart rate decreases regularly throughout adult life (Figure 15). Early studies suggested a drop to about 160 min^{-1} at age 65 (S. Robinson, 1938; Asmussen and Molbech, 1959), but more recent observations indicate that a sedentary North American who is pushed to an acceptable maximum effort develops a heart rate of at least 170 min^{-1} at the age of 65 (Lester et al., 1968; S.M. Fox and Haskell, 1968; S.M. Fox, 1969). The maximum heart rate is also lower at high altitudes (Figure 16), although an effect is not usually seen below 2000 metres in untrained subjects and sea level maxima are sustained to 4000 metres in athletes (Pugh, 1962; Stenberg et al., 1966; Kollias and Buskirk, 1974).

It is still unclear why there is a maximum heart rate, and why this should be lower in sustained than in brief activity. The influence of altitude suggests the possibility that oxygen lack is involved in some way, perhaps through a hindering of coronary flow at high heart rates, perhaps through the development of a cardiac work load that is excessive relative to flow through the coronary vessels.

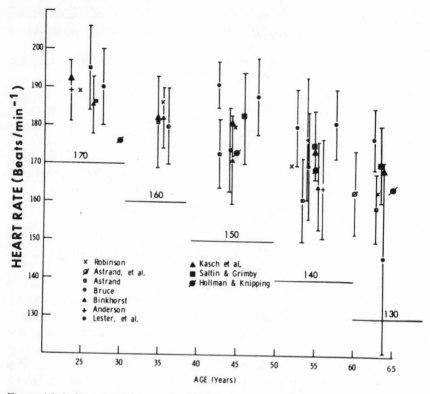

Figure 15 Influence of age on the maximum heart rate (collected data from the world literature, reproduced from S.M. Fox and Haskell [1968], by permission of the authors).

Unfortunately, for this hypothesis, the maximum heart rate of an older person cannot be restored to a youthful value by the administration of oxygen. A heart rate ceiling of 100–150 min^{-1} is set by problems of venous return when the resting heart is subjected to artificial pacing (Kissling and Jacob, 1973). On the other hand, there is no obvious relationship between the maximum heart rate of exercise and the work load at which the stroke volume of the heart begins to fail; P.O. Åstrand and Rodahl (1970) thus argue that there is no problem in filling the heart chambers even at rates as high as 200 min^{-1}.

Maximum stroke volume
The effect of exercise upon the stroke volume of the heart depends upon body posture. Rushmer (1959) aroused considerable controversy by concluding that

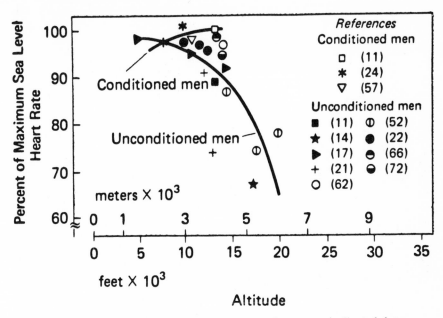

Figure 16 Influence of altitude on the maximum heart rate (collected data from world literature reproduced from Kollias and Buskirk [1974], by permission of the authors and publishers).

'increased stroke volume was neither an essential nor a characteristic feature of the normal cardiac response to exercise.' He based this conclusion on observations made in the supine position, and in the experiments cited the venous reservoirs of the legs as relatively empty prior to exercise. However, when subjects are sitting or standing, the leg veins are initially well filled. Exercise tends to empty these reservoirs, both through direct compression of the veins and also through an increase of thoracic suction. The increased return of blood to the right side of the heart, coupled with the increase of myocardial contractility, leads to an increase of stroke volume. A maximum is usually reached at a level of exercise corresponding to 30–50% of aerobic power (P.O. Åstrand, Cuddy, et al., 1964; Ekblom and Hermansen, 1968; Simmons and Shephard, 1971a); thereafter, any increase of cardiac output is dependent on an increase of heart rate. Some authors (Asmussen and Nielsen, 1955b; Mitchell et al., 1958; Åstrand et al., 1964) have suggested that there may be a further increase of stroke volume at the highest work loads. In Åstrand's dye-dilution experiments, the stroke volume plateaued at 90–100% of its maximum value between 40 and 100% of aerobic power, but 11 of the 23 subjects did not reach their maximum stroke

TABLE 5

Maximum cardiac output ($\dot{Q}_{max}$), heart rate (f_h), stroke volume (Q_s), arterio-venous oxygen difference ($C_{a,O_2} - C_{\bar{v},O_2}$), and maximum oxygen intake ($\dot{V}_{O_2}(max)$) during maximum exercise on treadmill (TM) or bicycle ergometer (BI); results for five Canadian endurance athletes and five control subjects (Simmons, 1969)

Age (yr)	Wt (kg)	Sex	Event	Mode of exercise	$\dot{Q}_{max}$ (l. min⁻¹)	f_h (min⁻¹)	Q_s (ml)	$C_{a,O_2} - C_{\bar{v},O_2}$ (ml l⁻¹)	$\dot{V}_{O_2}(max)$ (ml kg⁻¹ min⁻¹ STPD)
21	70.8	M	Swimming, 400 m	BI	30.4	183	166	153	65.8
21	93.2	M	Swimming, 400 m	TM	37.3	184	203	156	62.7
23	68.3	M	Field hockey	TM	32.2	187	172	154	70.7
40	63.5	M	Long distance running	TM	28.1	195	144	142	63.6
33	68.7	M	Long distance running	BI	30.2	170	177	159	70.0
Mean					31.6	184	172	153	66.6
29	78.9	M	Control	TM	27.5	195	141	141	47.4
25	69.8	M	Control	TM	24.5	173	141	128	47.2
27	63.2	M	Control	TM	22.7	191	119	126	44.6
34	75.3	M	Control	TM	28.3	173	164	136	52.3
23	76.3	M	Control	TM	25.7	187	137	136	50.1
Mean					25.7	184	140	133	48.3

TABLE 6

Maximum cardiac output, stroke volume, and arterio-venous oxygen difference for treadmill (TM) and bicycle ergometer (BI) exercise. Readings for eight healthy men, with mean and standard deviation (SD), as reported by Shephard, Allen, et al. (1968b)

Subject	Maximum cardiac output (l. min^{-1})			Stroke volume (ml)			Arterio-venous oxygen difference (ml l.$^{-1}$)		
	TM	BI	Δ	TM	BI	Δ	TM	BI	Δ
1	27.5	23.2	4.3	141	127	14	141	148	-7
2	24.5	24.6	-0.1	141	144	-4	128	128	0
3	22.7	21.5	1.2	119	114	5	126	124	2
4	32.2	26.1	6.1	172	140	32	154	142	12
5	28.3	25.6	2.7	164	149	15	136	140	-4
6	28.1	24.6	3.5	144	119	25	142	137	5
7	37.3	35.3	2.0	184	178	6	156	148	8
8	25.7	23.7	2.0	137	128	9	136	140	-4
Mean	28.3	25.6	2.7**	150	137	13*	140	138	2
±SD	±4.7	±4.2	±1.9	±21	±20	±11	±11	±8	±7

* Probability of occurrence by chance 0.01–0.001.
** Probability of occurrence by chance < 0.001.

volume until the maximum oxygen intake was attained. We have not seen this phenomenon either in acetylene-rebreathing experiments on fit young adults (Simmons, 1969) or carbon dioxide rebreathing experiments on children (Shephard, Lavallée, et al., 1974). Again, J.A. Faulkner et al. (1971) have reported a decrease of stroke volume at heart rates greater than 165 per minute. Nevertheless, it is conceivable that if the subjects are sufficiently stressed, a further surge of β-adrenergic activity plus the secretion of medullary catecholamines (adrenaline and noradrenaline) could boost myocardial contractility and (through an increase of venous tone) aid muscle contraction in returning blood from the venous reservoirs.

In our studies (Shephard, Allen, et al., 1968b), the maximum stroke volume has varied somewhat with the fitness of the individual and with the type of exercise performed; treadmill exercise gives a larger stroke volume than bicycle ergometer exercise (Tables 5 and 6), and leg ergometer values are in turn larger than data for the arm ergometer (Stenberg et al., 1967; Simmons and Shephard, 1971a). Values of 120–180 ml are typical of young men performing maximal treadmill exercise. Figures are lower for the female, but it is less certain that the stroke volume decreases with age (Niinimaa, 1976); most of the decrease in maximum cardiac output of the elderly is attributable to their lower maximum heart rate.

If work is prolonged, there is a progressive diminution of stroke volume, with a corresponding increase of heart rate. Various explanations have been offered for this 'cardiovascular drift.' Possible central factors include a mechanical slowing of ventricular systole (Ekelund and Holmgren, 1967), a reduction of vagal discharge (Hartley et al., 1970), and a heat-induced increase of heart rate (7 beats min^{-1} for a 1°C rise of rectal temperature, José et al., 1970). Among peripheral factors, Ekelund and Holmgren (1964) and Ekelund (1967a,b) suggested a progressive peripheral vasodilatation, with associated peripheral displacement of the available blood volume; greater filling of the superficial veins might be partly a passive consequence of an increasing blood flow to the skin, and partly a reflection of relaxation of venous tone (Zitnik et al., 1971). Saltin (1973) argued against the importance of peripheral mechanisms on the grounds that the progressive decrease of stroke volume occurred also in supine exercise (where venous pooling was presumably minimal); further, in his experience a normal stroke volume could be restored by a brief period of maximal exercise following prolonged heavy work.

Blood volume

As we have noted above, the stroke volume is markedly influenced by the availability of blood for pumping. This point was emphasized in one of the classical papers of physiology (Patterson and Starling, 1914): 'The circulatory problem in muscular exercise is not therefore how the heart drives the blood round, but the mechanism by which blood is brought rapidly from the peripheral parts of the body.' Although the filling of the heart depends directly upon the central blood volume (Asmussen and Christensen, 1939) and venous return, these are influenced in turn by the total blood volume. Some workers, for example Holmgren (1967b), have pointed out a close statistical correlation between maximum oxygen intake and blood volume or total haemoglobin; unfortunately, this does not prove a causal relationship, and others (Buskirk and Taylor, 1957) have dismissed the relationship as due to a mutual dependence of the two variables upon fat-free body mass. A further important consideration is the effectiveness of mechanisms regulating circulatory capacity. The tone of the cutaneous veins normally increases roughly in proportion to the severity of effort (Bevegard and Shephard, 1967; Hanke et al., 1969; Rowell, 1974), while exercise can also give rise to a 35% reduction in splanchnic blood volume (Wade et al., 1956). Failure of regulation impairs working capacity (the syndrome of vaso-regulatory asthenia [Holmgren, 1967a]).

Experimentally induced changes of blood volume have had varying effects upon oxygen transport and cardiac performance (Williams, 1974). Robinson et al. (1966) saw no acute increase of cardiac output when one litre of blood was returned to their subjects two weeks after a corresponding donation of blood. On the other hand, Kirschner (1972) found a 32% loss in the performance of a group of dogs one hour after withdrawing 10-12% of the total blood volume while Keroes et al. (1969) saw a marked increase of stroke volume when dogs were given a rapid intravenous transfusion. Rowell (1974) found only a 2-3% reduction in the aerobic power of human subjects three hours after the sudden withdrawal of 500 ml of blood, and Roberts et al. (1972) saw no change of maximum oxygen intake one hour after removal of 10% of the total blood volume. In contrast, Ekblom et al. (1972) found a reduction of maximum oxygen intake proportional to blood loss, with a diminution in the amount of work that could be performed at a specified submaximal heart rate, and a larger decrease of maximum effort than would be predicted from the change of $\dot{V}_{O_2}$(max). The main difference from the experiments of Rowell and of Roberts et al. seems to be that Ekblom et al. allowed a two-day delay prior to the measurement of $\dot{V}_{O_2}$(max). The blood was reinfused after an interval of 28-30 days had been allowed for regeneration of haemoglobin; contrary to the observations of B.F. Robinson et al. (1966), Ekblom and his associates then found a brief period of supranormal performance. Fears were naturally aroused that some endurance athletes might use this technique as an illicit method of augmenting their competitive performance. The effects of blood loss and reinfusion on both the heart rate/work load relationship and maximum oxygen intake probably arise mainly from changes in the haemoglobin content of unit volume of blood, and thus the solubility factor λ of equation (11). A second possible mechanism is a transient change in the circulating blood volume and thus the cardiac stroke volume.

The immediate effect of heat dehydration is a reduction in blood volume, with a diminished capacity to sustain a high work load (Saltin, 1964). With the exception of Klausen et al. (1967), most authors have found no immediate decrease of maximum oxygen intake in the heat (C.G. Williams et al., 1962; Saltin, 1964; Rowell, Marx, et al., 1966; Saltin, Gagge, et al., 1972). In the usual brief measurement of maximum oxygen intake, body temperature is not a limiting factor. However, a decrease of $\dot{V}_{O_2}$(max) is seen if the body is pre-heated before the test commences (Rowell, Brengelmann, et al., 1969b, Pirnay, Deroanne, and Petit, 1970). Aerobic power also seems limited in the period following heat dehydration (Pirnay, Petit, et al., 1968a).

Another group of subjects who may suffer a sudden change of blood volume are wrestlers who deprive themselves of fluid in an attempt to enter a lower weight category than that to which they are entitled by their body build. Dehydration brings about an immediate decrease of working capacity which persists for at least five hours after rehydration (W.G. Herbert and Ribisl, 1972).

Physical activity itself causes a 5–10% reduction of blood volume during the first few minutes of effort, with little change thereafter (Rowell, 1974). There is some evidence that exercise dehydration has a more adverse effect upon performance than heat dehydration (Costill, personal communication). However, Saltin (1964) found no change of maximum oxygen intake with an 11% exercise dehydration. Deterioration of performance may thus be attributable to other factors, including intramuscular water loss and associated glycogen depletion, fatigue, and inefficient use of available muscles.

In summary, it would seem that there are circumstances where a decrease of blood volume can impair both performance and oxygen transport, and that such a development is particularly likely if the capacity of the system is strained by a combination of heat relaxation of the venous reservoirs, loss of fluid from the circulation, and sustained exercise.

Maximum cardiac output

The maximum output of the heart is given by the product of maximum stroke volume and maximum heart rate. It amounts to 20–25 l. min^{-1} in normal young men and 30–35 l. min^{-1} in athletes (Table 5), falling to perhaps 15–20 l. min^{-1} at age 60 (Niinimaa, 1976). Over much of the range from rest to maximum effort, there seems a linear relationship between cardiac output and oxygen consumption (Pirnay, Dujardin, et al., 1972b), although P.O. Åstrand, Cuddy, et al. (1964) have presented evidence that there is a significant decrease of slope at loads demanding more than 70% of maximum oxygen intake. Certainly, as exhaustion is approached, one of the signs of a centrally limited maximum oxygen intake is a fall in cerebral perfusion, and a decline in cardiac output may be at least partially responsible for this (Shephard, Allen, et al., 1968b).

The conductance $\dot{Q}$ required for equation (11) is always a little less than the maximum cardiac output, since perfusion of the lungs is never 100% efficient. Part of the blood by-passes the lungs through venous-arterial shunts, and part perfuses poorly ventilated alveoli. The level of arterial oxygen saturation indicates the approximate magnitude of the problem. Arterial blood is usually at least 90% saturated with oxygen, and if mixed venous blood has a saturation of 15%, inefficiencies of perfusion cannot exceed 10–12% of the total cardiac output. Problems of diffusion make a small contribution to arterial unsaturation, and the effective conductance $\dot{Q}$ therefore amounts to 90–95% of the maximum cardiac output.

Distribution of cardiac output

Under resting conditions, muscle and skin blood flow together account for some 24% of the total cardiac output (about 1.5 l. min^{-1}), while the remainder (about

TABLE 7

Probable distribution of cardiac output in maximum exercise (from Shephard, 1968e)

	Volume of tissue (l.)	Oxygen consumption (ml min^{-1} STPD)	Maximum blood flow per unit volume of tissue (ml l.$^{-1}$ min^{-1})	Total blood flow (l. min^{-1})	Arterio-venous oxygen difference (ml l.$^{-1}$)
Muscle	28	4550	870	24.5	186
Skin	10	12	600	6.0	02
Other organs	32	138	47	1.5	92
All tissues	70	4700	457	32.0	147

4.6 l. min^{-1}) is distributed to other parts of the body. Most tissues are relatively well perfused, and on average less than a quarter of the available oxygen is extracted from the blood as it passes around the circulation.

During maximum exercise, the situation is very different. Almost all of the available oxygen is extracted from blood perfusing the active muscles (Table 7). Blood flow is also diverted from other parts of the body to the active muscles (Donald et al., 1954; Mitchell et al., 1958; Elsner, 1959; Wade and Bishop, 1962; Bevegard and Shephard, 1967, Haddy et al., 1968; Rowell, 1971, 1974), the reduction of visceral flow being proportional to effort expressed as a percentage of maximum oxygen intake (Grimby, 1965; Rowell, 1971). The greatest redistribution of flow occurs with a combination of severe exercise and heat exposure. The blood supply to the liver and kidneys may then be only 50% of normal resting values (Rowell, Blackman, et al., 1967; Rowell, 1971). The fractional extraction of oxygen from blood supplying the internal organs is necessarily increased by the flow redistribution, and a limit is set to circulatory adaptations of this sort by the susceptibility of the viscera to oxygen lack. If heavy exercise is performed in the heat, a mild tissue protest is often registered; enzymes from the liver are found in the blood stream, and red cells and protein make their way into the urine.

The percentage of the total cardiac output released by economies of visceral flow is relatively small (less than 10% of maximum output). A more important possibility is a reduction in the circulation to the skin. Several authors have recently shown skin flows of 7-10 l. min^{-1} with sustained heat stress (Koroxenidis et al., 1961; Folkow et al., 1965; Rowell, Brengelmann, et al., 1969a; Detry et al., 1972). During near maximum exercise, skin flow can again account for as much as a quarter of total cardiac output (Simmons, 1969), although the skin blanches as central exhaustion is approached (Shephard, Allen, et al., 1968a). Skin blood flow is reduced by exercise in the upright posture (J.M. Johnson et al., 1974), by heat acclimatization (Eichna et al., 1950) and by training (Shephard & Simmons, 1971b); heat tolerance is improved through earlier and more vigorous sweating (W.C. Adams et al., 1975), with an increased temperature gradient from the core of the body to the skin surface (Eichna et al., 1950; Leithead and Lind, 1964; Belding et al., 1966; Wyndham, Benade, et al., 1968; Rowell, 1974). Some authors (Whitney, 1954, but not Wood and Bass, 1960) have found a progressive restoration of venous tone with heat acclimatization. There is also some evidence for an increase of blood volume (Wyndham et al., 1968). In view of similarities in the adjustments which occur with chronic exercise and chronic exposure to heat, it is not surprising that there is some interaction between heat acclimatization and physical training (R.H. Fox et al., 1963; Piwonka et al., 1965; Marcus, 1972).

Although there is ample potential to redistribute blood flow from skin to muscle during exercise, the body sometimes adopts the alternative stratagem of reducing maximum cardiac output when the blood flow to the skin is restricted. Saltin (1973) found a cardiac output of 23.8 l. min^{-1} in a brief (3-4 min) maximum test, but a value of 26.7 l. min^{-1} with more protracted maximum effort (6-9 min). In the latter situation, it became necessary to dissipate heat by cutaneous vasodilatation. Systemic blood pressures were much lower in the protracted experiment (mean 111 mm Hg, 14.8 kPa, compared with 146 mm Hg, 19.8 kPa, in brief maxima). It is thus likely that the added cardiac output was achieved without increasing the work load of the heart.

THE OXYGEN EXPENDITURE OF THE HEART

It is theoretically possible to reach a point where a further increase of cardiac output causes an increase in the oxygen expenditure of the heart muscle that exceeds the gain in over-all oxygen intake. However, it is unlikely that such a situation arises in practice.

Many measurements of cardiac oxygen consumption have been made in dogs with opened chests, and there have been some observations on unanaesthetized animals; these are in agreement, showing that the resting heart consumes oxygen at a rate of about 10 ml min^{-1} per 100 g of tissue, with an increase to some 60 ml min^{-1} per 100 g in vigorous work (McKeever et al., 1958; Gregg and Fisher, 1964; Rowe et al., 1964; Van Citters and Franklin, 1969). Figures for the human heart seem of the same order (Lombardo et al., 1953; Holmberg et al., 1971; Jorgensen, 1972); thus, with a heart weight of 300 g, the resting oxygen consumption would be 30 ml min^{-1} and a maximum consumption of 180 ml min^{-1} would be reached during vigorous exercise.

The oxygen expenditure per litre of cardiac output (5-6 ml l.$^{-1}$) is similar during rest and exercise, and is small relative to the oxygen transported per litre (50 ml l.$^{-1}$ at rest, up to 150 ml l.$^{-1}$ in maximum exercise). Nevertheless, the oxygen needs of the heart make an appreciable charge on the over-all oxygen account, and can add to embarrassment caused by the increasing oxygen cost of respiration at large respiratory minute volumes.

THE SOLUBILITY COEFFICIENT λ

The value of the solubility coefficient applicable between arterial and mixed venous points ranges from about 1.2 to 2.4 (Figure 10; Hatch and Cook, 1955); however, since blood is almost fully saturated with oxygen during much of its time within the pulmonary capillaries, the integrated value of λ relevant to the interaction of pulmonary diffusion and blood transport is much smaller (0.3-0.4). A fall in the oxygen saturation of arterial blood increases the effective value of λ (Figure 10); this characteristic of blood oxygen carriage plays a large part in the ability of the body to withstand oxygen lack, both at high altitudes (Houston and Riley, 1947) and in congenital heart disease (Ernsting and Shephard, 1951). Early attempts to demonstrate adaptive changes in the oxygen dissociation curve of 'blue babies' were essentially negative (Ernsting and Shephard, 1951). More recently, it has been appreciated that changes in the 2:3 diphosphoglycerate levels of the red blood corpuscles (Dempsey et al., 1971) can modify the oxygen pressure needed for 50% saturation of haemoglobin (the P_{50} value). Boning et al. (1974) found a substantial rightward shift of the oxygen dissociation curve with training, caused not only by a change of 2:3 diphosphoglycerate levels but also by an increase of carbon dioxide pressures in the blood. However, Flenley et al. (1973) have queried how far such changes of P_{50} modify mixed venous oxygen pressures and thus oxygen transport.

The magnitude of λ varies directly with the oxygen carrying capacity of the blood, so that within certain physiological limits the haemoglobin level should be as important as the maximum cardiac output in determining the maximum rate of oxygen transport via the blood stream. In animals such as the cat and dog there is some evidence that stimuli such as exercise and fear cause a contraction of the spleen, thus increasing both the total volume of circulating blood and also the oxygen carrying capacity of unit volume (Ahlquist et al., 1954; Celander, 1954; Holtz et al., 1952). However, it is doubtful if the human spleen can contract in this way (Glaser et al., 1954; Wade et al., 1956; Brashear and Ross, 1968). Sustained exercise may give a small increase in the red cell count (5-10%), but this is due mainly to various forms of water loss such as sweating and exudation of fluid into the tissues. Prolonged exposure to oxygen lack (for example, congenital heart disease or life at altitudes greater than 10,000 ft, 3000 m) accelerates the formation of red cells, increasing the haemoglobin level by as much as 50%. Unfortunately, such increases lead to other less advantageous changes, particularly a greater blood viscosity. There has been much discussion regarding the possible value of altitude training for endurance athletes (Arch. d. Cabinet Medico del Comite Nacional de Deportes, 1947; Schilling et al., 1956; Shephard, 1974j). Top athletes commonly find their training schedules are interrupted in the unfamiliar environment, and the net result is a deterioration rather than an improvement of condition. Two studies reporting gains of maximum oxygen intake after a return to sea level (J.A. Faulkner, 1967; Mellerowicz et al., 1970) used subjects that were initially poorly trained; the changes that were seen could thus be due to training rather than the altitude residence itself. Certainly, the red cell count and haemoglobin level return rapidly to normal once the stimulus of a low partial pressure of oxygen is removed (Buskirk et al., 1967), and thereafter any residual gains of performance must reflect more general effects of the altitude training camp.

Endurance training increases the total amount of haemoglobin in the body, but it has a more variable influence on the haemoglobin content of unit volume of blood. Some well-trained athletes have a tendency to anaemia (Gilligan et al., 1943; Ekblom and Hermansen, 1968; Ekblom, 1969b; de Wijn et al., 1971), variously blamed on fads of diet (de Wijn et al., 1971), loss of iron in the sweat (Wheeler et al., 1973), a decreased formation of red cells (Kiiskinen et al., 1975), and an increased rate of destruction of red cells (Kiiskinen et al., 1975). Serum iron sometimes decreases over the course of sustained exercise (Kavanagh and Shephard, 1975b), but this may reflect a diminished delivery of iron from the reticulo-endothelial system; the high concentrations of iron found in sweat are due partly to contamination of the fluid by iron-rich epidermal cells (Shephard, Kavanagh, et al., 1976), and most authors now think the main problem of the athlete is an increased destruction of red cells.

In adult women, the haemoglobin level is 10-18% less than in men (Price-Jones, 1931; Vahlquist, 1950; Haekins et al., 1954). This causes a reduction in the oxygen solubility factor λ of equation (11), and contributes to the lower aerobic power of the female.

The practical importance of the oxygen carrying capacity of the blood is seen in carbon monoxide poisoning, where the resultant decrease of aerobic power is directly proportional to the percentage of red cell pigment converted to carboxy-haemoglobin (Apthorp et al., 1958; Ekblom and Huof, 1972; Vogel and Gleser, 1972). Some of the work on reinfusion of blood (see above) also indicates that an advantage is gained from increasing the blood haemoglobin level. However, observations on patients with anaemia have yielded conflicting results. In mild anaemia (11-12 g per 100 ml of blood) responses to submaximal exercise are normal and no reduction of aerobic power is found (Cotes et al., 1969b; Vellar and Hermansen, 1971), whereas in severe anaemia (5-8 g per 100 ml) maximum oxygen intake is reduced (Sproule et al., 1960; Davies, 1972c; Davies, Chukweu-meka, and Van Haaren, 1973), with gains of oxygen transport after correction of the condition (Davies and Van Haaren, 1973). One possible explanation of the discordant results is that in moderate anaemia a lower blood viscosity permits an increase of maximum cardiac output, thus sustaining a normal value of $\lambda\dot{Q}$.

TISSUE DIFFUSING CAPACITY

P.O. Åstrand (1952) argued that since an increase in the number of active mus-cles increased oxygen uptake, the main factor limiting performance was 'the local circulation within the working skeletal muscles.' However, he admitted that the distinction between central and peripheral circulatory factors was fine, and perhaps not physiologically correct. The need to exercise a substantial bulk of muscles in order to develop the maximum oxygen intake could reflect a peripheral limitation (such as the need for a minimum number of active capillaries) or a central limitation (such as a maximum tolerated systemic pressure, or a minimum demand for venous return).

More recently, the argument over central or peripheral limitation of oxygen transport has continued. Folkow et al. (1970) argued that the twin problems of muscle perfusion and venous return were best resolved by adopting a regular working rhythm, with contraction occupying 0.3 second of each second. In some forms of activity, such as vigorous cycling, contraction may be sustained for longer than a third of a repetitive movement, thus interfering with perfusion. Clausen (1973) found that in bicycle ergometer exercise, the blood flow to the vastus lateralis muscle (as indicated by the clearance of [133]xenon) reached a plateau at about 70% of maximum oxygen intake. In some subjects, flow apparently declined at higher work loads. The radioactive method of flow measurement is not very precise. It is also conceivable that at higher work loads blood flow is directed to muscles other than the vastus lateralis. Nevertheless, Clausen's observations support the view that one significant limiting factor in bicycle ergometry is a difficulty in pumping blood through the actively contracting muscles.

Kaijser (1970) has argued strongly that the main limiting factor is not the delivery of oxygen, but rather the ability of the tissues to utilize the oxygen that is transported. Some of the bases for this view are as follows:

1. *Variations of aerobic power with mode of exercise.* If aerobic power were centrally limited, it should be independent of the method of measurement. However, Bouchard et al. (1973) reported a correlation of less than 0.7 between the results of forearm, seated and supine leg ergometry, stepping, and treadmill data. In other words, less than 50% of the variance in scores reflected a common maximum oxygen intake. Closer analysis of their data shows that this seemingly poor result reflects the use of a rather homogenous population; their total coefficient of variation of 20% can be partitioned between inter-individual differences of maximum oxygen intake (10%), measurement errors (3%), and differences of maximum oxygen intake due to technique (7%, 0.21 l. min^{-1}). Stated in such a format, the experimental findings are less dramatic, and indeed agree well with previous comparisons of the various possible methodologies (Bobbert, 1960; Shephard et al., 1968a). It is generally agreed that the largest maximum oxygen intake is attained during uphill treadmill running, particularly if vigorous arm movement is permitted during the test. The treadmill value seems a stable maximum and cannot be increased appreciably by adding deliberate arm work (H.L.

Taylor, Buskirk, and Henschel, 1955; Stenberg et al., 1967; Pirnay, Deroanne, et al., 1971; Secher et al., 1974; Gleser et al., 1974). In young men, step test and bicycle ergometer tests yield data that are respectively 3-4% and 6-7% smaller (P.O. Åstrand and Saltin, 1961b; Damoiseau et al., 1963; Glassford et al., 1965; Wyndham, Strydom, et al., 1966a; Kasch et al., 1966; Shephard, Allen, et al., 1968b; Hermansen and Saltin, 1969; J.A. Faulkner et al., 1971; Ekblom, 1971; Taguchi et al., 1971); in older subjects with weak quadriceps muscles, the bicycle ergometer may yield proportionately even lower results (Kay and Shephard, 1969; Bailey and Shephard, 1976). Forearm exercise normally develops an oxygen consumption plateau that is only 70% of the treadmill maximum (Åstrand and Saltin, 1961b; Simmons and Shephard, 1971a, 1971b; Pirnay et al., 1971; Secher et al., 1974). However, it may approach or even exceed the treadmill figure in athletes such as canoeists who have well-developed arms (Saltin, 1966; Secher et al., 1974). If the trunk is immobilized by strapping, the arm value drops to only a third of that for the legs, although remaining high in proportion to the active muscle volume (Davies and Sargeant, 1974a).

During bicycle ergometer exercise, the cardiac output falls short of figures attained in treadmill running (Table 6), and to the extent that the body fails to call upon its known cardiac potential, we must accept that there is some peripheral limitation of effort while cycling. This view is supported by subjective complaints of leg fatigue (Shephard, Allen, et al., 1968b) and objective evidence such as the accumulation of blood lactate at quite low levels of submaximum work (Shephard, Allen, et al., 1968c; Hermansen and Saltin, 1969) with corresponding increments of systemic blood pressure. Nevertheless, application of conductance theory shows that if 70% of the treadmill maximum oxygen intake can be developed on an arm ergometer, the small muscle mass concerned in arm work still imposes only 43% of the resistance to oxygen transport due to central factors (Shephard, 1976c).

2. *Effect of variations in ambient pressure.* Kaijser (1970) reasoned that if circulatory transport of oxygen limited performance, then exposure to oxygen at a pressure of three atmospheres should augment performance. In fact, he found little change in a hyperbaric chamber. However, he judged performance on the subjective criterion of endurance time, making no direct measurements of maximum oxygen intake. It seems likely that the performance of his subjects was limited by an accumulation of carbon dioxide and other problems of exercise at high ambient pressures (Luft et al., 1972). Further, the oxygen pressure of venous blood was still only 65 mm Hg (8.6 kPa) when working in three atmospheres of oxygen, so that even in Kaijser's experiments the major part of the pressure gradient from inspired air (oxygen pressure 1800 mm Hg, 240 kPa) was occurring in the lungs and the circulation rather than within the tissues. Other experiments,

both before and after those of Kaijser, have shown gains of oxygen transport from quite modest increases of oxygen pressure (Nielsen and Hansen, 1937; Bannister and Cunningham, 1954; Margaria, Cerretelli, et al., 1961; L'Huillier et al., 1969; Taunton et al., 1970; Wyndham, Strydom, et al., 1970; Forgraeus, 1973; Shephard, 1976d). Again, although Kaijser found no shortening of endurance times when chamber pressures were reduced to subatmospheric values, there is now almost universal agreement that a substantial decrease of ambient pressure leads to a decrement of maximum oxygen intake (Goddard, 1967; Kollias and Buskirk, 1974).

3. *Specificity of training.* Clausen et al. (1970, 1973) claimed that a program of forearm training had a relatively small effect on the heart rate response to subsequent submaximum leg ergometry, while a program of leg training had little impact on the subsequent arm ergometer response. Such apparent specificity of training is hard to reconcile with a central limitation of oxygen transport (Shephard, 1975b).

By choosing an arm ergometer, Clausen undoubtedly biased his experiments towards the demonstration of a peripheral limitation of effort. Nevertheless, a repetition of the experiments with direct measurements of maximum oxygen intake (Clausen et al., 1971; Clausen, 1973) showed that leg training increased the aerobic power during arm work, the increase for the arms being 57% of that for the legs. This last finding seems very much in keeping with the postulate (Shephard, 1975b) that the small muscle mass of the arms imposes an additional 43% resistance on the transport of oxygen. Others demonstrated the treadmill training produced equal gains of maximum oxygen intake in subsequent treadmill and bicycle ergometer tests (Pechar et al., 1974), although the reverse was not true (Roberts and Alspaugh, 1972; Pechar et al., 1974).

4. *Effect of changes in cardiac output.* P.O. Åstrand and Saltin (1961a) found a higher cardiac output during long (6–10 min) than during brief (3–5 min) measurements of maximum oxygen intake. Oxygen transport was identical in the two types of experiment. This might seem to argue against a central limitation of effort. However, the paradox is readily explained by changes in the distribution of cardiac output, a greater proportion of flow being directed to the skin vessels during longer periods of effort. The heart works at a similar rate despite the small changes of maximum output. A similar explanation can be offered for the action of β-blocking drugs such as propranolol. These reduce cardiac output without changing maximum oxygen intake (Åstrand, Ekblom, and Goldberg, 1971); presumably, they alter the distribution of cardiac output between nutritional and shunt vessels.

5. *Effect of changes in muscle temperature.* Kaijser (1970) examined the effects of warming and cooling the limbs prior to maximal activity. His objec-

tive was to modify the rate of peripheral (muscle) metabolism, without changing the local blood flow or mechanical efficiency. He found an increase of oxygen consumption with warming, and a decrease with cooling. However, the magnitude of the change (less than 1 l. min^{-1} for a 10°C change of tissue temperature) was smaller than the usual metabolic effect predicted from the 'law' of Arrhenius (a doubling of oxygen consumption for a 10°C change of tissue temperature), and after limb cooling both the maximum heart rate and the maximum arterio-venous oxygen difference were substantially reduced. One may thus suspect that cooling reduced the normal exercise-induced vasodilatation within the active muscles. Kaijser interpreted the narrowed arterio-venous oxygen difference as clear proof of a reduction in the activity of tissue enzyme systems that normally were limiting oxygen transport. However, other tenable explanations include: (i) a greater relative dilution of blood that has perfused the active muscles by blood leaving the subcutaneous veins, and (ii) an increase of the diffusion pathway from the tissue capillaries to the active fibres, with a consequent augmentation of oxygen pressure gradients. Both of the latter explanations would implicate the muscle capillary system rather than tissue enzymes as a factor limiting performance.

6. *Biochemical responses to training.* Perhaps the strongest arguments in favour of a peripheral limitation of effort have come from the exercise biochemists. They have found close correlations between tissue enzyme levels and maximum oxygen intake (Howald, 1975), and an augmentation in the activity of supposedly rate-limiting enzymes such as phosphofructokinase and succinic dehydrogenase in response to training (Saltin, 1973; Holloszy, 1973). Enzyme activity is approximately doubled by a training program that increases maximum oxygen intake 15% (Saltin, 1973), and the teleologists demand some reason for this biochemical development.

The first point to stress is that endurance training is not the most effective method of augmenting the activity of tissue enzymes. Much larger changes can be induced by programs of isometric or anaerobic training (Gollnick and Hermansen, 1973). A second strand of evidence used to support the importance of the enzyme changes is the usual widening of maximum arterio-venous oxygen differences after training (Holloszy, 1973). It is argued that this reflects a peripheral limitation of oxygen transport in the untrained, with enhanced oxygen extraction after development of the tissue enzyme systems. However, the normal oxygen content of blood leaving the active muscles leaves little scope for further oxygen extraction with the development of tissue enzymes. L.H. Hartley and Saltin (1969), for example, found only 6 ml of oxygen per litre of femoral venous blood. Again, Doll et al. (1968) found no difference of femoral venous oxygen tensions between athletes and sedentary subjects. An alternative explanation of the widened arterio-venous oxygen difference in the trained group is that the habitually active individual directs a larger proportion of his total cardiac output to the active muscles (Simmons and Shephard, 1971b). This reflects not only an increase in the maximum cardiac output, but also an improvement of mechanisms for heat dissipation due to earlier sweating and a reduction of subcutaneous fat.

If we reject the view that there is significant limitation of oxygen transport at the tissue level, what alternative explanation can be offered to the teleologists to account for the doubling of tissue enzyme activity during endurance training? One possibility would be that compensation was occurring for an increase in the mean diffusion path. Endurance exercise produces little or no hypertrophy of muscles in the rat (Holloszy, 1967), perhaps because prolonged exercise markedly suppresses the appetite of small mammals (Stevenson, 1967). However, in Saltin's human experiments, the 15% gain of maximum oxygen intake was associated with a 37% increase of muscle fibre area, so that in the absence of other adaptations there would have been a substantial drop in oxygen pressure at the centre of the muscle fibres. Often hypertrophy is accompanied by an increase of capillarity, holding the oxygen diffusion distance relatively constant, but in the absence of such an adjustment, an increase of enzyme activities could serve the same purpose. Another advantage of the increased enzyme activity is that less phosphagen depletion is needed to 'turn on' mechanisms of oxygen transport at the commencement of vigorous exercise (Saltin and Karlsson, 1971). Lastly, with more active enzymes, the steady-state combustion of carbohydrate tends to be replaced by the utilization of fat (Holloszy, 1973), thus conserving glycogen in those muscles that contract too strongly – or too long per cycle – to permit unrestricted perfusion. In summary, there is no need to provide a 'reason' for the increases in enzyme activity during endurance training; nevertheless there are several convincing teleological explanations that can be offered without invoking a peripheral limitation of endurance performance.

Although there is some truth in a number of arguments advanced for a peripheral limitation of oxygen transport, calculations of tissue diffusing capacity and applications of the conductance equation support my thesis that the tissues do not normally offer a major resistance to the delivery of oxygen. The effective tissue diffusing capacity can be estimated from the known maximum oxygen intake and the probable gradient of oxygen tension from the tissue capillaries to the ultimate site of oxygen consumption within the active cells. Millikan (1937) observed the behaviour of myoglobin during tetanic stimulation of the soleus muscle; the saturation of the pigment suggested that the oxygen pressure within the muscle cytoplasm was between 3 mm Hg (0.4 kPa) and 5 mm Hg (0.66 kPa) (Landis and Pappenheimer, 1963; H. Barcroft, 1963; Coburn and Mayers, 1971).

Chance (1957) excited the fluorescence of diphenylnitrohydrazine (DPNH); from the oxidation/reduction status of this compound and other components of the respiratory chain (Granger et al., 1975), it was concluded that resting cellular metabolism dropped to 50% of its normal value when the oxygen pressure within the cell had fallen to 1 mm Hg (0.13 kPa); in the mitochondrion itself, where the majority of the oxidative chemical reactions occur, the critical oxygen pressure was perhaps two orders smaller than this (Chance and Pring, 1968).

Some early experiments with isolated muscle preparations indicated a rather higher critical oxygen pressure. However, this probably reflects inadequate perfusion of the muscle. More recently, Whalen and Nair (1967; 1970) have reported an intracellular oxygen pressure of 1–4 mm Hg (0.13–0.52 kPa) in the resting gracilis muscle of the pig, and Stainsby et al. (1960; Stainsby, 1966) have found a venous effluent oxygen pressure of 6–10 mm Hg (0.8–1.3 kPa) in muscle consuming oxygen at a rate equivalent to an oxygen consumption of 3 l. min^{-1}. Doll et al. (1968) found a femoral venous oxygen tension of 22 mm Hg (2.9 kPa) during maximum leg exercise in man, corresponding to an oxygen content of about 60 ml per litre of blood. Pirnay and Lamy, et al. (1971) also reported a figure of 16.6 mm Hg (2.2 kPa); these findings, although apparently confirmed by the more recent experience of the first laboratory (Keul and Doll, 1973), are somewhat surprising, since in some studies the oxygen content of *mixed* venous blood has dropped to 30–40 ml per litre during maximum exercise (Asmussen and Nielsen, 1955b; Sjöstrand, 1960; Saltin et al., 1969; Shephard, 1968e). Mixed venous blood is inevitably enriched by blood that has perfused the skin vessels, and an oxygen content of between 6 and 20 ml per litre (L.H. Hartley and Saltin, 1969; Shephard, 1968e) is likely in blood leaving the active muscles. It must be presumed that in the experiments of Doll et al. the femoral venous specimens were contaminated with substantial quantities of blood from skin rather than muscle.

The mean tension of oxygen within the tissue capillaries can be estimated graphically, using a procedure described by Bohr (1909). To the extent that the tissue oxygen pressure is non-uniform, the tissue diffusing capacity is underestimated by this approach. Given a pulmonary venous oxygen tension of 115 mm Hg (15.4 kPa), an oxygen tension of 5 mm Hg (0.66 kPa) in the muscle veins, and an average oxygen tension of 4.5 mm Hg (0.6 kPa) in the surrounding tissues, the Bohr integration indicates a mean oxygen tension of 17.5 mm Hg (2.3 kPa) in the tissue capillaries, with a gradient of 13 mm Hg (1.9 kPa) from the capillaries to the tissues. Given a maximum oxygen intake of 4 l. min^{-1}, the tissue diffusing capacity would thus amount to 308 ml min^{-1} $(mm\ Hg)^{-1}$ (2310 ml min^{-1} kPa^{-1}), or 219 l. min^{-1} in the units of our conductance equation.

THE OVER-ALL CONDUCTANCE EQUATION

It is useful by way of summary to incorporate the various constants we have defined into the conductance equation (11). Since tissue diffusing capacity is so large, the fourth term can be neglected except in patients with peripheral vascular conditons such as Burger's disease. In a healthy but sedentary young man, we may set the alveolar ventilation $\dot{V}_A$ at 73 l. min^{-1}; the corresponding value of $\lambda \dot{Q}$ is 24.9 l. min^{-1}. Applying the nomogram for integration of λ (Shephard, 1971a), we find that the cumbersome term $B/(1 - B)$ amounts to only 0.006, so that the over-all oxygen conductance equation reads

$$\frac{1}{\dot{G}_{O_2}} = \frac{1}{73} + \frac{0.006}{24.9} + \frac{1}{24.9} \; .$$

At normal ambient pressures this is equivalent to a maximum oxygen intake of 3.55 l. min^{-1}.

In a more athletic man $\dot{V}_A$ might rise to 91 l. min^{-1}, $\lambda \dot{Q}$ to 35.9 l. min^{-1}, and $B/(1 - B)$ to 0.010. The equation would then read

$$\frac{1}{\dot{G}_{O_2}} = \frac{1}{91} + \frac{0.010}{35.9} + \frac{1}{35.9} \; ,$$

equivalent to a maximum oxygen intake of 4.88 l. min^{-1}.

If these two solutions of the equations are taken at their 'face value,' then the main factor limiting oxygen transport is the third term of the conductance equation, $\lambda \dot{Q}$, effectively the product of the haemoglobin level and maximum cardiac output. However, such an analysis ignores the influence of the shape of the oxygen dissociation curve upon $\dot{V}_A$ and $\lambda \dot{Q}$; the effect is to limit further the increase of oxygen transport that can be accomplished by an increase of alveolar ventilation. The equation also takes no account of the possible increase of blood viscosity with red cell count, a response that could restrict maximum cardiac output and thus hold $\lambda \dot{Q}$ constant in the face of an increase in λ. Finally, it leaves unanswered such questions as the relative importance of central factors (cardiac power, depressor reflexes) and peripheral variables ('nipping' of major vessels in the fascia of contracting muscles, adequacy of the intramuscular capillary bed, and pooling of blood in the inactive limbs) as determinants of the maximum cardiac output $\dot{Q}$.

The calculated values for maximum oxygen intake – 3.55 l. min^{-1} in a sedentary young man, 4.88 l. min^{-1} in a more athletic individual – are plainly of the correct general order. Direct comparisons between the measured maximum oxygen intake and predictions based on the conductance equation show a good correspondence in children, but in young adults only about 84% of the predicted oxygen transport is realized (Shephard, 1970b): the explanation seems a substantial mismatching of diffusion and perfusion within the lungs (Shephard, 1971a), possibly a consequence of prolonged exposure to air pollutants and cigarette smoke.

Although the dominant role of blood transport is clearly established for the child and the young adult, it is less certain that other possible determinants of oxygen transport are unimportant in elderly men and women. Finally, it must be remembered that disease can cause sufficient deterioration in any term for it to become the main factor limiting oxygen uptake.

4
Methodology of fitness tests

In the physical sciences, the battles of standardization have already been largely fought and won. A metre is the same distance whether measured in Stockholm or in Philadelphia. But the same is by no means true of physiological measurements. For instance, if it is reported that subjects in Stockholm have a higher maximum oxygen intake than a similar population in Philadelphia, we immediately wonder whether there is a genuine difference between the two groups or whether the difference has arisen through some quirk of methodology or sampling in one of the two laboratories making the measurements. Regional comparisons of endurance fitness would be of particular interest in view of cultural variations in habitual activity and diet around the world, and it is unfortunate that at present many of the most interesting potential comparisons are vitiated by the lack of standard techniques of measuring and reporting data.

Fortunately the biologists are making progress in this area. Metrication has been followed by a move towards acceptance of the Système International d'Unités (SI units): hallowed traditions such as the calorie and the mm Hg of partial pressure are giving way to the kilojoule and the kilopascal (Ellis, 1971). Biochemical variables are starting to be expressed in millimoles per litre, with standardization of estimations against international reference preparations. Thus, any laboratory wishing to measure haemoglobin concentrations can obtain a reference solution of cyanmethaemoglobin from a central laboratory, and then calibrate its own secondary standards against this reference preparation (International Committee, 1965; 1967; Lewis and Burgess, 1969; British Medical Journal, 1972a). There is no fundamental reason why the gas analyses involved in the measurement of oxygen consumption should not be controlled in a similar manner. Cotes and Woolmer (1962) once distributed a single cylinder of a respiratory gas mixture to a group of established investigators in the United Kingdom, and noted an alarming inconsistency in the results reported. Oxygen concentrations were estimated at 15.70–16.21%, and reports of the carbon dioxide concentration ranged from 6.01 to 6.28%. Some of these errors might have been avoided if the investigators concerned had shown the humility to commence their labours by analysing room air; however, analysis of a standard mixture approximating the composition of expired gas provides an even more effective control of analytical technique, and it should be a normal feature of protocol in any trial involving the cooperation of several university centres (Cormack and Heath, 1974; Shephard and Kavanagh, 1975a).

Although many erroneous estimates of maximum oxygen intake can be traced to faulty gas analysis, this is by no means the only source of variation. Having perfected the chosen method of gas analysis, there remains a need to standardize experimental and environmental conditions, to decide upon the optimum mode of exercise (step, bicycle, or treadmill), and to specify the mechanical characteristics of the chosen exercise machine. An appropriate pattern of exercise (rhythm and duration) must be selected, and a choice made between direct and indirect measurements of oxygen intake. Finally, procedures for the measurement of individual variables (Phillips and Ross, 1967) must be specified in some detail.

Recognizing that resolution of these issues could prove controversial, the International Biological Programme convened a 'bench-level' working party in Toronto in the summer of 1967. The objectives set for a group of 15 representative work physiologists from leading laboratories were the comparison and evaluation of possible procedures, the recommending of an optimum protocol to the Human Adaptability Project of the International Biological Programme, and the making of a pilot trial of the chosen methodology on a population of school children.

The endeavour was widely publicized (Shephard, Allen, et al., 1968b,c; Weiner and Lourie, 1969; Shephard, 1970a, 1971b), but unfortunately its impact was blunted by vested interests. Some laboratories were reluctant to abandon other protocols by which they had accumulated substantial quantities of data. Further, although the IBP was the only international group to organize an experimentally oriented working party, a number of other national, regional, and international groups also attempted to review or legislate standard procedures, all with slightly different emphases. The IBP methodology was envisaged as particularly suited to the study of 'primitive' communities, industrial populations, and athletes. Proposals from expert committees of the World Health Organization (Rose and Blackburn, 1968; K.L. Andersen, Shephard, et al., 1971) were aimed largely at the patient with cardiovascular disease. The International Committee for the Standardization of Physical Fitness Tests (1969; Larson, 1974) recommended procedures that the physical educator could apply in the absence of medical supervision. A group of German-speaking physiologists formed the Internationales Seminar für Ergometrie, approaching the problem from the standpoint of measuring work output rather than physiological responses (Mellerowicz, 1966). The International Labour Organization sought a simple measure of fitness applicable to the relatively light loads encountered in modern industry (Cotes, 1966). Groups of physicians (Erb, 1970; Kattus, 1972) and physiologists (Faulkner and Stoedefalke, 1975) from the U.S. made further proposals, apparently in ignorance of the previous deliberations, and inevitably many textbooks of exercise physiology have yet to catch up with all this ferment of activity.

Although the millennium of a consensus on details of methodology has yet to be reached, very effective practical standardization can be realized by organizing a panel of volunteers of known aerobic power who are willing to travel to neighbouring laboratories to calibrate their technique and develop secondary reference standards. Bonjer (1966) reported an experiment of this sort; when the same subjects were tested by three cooperating investigators, the mean estimates of maximum oxygen intake ranged from 3.88 to 4.29 l. min^{-1}. G.R. Cumming (1970) found discrepancies as large as 25% when athletes were tested in several laboratories prior to the Winnipeg Pan American Games. Regular circulation of a panel of volunteers is a further desirable feature of protocol when exercise test data are to be pooled from several laboratories (Shephard and Kavanagh, 1975a).

EXPERIMENTAL AND ENVIRONMENTAL CONDITIONS

The ideal experimental and environmental conditions for the measurement of endurance fitness have been specified by an expert committee of the World Health Organization (Shephard, 1968a; K.L. Andersen, Shephard, et al., 1971), by a committee of the International Council of Sport and Physical Education (Mellerowicz, 1968), and by the Human Adaptability Committee of the International Biological Programme (Lange Andersen, unpublished report; Weiner and Lourie, 1969). The three statements agree closely, and in essence require the subject to be as near a true resting state as possible at the commencement of measurements.

It is recommended that observations be made in the morning, after a good night's sleep. A constant time of testing avoids difficulties due to circadian variations of heart rate (Voigt et al., 1967; K.E. Klein et al., 1968; Wojtczak-Jaroszowa et al., 1974; Davies and Sargeant, 1975). Strenuous muscular work should be avoided on the preceding day. A minimum of an hour's rest in a comfortable environment without food or tobacco is essential, and a longer period without stimulants, fatty food, or a large meal is desirable (Jones and Haddon, 1973).

However, the conditions that can be achieved in practice vary with the nature of the experiment. In a hospital, where a single test is being carried out for diagnostic purposes, it is possible to insist upon the ideal; but when a large population of volunteers is being tested for experimental purposes, certain compromises may be necessary. These need not invalidate the observations. Anxiety (Halicka-Ambroziak et al., 1975) is a greater source of difficulty than lack of rest, particularly in subjects who are unfamiliar with the laboratory. Pulse rates of 100 and even 120 per minute are not uncommon in those awaiting testing, and if the setting is a doctor's office fears of what the examination may reveal can precipitate a 'heart attack' (Shephard, 1976a). Time must be allotted for a careful and unhurried explanation of all that is planned. If such an 'indoctrination' is successful, the results obtained one hour after a meal may be more meaningful than those obtained after longer 'rest' in a forbidding environment. Repetition of the test is another effective method of overcoming anxiety. The rate of 'habituation' to an experiment is quite rapid (Glaser, 1966; Shephard, Allen, et al., 1968c; Shephard, 1969b), and much can be gained from a single practice of the proposed test. Other preliminaries include (i) the completion of a form of consent approved by a university committee on human experimentation, or similar ethical guardian (Shephard, 1967e; Shephard, 1972b), and (ii), depending on the age and physical condition of the subject, a medical examination with review of the electrocardiogram before and during the first period of exercise (Cooper, 1970; J.A. Faulkner, 1973; G.R. Cumming, 1973, 1975; Shephard, 1976a). In the United States, traditional wisdom has been to insist on medical supervision of every exercise test conducted on patients over the age of 35 years. Several Canadian authorities have recently suggested that this is an unrealistic position in the context of the universal delivery of health care; no nation has either the budget or the medical manpower to permit such an approach except for 'high-risk' patients. The cumulative cost of indiscriminate supervision could run as high as $20 billion per successful resuscitation (Shephard, 1976a)! One interesting alternative possibility is the training of fire department or ambulance workers in cardiac resuscitation and other forms of primary care. In Seattle, such a scheme is already in effect, and well-equipped and trained teams can reach an emergency in one to five minutes, with a cost of less than $2000 per resuscitation (L. Cobb, personal communication, October 1975).

Irrespective of decisions regarding the use of medical personnel, the tests should be conducted in a quiet room, with a minimum of staff. Nothing is more calculated to give falsely high heart rates, abnormalities of rhythm, and the occasional myocardial infarction than a large team of over-zealous assistants handling an excess of complex apparatus. The room temperature should be between 18 and 22°C (Rowell, Taylor, and Wang, 1964), with a relative humidity of less than 60%, and the subject should wear a minimum of clothing. Women co-operate much more whole-heartedly in such items as the recording of chest electrocardio- grams if they are advised to bring a brief but attractive bikini top.

It is sometimes difficult to achieve the desired range of temperatures under field conditions; some of the International Biological Programme teams had to set up their equipment in jungle clearings where temperatures were 25-30°C (Thinkaren et al., 1975), and despite the oil crisis North American schools still offer test rooms in the same range! The influence of environmental temperature on human performance will therefore be noted briefly. At 20°C, most of the sub- cutaneous blood vessels are constricted. However, if effort is prolonged or the room temperature is raised, vessels progressively dilate, until at a room tempera- ture of about 30°C all of the subcutaneous vessels are widely patent. A warm room does not affect the maximum oxygen intake during brief periods of ex- hausting exercise (Saltin, 1964; Pirnay, Petit, et al., 1968a; 1969a), but the maxi- mum cardiac output is greater than in a cool environment, and there is a parallel reduction in the maximum arterio-venous oxygen difference (Saltin, 1973). The heart rate in rest and submaximum exercise is substantially increased, although contrary to classical teaching (Figure 17), much of the change in response may occur between 20 and 30°C. Heat reduces muscle viscosity, and thus tends to lower the oxygen cost of the activity itself. Over the usually encountered range of body temperatures this effect is offset by an increase of metabolism in other body organs, so that there is little change of over-all oxygen consumption (Con- solazio et al., 1963; Gold et al., 1969). However, exposure to heat can cause non- linearity of the heart rate/oxygen consumption line (Davies, Barnes, and Sargeant, 1971), and thus underpredictions of maximum oxygen intake from the responses observed during submaximum exercise (see page 129); possibly, the over-heating of North American laboratories may account for the difficulties that some auth- ors have encountered with prediction procedures (Rowell et al. [1964] reported an *average* room temperature of almost 26°C). At room temperatures of 22-30°C, the body can lose heat by convection, the main barrier to such loss being a layer of still air in immediate contact with the skin. The limitation of effort and the dis- tortion of test results caused by a hot environment can thus be mitigated if air movement is increased by a fan. Heating and ventilation engineers have derived scales of 'effective temperature' that take into account not only air temperature, but also radiant heat, relative humidity, and the speed of air movement (Figure 18). Under typical warm and humid conditions, a small desk fan produces an effec- tive temperature about 2°C lower than the reading of an ordinary mercury ther- mometer, and since it is the effective temperature that determines human com- fort and performance, this figure should be recorded in experimental protocols.

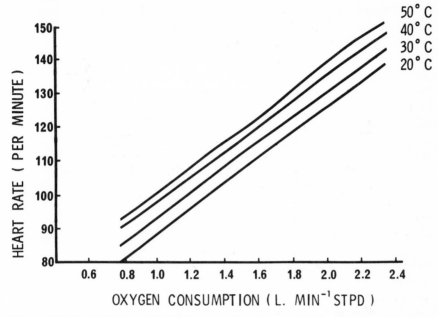

Figure 17 Classical view of the influence of environmental temperature upon the heart rate/oxygen consumption line during brief exercise (based on the data of Dill, 1942). More recent data suggest that a large part of the increase in heart rate occurs between 20 and 30°C.

In some large cities altitude is also an important variable. Thus in Mexico City (altitude 7350 feet, or 2240 metres), more than six million people exercise daily at a barometric pressure of about 580 mm Hg (77 kPa), some three-quarters of the sea level figure. A reduction in the oxygen pressure of inspired air leads in turn to a reduction in the oxygen content of the arterial blood. In rest and mild exercise, the body is able to transport the same quantity of oxygen to the tissues at the expense of a faster heart rate, but during maximum effort the oxygen intake is reduced. An effect is first detected at about 6000 ft (1800 m); in Mexico City, the impairment is 5–10%, and the functional loss increases progressively to about 40% at 18,000 ft (5500 m) (Shephard, 1967f; Goddard, 1967; Kollias and Buskirk, 1974). There is an associated decrease of maximum heart rate (Pugh, 1962; Stenberg et al., 1966; Kollias and Buskirk, 1974) which can cause errors in the prediction of maximum oxygen intake from responses to submaximal effort.

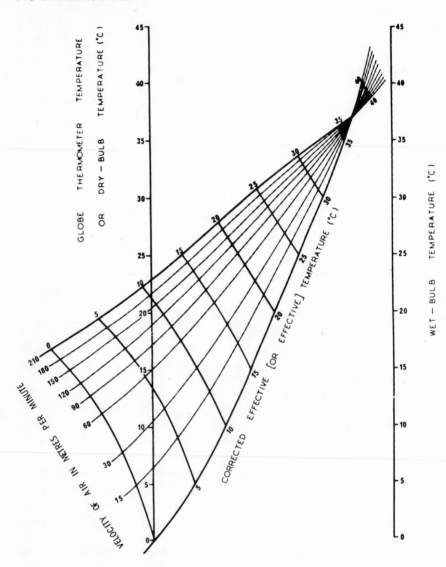

Figure 18 Nomogram for the calculation of corrected effective temperature. Based on data of American Society of Heating, Refrigerating and Air Conditioning Engineers, as quoted by Bedford (1948). Curves take into account humidity, air movement, and (if globe thermometer is used) radiant heating; they are applicable to men stripped to the waist.

MODE OF EXERCISE

Almost all tests of endurance fitness include either a short period of maximum exercise (3-8 min) or a slightly longer period of submaximum effort (5-18 min). The athlete may be evaluated while performing his chosen sport, either in the field or in a simulating device such as a rowing ergometer (di Prampero et al., 1971; Carey et al., 1974; Cunningham et al., 1975), a swimming 'flume' (Holmer, 1972), or an arrangement for tethered swimming (Magel, 1971; McArdle et al., 1971). The commonest devices for testing the general population are the treadmill, the bicycle ergometer, the step, and the hand ergometer; one laboratory has also experimented with a 'laddermill' (Ramanathan and Kamon, 1974). The relative merits of these several forms of apparatus will now be considered in personal, physiological, and practical terms (Shephard, 1968a; Shephard, Allen, et al., 1968b,c; H.L. Taylor, Haskell, et al., 1969; K.L. Andersen, Shephard, et al., 1971; Kamon and Pandolf, 1972).

Personal factors
Neither the bicycle ergometer nor the step test is particularly convenient for maximum exercise. Most bicycle ergometers have Edwardian roadster frames and bear little resemblance to a modern racing cycle; the typical ergometer saddle is designed for a quiet country ride, and becomes acutely uncomfortable at high intensities of effort, while few ergometers provide the toe-clips needed for efficient use of the pedals. The step test is especially difficult for the very fit subject. In order that such a person may reach maximum effort, it is necessary to use either a large step or a very fast rate of stepping; the required exercise becomes an unnatural and undignified gallop, and stumbling is frequent, particularly as the subject nears exhaustion. Very short subjects, including children under the age of 10, find the 18-inch (45 cm) step too tall to climb with comfort.

The main objective of a maximum test is to measure cardio-respiratory power, and the end-point of the test should thus be shortness of breath and general circulatory exhaustion rather than local muscle weakness. Respiratory and cardiac symptoms almost always limit effort when subjects are running on the treadmill, and they usually do so when stepping. However, performance on the bicycle ergometer is commonly halted by weakness of the knee muscles, especially the quadriceps.

Submaximum exercise should be familiar and easy to carry out. If the task is unfamiliar, the heart rate is increased by anxiety, and the oxygen consumption is also high because the subject is clumsy in his performance. Unfortunately, no type of vigorous activity is really familiar to the present generation of sedentary office workers. Any form of running is unusual; restricted running on the hard and slippery incline of a treadmill thus seems a very abnormal pastime and is somewhat frightening to many subjects. If a treadmill is to be used, middle-aged and elderly subjects respond better to a walking than to a running protocol. Despite booming sales in North America, bicycles are also rarely used by the adults of western nations. Children enjoy the novelty of a bicycle ergometer machine, but many older adults find cycling an unnatural form of exertion and complain of local muscular tiredness after riding for only a short period. A recent Canadian comparison of submaximum bicycle ergometer and step tests showed that in the oldest age group (60–69 years) local fatigue caused a 30% underestimate of maximum oxygen intake by the bicycle ergometer technique (Bailey, Shephard, and Mirwald, 1976). Stepping is still perhaps the most universal form of exercise, but the step used in daily life is shallow (commonly 8 inches, 20 cm), unlike the monstrosity of 17-22 inches (43–56 cm) beloved by many physiologists. Further, as an ever increasing proportion of the population moves to high-rise apartments, even the humble step is being supplanted by the elevator.

From the viewpoint of the investigator, the treadmill has an important advantage over other tests in that the intensity of effort is predetermined. The subject must keep pace with the belt if he is not to fall flat on his face. In most bicycle and step tests that intensity of effort is dependent on rhythm, and the cooperation of the subject is needed to achieve the desired work-load. Some bicycle ergometers indicate the correct rate of pedalling by means of a large pointer that the subject must hold in the vertical position; the pointer is linked to both the pedals and a synchronous motor through a differential gear. Simpler models merely have a small counter that indicates the number of pedal revolutions completed from commencement of the test. Some electrically braked ergometers have a 'feedback' device that maintains the external work-load relatively constant over a substantial range of pedalling rates (for example, 40–60 revolutions per minute). The subject of a step test adjusts his pace to correspond with a metronome, flashing lights, or in the case of the Canadian Home Fitness Test with appropriately structured gramophone music (Bailey and Shephard, 1976). Most people find it relatively easy to maintain the correct speed at moderate rates of climbing (50-150 paces per minute). At the very slow rates used in a South African test (initial load 6 ascents, 24 paces per minute), the subject may stand poised awaiting the beat of the metronome, and the test becomes markedly weight-dependent (Wyndham and Sluis-Cremer, 1968b; Shephard and Olbrecht, 1970). At very fast rates of stepping, stumbling (Kasch et al., 1965) and/or lagging may occur. Stumbling is particularly likely in older subjects with some arthritis of the knee joints, and for such subjects a padded hand-support is helpful.

Physiological factors

If maximum oxygen intake is to be measured, then the result reported should be the largest oxygen consumption the individual can achieve with any form of exercise. Unfortunately, a true maximum is difficult to define, and as we have seen (page 97) average values differ somewhat between the several standard modes of laboratory exercise. A comparative study of treadmill, step, and bicycle tests has shown that in young Canadian men the largest figures are obtained during uphill treadmill running, with results 3.4% smaller during a step test and 6.6% smaller when exercising on a bicycle ergometer (Shephard, Allen, et al., 1968b). Trained cyclists probably perform at least as well on the bicycle ergometer as on the treadmill, but in older subjects the deficit of performance on the bicycle ergometer can be much larger than 7%.

There are at least two physiological problems that hamper the cyclist. First, local muscle groups are exercised at a sufficient fraction of their maximum voluntary force (Royce, 1959; Hoes et al., 1968) to restrict perfusion of the active fibres (H. Barcroft and Dornhorst, 1949; Glassford et al., 1965; Wyndham, Strydom, et al., 1966b; Cumming and Friesen, 1967; Kay and Shephard, 1969; Moody et al., 1969; Davies, Tuxworth and Young, 1970; F.I. Katch, Girandola and Katch, 1971; Rowell, 1974). Several strands of evidence support the view that effort on the bicycle is limited by weakness of the most active muscles rather than by general exhaustion. Ekblom and Goldbarg (1971) found that the rating of perceived exertion (Borg, 1971) was greater on the bicycle ergometer than at an equivalent oxygen consumption on the treadmill, and a cluster analysis of fatigue symptoms (Weiser et al., 1973) showed that bicycle ergometer exercise at more than 50% of aerobic power induced leg rather than general fatigue. An increase of muscle force induced by tying weights to the legs further reduces maximum oxygen intake (Bottin et al., 1971). Lactic acid also accumulates more readily in bicycle than in step or treadmill exercise (Figure 19; Saltin and Åstrand, 1967; Dujardin et al., 1967-8), the phenomenon being similar to that encountered when exercise is performed by the small muscles of the arm with the part raised above the head (Freyschuss and Strandell, 1967; I. Åstrand, Gahary, and Wahren, 1968). Since the critical determinant of muscle flow is the percentage of maximum force that is exerted, an advantage might be anticipated from a strengthening of the thigh muscles. MacNab and Conger (1966) found a positive correlation between knee extension strength and the maximum oxygen intake of female university students, and Davies (1973) noted a close relationship between leg volume (muscle plus bone) and aerobic power. Kay and Shephard (1969) further reported that the accumulation of arterial lactate two minutes after performance of a standardized ergometer test (80% of aerobic power) was

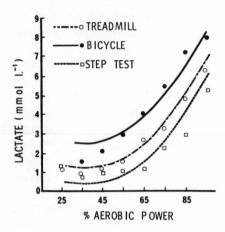

Figure 19 The lactic acid content of arterial blood two minutes after performance of three forms of submaximum exercise. Based on data of Shephard, Allen, et al. (1968c).

inversely related to the maximum voluntary force of the quadriceps muscle, while Klausen et al. (1974) demonstrated a decrease of arterial lactate if the effort was carried out by trained muscles. Katch, McArdle, and Pechar (1974) found no correlation between the peak isokinetic force measured during a bicycle ergometer test and the discrepancy between maximum oxygen intake on the bicycle and the treadmill; however, this discordant finding probably reflects (i) the measurement of peak forces rather than the integrated muscle force and (ii) failure to interpret the observations as a percentage of the maximum possible force for the same group of muscles.

A second problem of the cyclist is that blood pools in parts of the body that are immobilized, particularly the arm veins, and the resultant restriction of venous return prevent the rider from reaching a true maximum cardiac stroke volume. Both the stroke volume and the maximum cardiac output are thus appreciably smaller for bicycle than for treadmill exercise (Table 6, and J.A. Faulkner et al., 1971). Opinions have differed markedly on the usefulness of the arm ergometer. Most authors (page 97) have found a much smaller maximum oxygen intake for arm than for leg ergometers, but there have been occasional reports of substantially similar results for the two devices (Nowacki, 1966). The arm ergometer has yielded poor results under conditions where the faults of the normal bicycle ergometer were exaggerated. The subjects were sitting, turning a short crank that exercised only the muscles of the forearm, and the rest of the body was immobilized. The best results were obtained with the subjects standing, turning a large crank to which the full force of the upper half of the body could be applied. The arm ergometer finds particular application to the testing of amputees (Kavanagh, Pandit, and Shephard, 1973) and paraplegics (Zwiren and Bar-Or, 1975).

An interesting variation of the muscle mass theme is provided by single-leg bicycle ergometry (Düner, 1959; Freyschuss and Strandell, 1968; Davies and Sargeant, 1974c). Under such circumstances, the cardiac stroke volume is somewhat reduced relative to two-leg exercise, but the maximum cardiac output is almost unchanged, and the maximum oxygen intake is more than 50% of the two-leg value. This provides further evidence that the crucial factor limiting oxygen transport is circulatory rather than a problem of utilization within the active tissues.

In submaximum tests, perhaps the most important consideration is the extent of anxiety induced by the test procedure (Shephard, 1966d, 1969b; Antel and Cumming, 1969). Endurance fitness is usually assessed from the relationship between heart rate and oxygen consumption, and if the heart rate is increased by anxiety, then the fitness will be underestimated. In our experience (Shephard, Allen, et al., 1968c), anxiety has been most marked in treadmill exercise; the heart rate during treadmill running has averaged 5 beats per minute faster on the first than on subsequent days of testing. Changes of heart rate with repetition of the test have been less marked for stepping exercise, and least for bicycle ergometer exercise. H.L. Taylor, Haskell, et al. (1969) remarked that about a quarter of their railroad workers were very anxious when first tested on the treadmill; repetition of the measurements at a constant moderate work load was associated with a decrease in average heart rate from 124 to 111 min^{-1}.

Problems can also arise from an unmeasured oxygen debt. The oxygen consumed during submaximal exercise is usually measured during the fourth or fifth minute of activity. Some laboratories check that a steady state has been reached, but it is more usual to assume that oxygen intake and expenditure are equal at this stage of exercise. However, a substantial oxygen debt is accumulated when bicycle ergometer exercise exceeds 50–60% of aerobic power (Figure 19), lactate accumulation continuing for many minutes (Kay and Shephard, 1969). Thus, unless the investigator goes to the inconvenience of measuring the oxygen debt, his figures for the energy cost of the activity will be correspondingly in error. Oxygen debt accounts for a particularly large proportion of the energy expenditure of patients debilitated by long periods of bed rest, and as rehabilitation proceeds there is a diminution of reliance on anaerobic energy sources, with corresponding changes in estimates of mechanical efficiency and predictions of maximum oxygen intake (Kavanagh and Shephard, 1973).

It is sometimes necessary to estimate oxygen consumption from the work performed rather than from an analysis of expired gas. The assumption is then made that exercise is performed with a mechanical efficiency that is constant both for the individual concerned and for the population as a whole. The bicycle ergometer is most commonly used in this way, since it is widely believed that all subjects cycle with a mechanical efficiency close to an average figure of 23%. Unfortunately, this belief is not well founded. Even among healthy young men who are accustomed to cycling, the coefficient of variation* of mechanical efficiency is 4–5% at any given rate of pedalling. There are also substantial changes of efficiency with the frequency of pedalling, many subjects reaching a minimum of oxygen cost at 60 or 70 pedal revolutions per minute rather than the 50 per minute advocated by the makers of one popular mechanically braked bicycle ergometer (Dickenson, 1929; H.C. Burger et al., 1967; Banister and Jackson, 1967; Heinrich et al., 1968; Knuttgen et al., 1971; R.H.T. Edwards, Melcher, et al., 1972; Pandolf and Noble, 1973; Gaesser and Brooks, 1975; Hagberg et al., 1975; Gueli and Shephard, 1976). There is also a progressive increase of efficiency in any one individual as the task is learned; efficiency is low in children (Shephard, 1971c) and in 'primitive' groups such as the Eskimo (K.L. Andersen and Hart, 1963; Rode and Shephard, 1973b; Shephard, 1975a) and the Ainu (Ikai et al., 1971), but more normal in acculturated Kautocheino Lapps (K.L. Andersen, Elsner, et al., 1962). One paper sometimes quoted as showing a constant mechanical efficiency of cycling among indigenous populations (Van Graan and Greyson, 1970) in fact reports data equivalent to efficiencies of 17.3% for Bantu and 21.0% for 'Kalahari bushmen' who were no longer nomadic. These examples are sufficient to show that the assumption of a constant efficiency of 23% during bicycle ergometry can lead to serious errors in the prediction of maximum oxygen intake; whenever possible, the oxygen consumption should be measured directly rather than estimated from the work load.

Some authors have made the further assumption that if oxygen consumption is to be estimated from the work performed, this is only possible when a bicycle ergometer has been used. However, this assumption also is untrue. If a step test is carried out carefully, the oxygen consumption can be predicted with a precision that is little poorer than that achieved on the bicycle; one recent study has shown a correlation of 0.9 between scores for the Canadian home fitness test and the directly measured maximum oxygen intakes for the same group of subjects (Jetté et al., 1975). In order to obtain good predictions during a step test, it is important to weigh the subject in the clothing worn during the exercise, to ensure that he maintains the intended rate of stepping, and to check that he climbs fully at each step. Nomograms are also available to predict the oxygen consumption during treadmill running (Figure 20; see also Margaria et al., 1963; Workman and Armstrong, 1964; Shephard, 1968c); these are accurate to about 10%.

---

* When the standard deviation of a measurement is expressed as a percentage of its mean value, the result is described as the coefficient of variation. This coefficient provides a convenient basis for comparing the variability of data obtained by differing techniques.

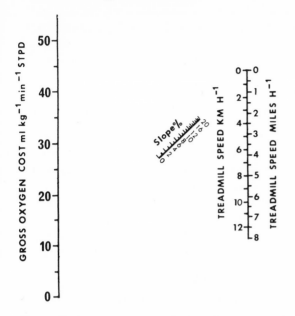

Figure 20 A nomogram to calculate the gross oxygen cost of treadmill running of non-athletic men from the treadmill slope and speed (based on data of Shephard, 1968c).

Practical factors
Both personal and physiological considerations are often outweighed by practical problems when choosing appropriate apparatus for a particular experiment. A treadmill is bulky, heavy, costly, often noisy, and requires a source of electrical power (commonly special three-phase wiring). A bicycle is less bulky, but in its more accurate forms is relatively expensive and often requires electrical power either for the braking system or the pacing device. Furthermore, frequent and careful calibration is essential if valid work measurements are to be obtained (Cumming and Alexander, 1968; Stein et al., 1967); 8–10% of the energy developed by the subject is lost in 'unmeasured' friction at the chain and pedal-bearings, and the true rate of working can only be determined if a torque calibrator is coupled to the pedal shaft. The basic step is simple, needing neither electricity nor elaborate calibration. The Canadian home fitness test can be carried out on an ordinary domestic staircase (Bailey, Shephard, and Mirwald, 1976), and an equivalent laboratory device is readily made in the workshop at little cost. More complicated designs of step have been suggested by some authors (Nagle et al., 1965; Wyndham and Sluis-Cremer, 1968b; Erb, 1970), but these are less suitable

for field use, and they strike at the simplicity which is the great virtue of the stepping procedure.

Account must also be taken of the ease with which intended observations can be made. The quality of the chest electrocardiogram is usually good during stepping, fair during cycling, and much poorer during treadmill running; on the treadmill, an obese subject may develop large movement artefacts that the novitiate has difficulty in distinguishing from electrocardiographic abnormalities such as ST segmental depression and extrasystoles (page 137). The clue to interpretation on the treadmill is that the abnormal appearances are in phase with the runner's pace rather than the heart rate. With all three types of exercise, the records are adequate to measure heart rate, and treadmill electrocardiograms can often be made interpretable if 16 or 32 successive complexes are averaged by a suitable digital or analogue computer (Rautaharju et al., 1971). The relative freedom from arm movement during bicycle ergometer exercise may be helpful if it is necessary to measure blood pressures or to introduce catheters into the arm vessels, but if advantage has been taken of the subject's immobility to attach several devices to him, it is then difficult for him to dismount in an emergency.

No one form of exercise can be commended as meeting the needs of every experimental situation. If the maximum oxygen intake of a young adult is to be measured directly in the laboratory, uphill treadmill running seems the procedure of choice. For many older subjects, uphill treadmill walking (Moody et al., 1969) is a preferable alternative. Very young children may refer a brief period of 'supramaximal' bicycle ergometry, or the operation of a suitably modified pedal-car. If maximum oxygen intake is to be measured in the field, a step test may be the most practical technique. The choice for submaximum exercise lies between the bicycle and the step test; in the laboratory, where many ancillary measurements are to be made, the bicycle ergometer may be preferred, but in the field a step test again seems more suitable.

MECHANICAL CHARACTERISTICS OF EXERCISE MACHINES

Treadmill

Treadmills vary greatly from the mighty giants of some physical education departments that roar into action at 25 miles per hour (40 km h^{-1}), to humble portable devices that reach 6 miles per hour (9.6 km h^{-1}) with something of a struggle. Very high speeds are needed to test and analyse the performance of sprint athletes, but if the sole objective of a laboratory is to examine the maximum oxygen intake and exercise responses of the average citizen, the desired work load can be obtained at quite moderate speeds through a tilting of the belt. The majority of subjects will reach exhaustion on a treadmill capable of running at

7 miles per hour (11.2 km h^{-1}) with an 18% slope. The smaller treadmills do not maintain speed when the subject jumps onto the belt; if the slope is shallow, the machine tends to slow down, and if the slope is steep it may speed up. It is thus necessary to check the speed during use by counting the number of belt revolutions per minute. Stumbling is a real danger, and no sharp objects should be placed in the possible trajectory of a flying subject! A safety rail should be available for grasping if necessary, and matting should also be fitted around the treadmill during maximum effort tests. Some workers provide their subjects with a waist harness, loosely suspended from the ceiling. However, this makes the subject excessively anxious and can promote carelessness in the observers; cases are on record where an exhausted subject has been dragged along the belt, supported by the harness, but sustaining serious friction burns of the legs. It is better for the observer to assume the responsibility of giving equal and less obtrusive support to the subject as the limit of exercise tolerance is approached. Many treadmills are rather noisy, and although this may not worry the immediate investigator, a busy running schedule can give much annoyance to other users of a building. The extra cost involved in providing a relatively silent treadmill is thus a good investment in public relations.

The basic controls needed on a treadmill are an easily accessible emergency switch, a smoothly operating speed regulator and braking system, and a mechanically operated worm drive for varying the slope. Maintenance for this type of machine is minimal. The only problems seem correct alignment of the rollers (to avoid a sideways movement of the belt) and a suitable choice of belt tension (if the tension is too great the belt creases longitudinally, and if the tension is too small slipping occurs). Some treadmills can be 'programmed' to deliver a sequence of speeds and slopes at the whim of the investigator or in response to the heart rate of the subject. Such 'refinements' are to be avoided since they greatly increase maintenance costs and reduce the likelihood of safe and careful observation of the subjects.

Bicycle ergometer
There are two distinct types of bicycle ergometer. In one, the braking system is electrical, while in the other it is mechanical. With most electrical devices, the subject operates a dynamo to generate electrical power at a known rate. Despite the low price of suitable dynamos, commercially available machines are very expensive, some costing $3000-$4000. With the more refined models, a 'feedback' device varies the voltage supply to the field coils of the dynamo inversely with pedalling speed, giving the doubtful advantage that the mechanical work load imposed on the subject is almost independent of the speed of pedalling (this ignores the problem that the mechanical efficiency of effort varies with pedal speed; see

page 116). The main difficulty with electrical machines, irrespective of their price, is that calibration procedures are tedious and exacting. With most machines, the labour of the calibrator is lost if the windings are jarred on the journey back from the calibrating laboratory.

The usual mechanically braked device has a leather or fibre friction belt applied to a heavy rear wheel; the work performed is calculated rather simply from the number of pedal revolutions per minute, the gear ratio, and the change in tension of the belt as it passes over the flywheel (Von Döbeln, 1954). There are two main difficulties with the standard type of apparatus. First, the brake belt becomes hot as the subject rides; friction thus diminishes and the intended effort is no longer maintained. Secondly, the system of springs, weights, and levers forms a wonderful complex oscillator, and if the belt is worn the spring balance or load indicator does not remain steady enough to permit accurate readings. Both problems are overcome in the Fleisch machine at the expense of a considerable increase in weight and price. With most designs of bicycle ergometer, it is necessary to change a series of slotted weights or to adjust the tension of a spring in order to increase the work performed. Neither procedure is easy to carry out smoothly during a progressive exercise test. Müller developed a system where the loading of the flywheel is increased automatically from 60 to 600 kg-m min^{-1} (10-100 watts) over the course of ten minutes of exercise; this pattern of effort is particularly suitable for the measurement of his *Leistungspulsindex* (see page 280). Another interesting variant is the Schwinn bicycle, where an elctromagnetic device controls belt friction. The total number of pedal revolutions per minute must be known accurately for all mechanical ergometers except the Schwinn device. A simple digital counter can be used, or the subject can be paced by a synchronous motor geared to run at the intended speed.

Desirable features rarely provided in commercially available apparatus include a narrow but comfortable saddle and toe straps, with saddle and handlebar pillars appropriately angulated and rapidly adjustable for different sizes of subjects. The frame and bearings should be rigid enough to withstand the forces developed by heavy subjects during maximum exercise, and the flywheel should be heavy enough to ensure an even rhythm of pedalling without imposing an excessive inertial load at the beginning of a test. If testing small children, the cranks should be of adjustable length (Klimt and Voigt, 1971, 1974); the optimum size of foot crank increases from 14 to 16 cm between the ages of six and ten years.

Step

Few comments are necessary on the optimum design of step for exercise testing. Elaborate escalators (M. Richardson, 1966) and steps (Nagle et al., 1965; Erb, 1970; Sharrock et al., 1972) have been described at various times. These have

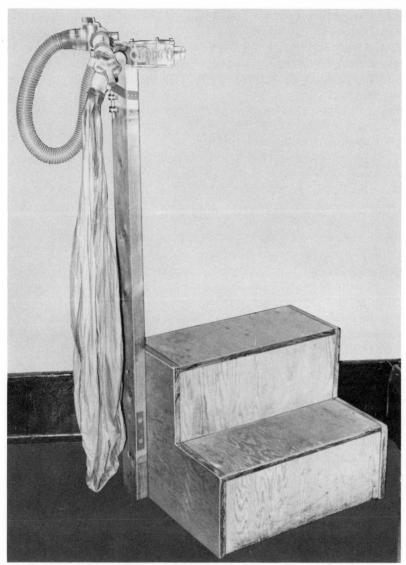

Figure 21 Design of step for maximum and submaximum exercise tests. In maximum tests, the 18-inch (45-cm) face is climbed with two paces. In submaximum tests, the two 9-inch (22.5-cm) steps are climbed with three paces. The post is used to support the gas-bag and also provides a light hand-rest if desired.

application to specific laboratory problems, but are unnecessary in most places where the step is likely to be used. The only essential requirements are rigidity, an adequate width of tread, and a non-slippery surface. For many purposes, the ordinary domestic or laboratory staircase may prove quite suitable. Thus, Margaria (1966) has used the staircase of his Institute very successfully to measure the rate of working that a subject can develop at the start of exercise, and the domestic staircase provides the basis of the Canadian home fitness test (Bailey, Shephard, and Mirwald, 1976); for the latter, an age-related stepping pace and timing of post-exercise pulse counts is provided by a long-playing gramophone record. Even in the laboratory, a step test of endurance fitness requires only a single or a double wooden step built by an ordinary handyman.

The height of the step selected should be both natural and comfortable to the subject. It should also permit the desired range of work loads without asking the subject to adopt too slow or too fast a rate of climbing. The ideal dimensions thus depend to some extent upon age, sex, fitness, and body weight. However, leg length is surprisingly unimportant (Shephard, 1967g; Howe et al., 1973), and the average adult can be tested quite satisfactorily using a box built with a single 18-inch (45-cm) step on one face and two 9-inch (22.5-cm) steps on the opposite face (Figure 21). If submaximum exercise is required, the two 9-inch steps are climbed and descended with a total of six paces (the same pattern of climbing as is used in the Canadian home fitness test), but if maximum exercise is required, the single 18-inch step is climbed and descended with a total of four paces.

PATTERN OF EXERCISE

Rhythm
There is a natural rhythm that is suited to the performance of any given type of exercise. Success in approximating this optimum rhythm is important not only to the comfort of the test, but also to the validity of any assumptions that are made regarding the mechanical efficiency of exercise. Efficiency deteriorates if the rhythm is too fast or too slow for a given load.

During treadmill exercise, the subject is usually allowed to choose a comfortable frequency of stride, and adjusts the length of each pace according to his leg dimensions and the speed of the belt. However, the oxygen consumption of treadmill effort is not usually predicted from the running speed, so that minor variations of rhythm are unimportant. During bicycle and stepping exercise, it is by no means uncommon either to report the work performed as such, or to use performance to predict the individual's oxygen consumption; an appropriate choice of rhythm is then vital. In the case of the bicycle ergometer, we have already commented that when a young man is performing submaximum exercise,

TABLE 8

Efficiency of progressive step test at increasing rates of climb.
Data obtained on Canadians by author and his associates, using double 9-inch (2 x 22.5 cm) step. Mean ±SE of data

Number of paces per minute	10 male laboratory workers, average age 29 years	122 young men, average age 20 years	44 older men, average age 46 years	30 Eskimo men aged 20–30 years
60	16.5 ± 0.4	14.5 ± 0.2	16.6 ± 1.0	14.3 ± 0.3
90	17.2 ± 0.4	15.8 ± 0.2	16.3 ± 0.3	14.7 ± 0.3
120	16.6 ± 0.3	15.7 ± 0.2	17.1 ± 0.7	15.1 ± 0.3
150	15.4 ± 0.4	16.1 ± 0.6	15.4 ± 0.6	14.2 ± 0.3

the most efficient speed of pedalling is 60–70 revolutions per minute; however, it is conceivable that 40 or 50 revolutions per minute may be more appropriate for those who are less fit, and a speed as high as 90 revolutions per minute may be necessary if an endurance athlete is to reach maximum effort. In the case of the step test, a cadence of from 60 to 150 paces per minute is acceptable, and over this range the efficiency of effort is relatively constant (Table 8).

Duration

Exercise is generally continued at a single intensity until the variables to be measured, such as heart rate and oxygen consumption, are close to new steady values. The physiologist would like to see a 'steady state' reached rather than approached, but in practice vigorous exercise cannot be carried to complete equilibrium. In submaximum tests, a slow increase of heart rate continues for many minutes (Shephard, 1970c). This reflects such factors as a progressive heating of the body and a depletion of the central blood volume, and as such does not constitute a part of the immediate response to exercise. It is thus necessary to record data at an arbitrary point such as the fifth or the sixth minute of effort, even though the heart rate is still increasing by two or three beats in each minute. In maximum tests, the duration of exercise is often limited by sudden exhaustion of the subject; in those who are poorly motivated, it is sometimes necessary to accept readings from the third minute of maximum effort, but fitter and better-motivated subjects may progress through five to eight minutes of maximum and 'supramaximum' effort. Fortunately, there is some evidence that during very intense exercise equilibrium is reached more quickly than during less vigorous activity (P.O. Åstrand and Saltin, 1961a). Valid answers are thus often obtained even if the subject halts the test relatively quickly; however, it is necessary to evaluate the success of individual experiments in terms of standard criteria of maximum effort (page 127).

Whether measurements of maximum or submaximum effort are planned, it is usually necessary to collect data at several intensities of exercise. The traditional approach has been a series of discontinuous tests, and ideally such tests should be separated by rest periods of at least 48 hours. In practice, few subjects are prepared to make repeated visits to the laboratory. Brief intervals of rest are not a satisfactory substitute, and if the subject does not have unlimited time available there is much to commend the use of a progressive test, where the intensity of exercise is increased at regular intervals without intervening rest periods.

In maximum testing, experiments where the load is increased at two-minute intervals yield a slightly higher maximum aerobic power and a slightly smaller oxygen debt than that found in discontinuous tests, where exercise is repeated with slightly differing loads on separate days (Shephard, Allen, et al., 1968b).

TABLE 9

The prediction of maximum oxygen intake from the response to four levels of submaximum exercise – a comparison of discontinuous and progressive tests*

	Step test	Bicycle test	Treadmill test
Series of four			
discontinuous tests	3.75 ± 0.87	3.57 ± 0.81	3.83 ± 0.90
Single progressive test	3.73 ± 0.93	3.64 ± 0.86	3.79 ± 0.89
Δ	–0.013 ± 0.34	+0.069 ± 0.29	–0.043 ± 0.61

* Results are in each case based on linear extrapolation of oxygen consumption to the predicted maximum pulse rate. Mean ±SD for 24 young Canadian men, as reported by Shephard, Allen, et al. (1968c).

Several authors (Moody et al., 1969; Horvath and Michael, 1970; Falls and Humphrey, 1973; McArdle et al., 1973; Molnar et al., 1974) have found little difference in results with changes in the pattern of exercise loading. Åstrand and Saltin (1961a) found the same maximum oxygen intake with two and eight minutes of exhausting exercise. Glassford et al. (1965) obtained very comparable results with two treadmill protocols (H.L. Taylor, Haskell, et al., 1969; Mitchell et al., 1958). Pirnay, Petit, et al. (1966) found a slightly higher aerobic power with continuous than with discontinuous tests, although results were the same whether the load was increased every second or every third minute (Bottin et al., 1968). Froelicher et al. (1974) suggested that slightly higher results were obtained with a 'progressive' test if five-minute rest intervals were allowed between stages, in the manner originally suggested by H.L. Taylor.

The usual submaximum test comprises three or four individual loads, selected to produce heart rates that are widely spaced over the range 120–170 per minute in young subjects and 100–150 per minute in older subjects. The duration of exercise at any one intensity can be reduced in a progressive test, partly because each increment of energy expenditure is smaller than in a discontinuous test, and partly because the longer total period of effort tends to warm the body, thus pushing heart rates more rapidly towards the equilibrium values found in discontinuous tests. In young and healthy subjects, the results of a series of four discontinuous submaximum tests can be approximated very closely by a single progressive test that involves three minutes of exercise at each of the four graded intensities of effort (Table 9). In older subjects, where the circulation is more sluggish, three minutes is barely adequate, and four minutes at each of three intensities may be preferable. Other authors (Rutenfranz, 1964; Bonjer, 1968; K.L. Andersen, Shephard, et al., 1971; S.M. Fox, 1974) have reviewed possible submaximal test schedules. As with maximum testing, it is possible to use quite a wide range of protocols and yet achieve very similar results. The one exception seems the *Leistungspulsindex* of Müller (1950); this test extends the idea of the progressive test to its logical conclusion, with the load increased continuously. Unfortunately, such an approach cannot be recommended. No steady state is then possible, and the apparent response of such variables as heart rate to a given load are underestimated by an amount that varies with the sluggishness of the circulation.

A recent variant of Müller's procedure uses a programmed treadmill, with the increment of work load adjusted to produce a 5 beat per minute increment of heart rate (Arstila, 1972). The author argues that the work of the heart depends mainly on heart rate rather than external loading, and that when examining electrocardiographic changes it is preferable to use heart rate as the independent variable. However, the continuously increasing effort again gives problems due to the absence of a steady state.

DIRECT AND INDIRECT ESTIMATIONS OF MAXIMUM OXYGEN INTAKE

Direct measurements

The least controversial method of assessing aerobic power is to measure the maximum oxygen intake directly. The subject is given a 'warm-up' at between 50 and 70% of his maximum, and a prediction of the maximum oxygen intake is made from the heart rate and the oxygen consumption during this warm-up period. Current wisdom is that such a preliminary reduces the likelihood of muscle tears and abnormalities of heart rhythm (Barnard, Gardner, et al., 1973; Barnard, MacAlpin, et al., 1973), while giving a small augmentation of maximum oxygen intake relative to a 'cold' start (H.L. Taylor, Buskirk, and Henschel, 1955; Pirnay, Petit, et al., 1966; B.J. Martin, Robinson, et al., 1975).

If a progressive maximum test is to be performed, the test proper commences at a loading that will produce an oxygen intake 90–100% of the predicted maximum for the individual. The intensity of exercise is then increased by 5–10% at two-minute intervals until the subject is exhausted or there are clinical indications to halt the test (the latter yielding what has been termed a 'symptom-limited' maximum test [Kasser and Bruce, 1969]). Physiological observations are made during the final 30 seconds at each level of exercise.

If a discontinuous series of maximum tests is planned, the first test is commonly set at a load corresponding to 110% of the predicted maximum oxygen intake, on the basis that the usual method of prediction (the Åstrand nomogram, page 130) underestimates the true maximum. The intensity of effort in subsequent tests is adjusted in the light of responses to the first test. It is accepted that the maximum oxygen intake has been reached when the oxygen consumption increases by less than 2 ml kg^{-1} min^{-1} for a sufficiently small (Milic-Emili et al., 1959; H.L. Taylor, Haskell, et al., 1969) increase of work load such as a 1-2% increase of treadmill slope. Subsidiary criteria of a true maximum include: (i) obvious exhaustion of the subject (blanching or cyanosis (blueness) of the extremities, an unsteady gait, breathlessness, and perhaps some impairment of consciousness); (ii) physiological evidence of tissue oxygen lack (a respiratory exchange ratio* of 1.15-1.20 during exercise, and an arterial lactate concentration of 11 mmol l.$^{-1}$ in young adults, 9 mmol l.$^{-1}$ in children, and 7 mmol l.$^{-1}$ in the elderly [Cumming and Borysyk, 1972]); (iii) a heart rate close to the expected maximum value (Asmussen and Molbech, 1959; Figure 15).

Although a plateau of oxygen consumption is a clear theoretical concept, there are a number of practical difficulties in applying it. Wyndham, Strydom, et al. (1959) and Glassford et al. (1965) cautioned that an apparent plateau could underestimate the true maximum value in subjects who approached their peak reading slowly, and Wyndham suggested as an alternative the fitting of a statistical curve to the work load/oxygen consumption relationship. A fixed criterion such as 2 ml kg^{-1} min^{-1} is unsatisfactory when applied to subjects with a very low aerobic power. It can also be quite difficult to define a plateau in children (P.O. Åstrand, 1952; Cumming and Friesen, 1967), and in very young subjects better results can sometimes be obtained by requiring three minutes of 'supramaximal' work, determined by extrapolating the linear portion of the heart rate/work load relationship to a theoretical heart rate of 247 per minute. The anaerobic work involved in a standard maximum test may also be undesirable in older patients with suspected ischaemic heart disease. Here, a possible alternative seems a very rapid increase of work load, with either a continuous record of oxygen consumption (Auchincloss and Gilbert, 1973) or collection of a brief (15-20 second) expired gas sample after about one minute of 'supramaximal' effort (Niinimaa et al., 1974).

Direct measurements of maximum oxygen intake are unquestionably the best approach in well-motivated subjects, and are being used increasingly in the evaluation of clinical material such as post-coronary patients (Kavanagh and Shephard, 1976a) and populations such as arctic Eskimos (Rode and Shephard, 1971a). One factor deterring universal adoption of direct measurements is the possible danger of the test to the patient and the consequent need for special staff and emergency equipment. Adequate statistics on the likelihood of death during maximum exercise have yet to be obtained. McDonough and Bruce (1969)

---

* The ratio of carbon dioxide output to oxygen intake, measured at the mouth.

tested a mixture of cardiac patients and middle-aged subjects enrolled in the Seattle 'Heart Watch' program; they found the risk of ventricular fibrillation or cardiac arrest to be about 1 in 3000 for 'symptom-limited' maximum tests, and 1 in 15,000 for submaximum test procedures. Rochmis and Blackburn (1971) encountered 16 cardiac emergencies in accumulated data on 170,000 exercise tests performed in North American laboratories; almost all of the victims had evidence of cardiac disease, but the status of the remainder of the population was uncertain. In the material of Rochmis and Blackburn, there was no obvious difference of risk between maximum and submaximum tests. If such figures are confirmed, a vigorous exercise test would remain acceptable as a necessary part of a clinical investigation, but might be rather risky to justify when research data are being collected without immediate benefit to the patient. Fortunately, more recent analyses suggest that when the stress of a medical consultation is removed, a brief maximum exercise test is only about twice as dangerous to a middle-aged person as sitting in an armchair (Shephard, 1976a). All forms of vigorous exercise undoubtedly have a small immediate adverse effect upon the chances of injury and death, although in the long term they are probably beneficial to health. It seems logical to assume that risks are increased somewhat when the exercise is pushed to maximum effort. Conversely, one might imagine that the risks would diminish almost to vanishing point if full medical precautions were taken, including the monitoring of the exercise electrocardiogram by a qualified cardiologist and the provision of facilities for restoring a normal heart rhythm (a dc or battery-operated defibrillator and a well-equipped emergency room). Considerations of cost and staffing make such a recommendation impractical for every middle-aged person who needs an exercise test prior to joining a physical activity program. Further, there is some possibility that the precautions may 'back-fire,' interaction of the subject with an over-zealous test staff increasing the chances of his developing fibrillation (Shephard, 1976a). While the research worker may welcome the protection from possible litigation associated with medical coverage of all tests, the risk to the average middle-aged person of a brief, carefree burst of maximum effort is probably only about one in 50 million; insurance of $500,000 should thus be possible for one cent per test!

Another objection to maximum tests, particularly in children (Kramer and Lurie, 1964; Cumming, 1974), women, and older men, is the difficulty experienced in pushing subjects to a plateau of oxygen consumption. Individuals who normally take no more exercise than an occasional slow walk are not easily persuaded to undertake maximum exertion, and such data as can be obtained are often of unsatisfactory quality. Patients complain of breathlessness and muscular weakness, and give up the test before the necessary gas samples have been collected. Thus there is much to commend the initial use of indirect measurements

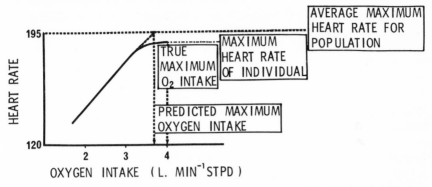

Figure 22 The relationship between heart rate and oxygen intake in an athletic subject. The heart rate reaches a maximum value before the oxygen intake, so that when the oxygen intake/heart rate line is extrapolated to the average maximum heart rate for the population, the predicted maximum oxygen intake is an underestimate of the true value. This error is partially compensated by the fact that the maximum heart rate is less than the average for the population in the individual under consideration.

when testing those who are relatively unfit; it may be practical to switch to direct measurements six to eight weeks later if the individuals concerned have been persuaded to enter a physical activity program (Sidney, 1973).

Indirect measurements

Most indirect measurements of maximum oxygen intake are based on two assumptions: (i) that the heart rate is linearly related to oxygen intake at work loads between 50 and 100% of oxygen consumption, and (ii) that there is a constant maximum heart rate for a given population. Debate continues on the validity of these assumptions. Maritz et al. (1961) suggested that the heart rate commonly reached a maximum a little before oxygen intake; this asymptote tended to cause a slight underestimation of the true maximum oxygen intake (Figure 22). Age (Figure 15) and altitude (Figure 16; Flandrois and LaCour, 1971) are known to influence the maximum heart rate, but allowance can be made for the effects of these two variables. Anxiety and a high environmental temperature both increase the heart rate during submaximum work, causing further underestimation of the true aerobic power. Finally, a problem may be presented by the negative relationship between maximum oxygen intake and maximum heart rate; acceptance of a common maximum heart rate for individuals differing in fitness could cause an overestimation of maximum oxygen intake in athletes and a further underestimation in sedentary subjects (Davies, 1967).

TABLE 10

Percentage discrepancy between the directly measured maximum oxygen intake and the value predicted from the Åstrand nomogram

Population	Error (%)	Authors
White-water paddlers	3.4	Sidney and Shephard (1973)
Distance rowers	-2.7	Wright, Bompa, and Shephard (1975)
University swimmers	-1.3	Shephard, Godin, and Campbell (1973)
Men aged 65 years	5.7	Sidney (1973)
Eskimos	8.0	Rode and Shephard (1971a)

Note. Testing of the Eskimos was by a stepping procedure. The treadmill was used for both submaximum and maximum tests on all other subjects.

These various problems limit the precision of indirect estimations of maximum oxygen intake. Unfortunately, such 'predicted' values lack the accuracy needed to advise an individual on his current fitness level, but they can be useful in motivating him to greater activity since gains of score can be demonstrated in response to training. Further, average values for populations often agree surprisingly well with direct measurements (Table 10). Various techniques are adopted to extrapolate the oxygen consumption/heart rate line to the maximum heart rate for the population under study. Data can be obtained at four or more submaximal work loads, and a line fitted to the observations by computer (Maritz et al., 1961). Alternatively, a nomogram may be used. That of Margaria, Aghemo, and Novelli (1965) is based on observations at two work loads, while that of P.O. Åstrand and Ryhming (1954) requires observations at only one work load.

Nomograms give an apparent sophistication to very simple formulae and often lead to unnecessary errors in the final data. The widely used Åstrand nomogram is a case in point. If the observed oxygen consumption is $\dot{V}_{O_2(obs)}$, and the corresponding pulse rate is P, then the maximum oxygen intake $(\dot{V}_{O_2(max)})$ obtained from the nomogram is given equally well by two formulae:

(1) for men, $\dot{V}_{O_2(max)} = \dfrac{195 - 61}{P - 61} \ \dot{V}_{O_2(obs)}$;

and

(2) for women, $\dot{V}_{O_2(max)} = \dfrac{198 - 72}{P - 72} \ \dot{V}_{O_2(obs)}$.

Desk computers such as the Olivetti Programma 101 can now carry out calculations of this sort automatically, applying necessary corrections for the age of the subjects (Shephard, 1970d); and except in the smallest laboratories the day of the nomogram has probably passed.

It might be assumed that the accuracy of the maximum oxygen intake prediction would vary with the number of observations on which it was based, the order of precision being Maritz et al. > Margaria et al. > Åstrand and Ryhming. This would certainly be the case if the heart rate was equally variable at all intensities of exercise. However, there is evidence that anxiety has a larger relative and probably a larger absolute effect during light work; partly for this reason and partly because of non-linearity in the heart rate/oxygen consumption relationship (Davies, 1968; Lindemann et al., 1973) a single paired measurement of oxygen consumption and heart rate during vigorous exercise may yield as accurate a prediction as an extended series of observations at more moderate work loads (Shephard et al., 1968b), particularly if the single pair of observations is made at a relatively high work load (Shephard, 1967i; Bottin et al., 1966).

The scatter of all three predictions is considerable, the standard deviation amounting to 10-15% of the mean value. In addition to this random variation, there can be a systematic underestimation of the true mean value, particularly if the subject is anxious or the test laboratory is over-heated. Partly for these reasons, and partly because the amount of information is not increased by extrapolation, some authors have preferred to report submaximal measurements more directly, as the predicted work rate (PWR or PWC) at a specified heart rate (170 per minute in younger subjects, 150 per minute in older subjects [Sjöstrand, 1947]), as the heart rate at a specified oxygen consumption (1.5 l. min^{-1} [Cotes, 1966], 0.75 and 1.0 l. min^{-1} [Spiro et al., 1974)], or as the slope of the oxygen consumption/heart rate line (the oxygen pulse [Müller, 1950; Spiro et al., 1974]). The main advantage of more direct reporting is that extrapolation or interpolation is minimal. The disadvantage is that no correction is possible for the decrease in maximum heart rate with aging. Values from young subjects are thus not comparable with those for older subjects; furthermore, the chosen oxygen consumption (1.5 l. min^{-1}) or heart rate (170 min^{-1}) presents little challenge to a fit young man, yet is beyond the reach of some healthy older people (Brown and Shephard, 1967; Sidney, 1973). These various problems are overcome through the use of age-related target heart rates. One variant on this approach is the Canadian home fitness test (Bailey and Shephard, 1976), where all subjects exercise at 70% of their anticipated age and sex specific aerobic power, and fitness is assessed from an age-specific pulse response (Table 11).

In view of the subjective cooperation needed for direct maximum tests, and difficulties in interpreting responses to submaximum effort, there has been some interest in assessing endurance fitness from anthropometric data, including skinfold thicknesses, muscle circumferences, and more sophisticated estimates of body composition such as underwater weighing and body potassium determinations (Shephard, Weese, and Merriman, 1971; Davies, 1972a,b; Cotes et al., 1973).

TABLE 11

Use of target heart rates in the testing of endurance fitness. Rates of ascent of double 9-inch (2 x 22.5 cm) staircase needed to attain 75% of maximum oxygen intake, with corresponding anticipated (target) heart rate (Bailey, Shephard, and Mirwald, 1976)*

Age (yr)	Ascents (min^{-1})		Cadence (min^{-1})		Target heart rate (min^{-1})
	M	F	M	F	
25	24.2	19.1	144	114	160
35	21.9	19.7	132	114	150
45	19.1	17.4	114	102	140
55	16.3	14.6	96	84	130
65	12.9	11.2	78	66	120

* On a domestic (8-inch) staircase, the loading is 70% of aerobic power.

Current evidence suggests that predictions of maximum oxygen intake derived in this way are approximately as accurate as those obtained from submaximum exercise tests.

TESTING OF SPECIFIC VARIABLES

Oxygen consumption
The accurate measurement of oxygen consumption is the keystone of the assessment of endurance fitness. The usual approach is to collect expired gas for a specified period and determine the volume and oxygen concentration of the expirate. Careful attention to detail is important if valid measurements are to be obtained at the high ventilation rates of maximum exercise, and some textbooks still contain photographs of apparatus that is hopelessly inadequate.

The essentials for the collection of expired gas are a mouthpiece, a box-valve, and a balloon. The mouthpiece should have wide flanges, since some subjects find difficulty in gripping the bite-plates during maximum effort. The box-valve should have a low resistance to airflow; two or three flap-valves should be provided for both inspiration and expiration, and these should be checked for free movement at the beginning of each experiment. The dead space between inspiratory and expiratory valves should be as small as possible, and sharp angulations of the airstream should be avoided as these greatly increase the work of breathing. One of the best commercially available valves is based on a design of McKerrow (Figure 23). The tubing connecting the box-valve with the balloon should be as short as possible (preferably not longer than one metre); it should have a large

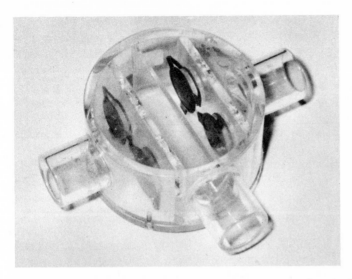

Figure 23 The McKerrow box-valve for the collection of expired gas. Airflow resistance is minimized by the provision of duplicate inspiratory and expiratory valves. The dead space between the valves is reduced by means of a central partition.

internal diameter (at least 3.2 cm) with a smooth interior (since internally corrugated tubing presents a high resistance to airflow). The balloon should have a broad neck (the neck of the traditional Douglas bag is too narrow), and it should be fitted with a Y rather than a T tap.

Expired gas is collected for a half to one minute. It is preferable to collect (say) 12 whole breaths over 32 seconds than 11 and a part breaths over an exact half minute, since in the latter case the measured volume depends on whether collection was begun during inspiration or expiration; the necessary timing is made easier if stop-watches are 'ganged' with the respiratory valves. Carbon dioxide diffuses quite rapidly from the average balloon (Shephard, 1955), and samples should be taken immediately into glass syringes or sampling bottles. The oxygen and carbon dioxide concentrations in such samples have traditionally been determined by chemical absorption, using a Haldane, Lloyd-Haldane, or Scholander apparatus, and these methods remain standard procedures against which other techniques are judged and calibrated. However, chemical analysis is time-consuming, and needs well-trained staff. Physical methods of oxygen analysis are thus very popular. The commonest of such techniques is based on the paramagnetic effect, the alteration in strength of a magnetic field that occurs with a change in oxygen concentration. A paramagnetic analyser can yield results that are accurate to about 0.4% of full-scale, that is 0.04% for a machine analysing over the range 12–22% oxygen (Shephard, 1966b). Skilful chemical analysis is reproducible to 0.01–0.02%, although a close watch must be kept for systematic errors. During maximum exercise, the difference of oxygen concentration between inspired and expired gas is no more than 2–3%, so that a 1–2% error of oxygen consumption measurements inevitably arises during oxygen analysis. Carbon dioxide concentrations are commonly estimated from the infra-red absorption of this gas; the linearity of the analysers has been improved in recent years, but it still leaves something to be desired. Nevertheless, most laboratories regard the infra-red estimate of CO_2 concentration as adequate for the determination of respiratory gas exchange ratios. The volume of expired gas is best determined by transferring the contents of the balloon to a large gasometer such as a 150-litre 'Tissot spirometer.' However, both water-sealed and bellows gasmeters are adequate means of measuring volumes if they have been calibrated recently, and the permitted rate of gasflow is not exceeded. Many physiologists are sorely provoked by a well-filled balloon, and expel air at much too rapid a rate; this causes bubbles to pass the water seal if a wet gasmeter is used and induces pressure artefacts if a dry gasmeter has been selected.

If many subjects are to be tested in a well-equipped base laboratory, there are obvious attractions to the continuous monitoring of oxygen consumption and other variables, data being processed through an analogue computer or an analogue/digital converter. One commercially available device uses a heated wire to measure airflow, and multiplies this with an estimate of oxygen concentration derived from an oxygen electrode. Unfortunately, the methods used in this equipment lack the accuracy needed for good determinations of oxygen consumption. Alternative electrical methods of monitoring gas flow, such as the integration of the pressure signal from a gauze screen, are rather unstable for continuous use. Many subjects also breathe too vigorously to pass the expired air directly through a gasmeter; one way of bringing the flow rate within the range of a good gasmeter is to collect the expired air in a small spirometer or bellows, pumping it through the gasmeter during both inspiration and expiration. Continuous monitoring of the oxygen concentration can also be something of a problem. The most widely used paramagnetic device (the Beckman E-2 apparatus) is designed for the analysis of spot samples rather than a continuous gas flow, and several continuous analysers (based on the paramagnetic principle, the thermal conductivity of oxygen, and the use of a platinum electrode) all respond rather slowly to a change in oxygen concentration. A fuel cell, designed for the testing of rocket propellants, has a more rapid response (measured in milliseconds rather than seconds), but unfortunately the basic calibration curve for this apparatus has a logarithmic rather than a linear form, and the high operating temperature creates other technical problems in use of the equipment. The only practical method for the continuous analysis of the respiratory gases at the present time is thus the mass spectrometer; although costly (around $17,000), it seems reliable and accurate, providing a fast and matched response time for carbon dioxide and oxygen.

Heart rate
It is desirable that the heart rate should be measured during rather than following exercise. However, if readings are taken within the first 15 seconds of stopping exercise (as in the Canadian home fitness test), there is a fair correspondence with measurements taken in the final few seconds of exercise. If observations are delayed for 30 seconds or more, the correlation between the two sets of data falls to about 0.8 (Ryhming, 1954; Shephard, 1966f, 1967g), implying that about 36% of the variation in the recovery heart rate is attributable to extraneous factors (page 51). This unavoidable contamination of data seriously limits the usefulness of all but immediate post-exercise readings in the study of endurance fitness.

The pulse rate can be estimated by palpation of the carotid artery at the root of the neck, although care must be taken not to press so firmly on the carotid sinus as to cause a drop in blood pressure and loss of consciousness. Alternatively, a stethoscope can be strapped to the chest to listen to the heart sounds. However, considerable experience is necessary to obtain accurate readings by either method while a subject is actually exercising. Most observers thus prefer to record the electrocardiogram; this not only gives an accurate indication of heart rate, but allows the condition of the heart muscle to be monitored throughout the exercise period. The electrocardiograph equipment should meet minimum frequency-response specifications (Berson and Pipberger, 1966; American Heart Association, 1967). If a single set of recording electrodes is to be used, the recommended placement for maximum detection of cardiac abnormalities is the CM_5 position (Blackburn et al., 1967); one electrode is fitted over the manubrium sterni and the other is placed in the space between the fifth and the sixth ribs a little to the left of where the apex beat of the heart is most readily palpated (Figure 24). The third (neutral) electrode is placed on the back of the chest or on the forehead. Some authors now prefer to record three leads from different parts of the chest (for example CM_2, CM_4, and CM_6). The likelihood of detecting local areas of oxygen lack in the heart muscle is somewhat increased at the expense of a considerably more complex recording; it is also arguable that the single lead system gives the information that is needed to predict the future health of the patient.

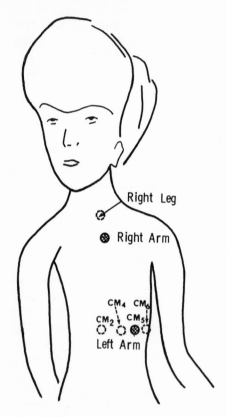

Figure 24 To illustrate the recommended placement of electrodes for exercise tests (lead CM_5). The lead labelled 'right arm' is attached over the upper part of the sternum (manubium sterni). The lead labelled 'left arm' is attached over the apex beat (in the space between the fifth and sixth ribs, 3–4 inches to the left of the mid-line). The lead marked 'right leg' is attached at the back of the neck. Alternative placements for leads CM_2, CM_4, and CM_6 are also indicated.

The electrodes used can be either suction cups or the newer light plastic type. The former are more durable and thus cheaper, but owing to their weight they may displace pendulous skinfolds, giving rise to movement artefacts during running. The suction itself can cause small capillary (petechial) haemorrhages; these have no great medical significance, but may alarm an anxious subject. Difficulty is sometimes encountered because the baseline of the electrocardiograph signal wanders across the recording chart in phase with respiration. Such changes in mean signal voltage are particularly troublesome when studying details of the tracing such as depression of the ST segment (Figure 25). They reflect variations in electrode contact and thus impedance at the skin surface, and can be minimized by careful preparation of the skin and taping of the electrodes. Residual disturbances can be counteracted by electronic averaging of a succession of ECG complexes (Rautaharju et al., 1971).

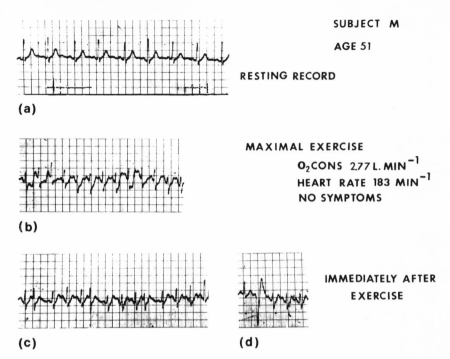

Figure 25 Abnormalities of the electrocardiogram during and following maximal exercise: (a) normal resting record, (b) depression of the ST segment, the commonest sign that the heart muscle is short of oxygen, (c) extra beats arising in the atrio-ventricular node (normal QRS complex, but no preceding P wave), and (d) extra beats arising in the left ventricle (abnormal form of QRS complex). Illustration from Shephard (1968b)

A telemeter can be used to transmit the ECG signal to a recording device across a room or a field (Goodwin and Levitt, 1962). This can be helpful in analysing obscure symptoms that develop in 'post-coronary' patients while they are in the gymnasium. In the laboratory, a telemeter avoids the inconvenience of a trailing cable, but is by no means essential for a standard exercise test on a sensible subject.

A horizontal or downward-sloping depression of the ST segment of the electrocardiogram can be an important danger sign of developing oxygen lack in the heart muscle (Figure 25). Almost all subjects show a slight ST depression during maximum exercise, but a depression greater than 0.1 millivolt indicates an increased risk that the subject may develop overt coronary vascular disease in later life; an asymptomatic man over the age of 40 who shows such a picture is 3-10 times as likely as an average person to sustain a coronary event over the next five years. False positive tests due to drugs (digitalis, quinidine), potassium deficiency, anxiety, over-breathing, and postural factors must be ruled out. The incidence of abnormal records also varies with the test format, some 'positive' records being missed if only a submaximal or a recovery ECG is examined (Cumming, 1972). Some 10% of men over the age of 40, at least 20% of men over the age of 60, and as many as 50% of women over the age of 60 show significant ST depression (Cumming, 1972; Cumming, Borysyk, and Dufresne 1972; Froehlicher et al., 1975). The majority of the patients concerned also develop deep ST depression during normal daily living, as can be demonstrated by 24-hour tape recordings of the ECG (Wolf et al., 1974).

Current wisdom suggests that an exercise test should be stopped if the average ST depression in a sequence of 10 beats exceeds 0.2 millivolt. The other main electrocardiographic indication for stopping exercise is a chain of extra beats (extrasystoles) arising in the ventricles (Figure 25). These are particularly dangerous if they are arising at several sites (as shown by differences of waveform) and occur soon after the preceding T wave of the ECG. Early extrasystoles allow repolarization of the ventricles, with a potential for perpetuation of the abnormal pattern of electrical discharge (Harrison and Reeves, 1968). If the warning signs are ignored, there is a risk that one of the irritable areas of heart muscle may initiate the completely incoordinated and rapidly fatal writhings of ventricular fibrillation. Irritability usually reflects a patchy oxygen lack, and is thus a further indication of coronary vascular disease. Some authors maintain that extrasystoles that first appear during exercise are a more serious sign than occasional resting extrasystoles (McHenry et al., 1972; Beard and Owen, 1973; Blackburn et al., 1973; British Medical Journal, 1973a); others maintain that both types carry an above average risk of overt heart disease in the future (Chiang et al., 1969; Hinckle et al., 1969; Kohn et al., 1971; Sharma et al., 1974).

Blood pressure
Accurate measurement of pressures in either the systemic or the pulmonary circulation during exercise requires the introduction of a recording needle or catheter into one of the major blood vessels of the body. This carries various risks that are not justified in most investigations of endurance fitness. The systolic pressure in the systemic circulation can be estimated with a standard clinical Riva-Rocci sphygmomanometer cuff; the observer records the pressure at which Korotkov sounds can be heard in the brachial artery at the elbow or pulsations can be detected in the radial artery. Occasionally errors of 10-20 mm Hg (1.3-2.7 kPa)

and more can arise during exercise (Rowell, Brengelmann, et al., 1968; Kleinhauss and Franke, 1971). Even greater difficulty is found in measuring the diastolic pressure during exercise, since there is usually no clear point at which the Korotkov sounds become muffled. For some calculations, it is possible to make the convenient (and not grossly incorrect) assumption that the diastolic reading remains at its resting level during rhythmic exercise. The systolic pressure climbs progressively throughout sustained activity, and can finally reach levels of 200 mm Hg (27 kPa) and more. Some clinicians warn against producing an 'excessive' rise of blood pressure during exercise, although no one seems to have defined what is excessive, and there is no very strong evidence that rises occurring during physical activity increase the risks of such catastrophes as a rupture of the cerebral blood vessels. Occasional failure of the blood pressure to rise, or a sudden drop of pressure during effort, is of more serious portent; it may indicate a narrow aortic valve, with failure of an overworked heart to pump blood past the point of narrowing.

Other measurements
Other more detailed physiological measurements are possible in well-equipped laboratories. The cardiac output can be measured by rebreathing a gas mixture containing 1%* acetylene (Simmons, 1969) or 5-15% carbon dioxide in oxygen (Defares, 1956; Jones et al., 1967; Bar-Or and Shephard, 1971; Cunningham and Paterson, 1976). With either gas mixture, the results agree with more complicated methods that involve blood-letting to within about 10%. It is now generally accepted that the main problem with rebreathing methods is the recirculation of gas (Cumming, 1976); to minimize such effects, individual measurements should be completed within 7-10 seconds. With the CO_2 rebreathing method, the answers obtained also depend on assumptions regarding the carbon dioxide carrying properties of the blood and allowances made for systematic errors in the estimation of arterial and venous carbon dioxide pressures from examinations of alveolar gas (Cunningham and Paterson, 1976).

The heart volume may be estimated if facilities are available for taking good-quality frontal (postero-anterior) and lateral X-rays of the chest (Musshoff and Reindell, 1956). The formula adopted is usually that of Reindell et al. (1966):

Heart volume = $0.4 \times L \times B \times T$ ml,

---

* The classical studies of Grollman (1929) used 20-30% acetylene. This was necessary to obtain accurate chemical analyses, but with current developments in gas chromatography mixtures of 1% acetylene can be analysed quite precisely. Higher concentrations are no longer admissible. They are unpleasant for the subject, ultimately anaesthetic, and sufficiently explosive to have caused the death of more than one unfortunate volunteer.

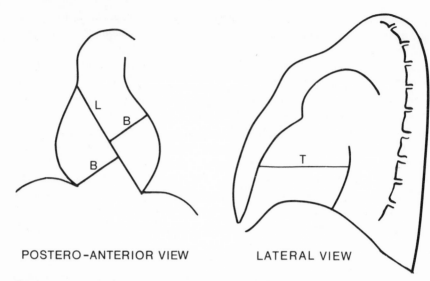

POSTERO-ANTERIOR VIEW   LATERAL VIEW

Figure 26 Estimation of the heart volume from X-ray pictures of the chest. The maximum length L is measured from the origin of the great vessels to the apex of the heart. The maximum breadth B is measured at right angles to this. The maximum depth T is measured in the lateral view. The heart volume is then $0.4L \times B \times T$ cm^3.

where L (cm) is the maximum length of the heart shadow, measured from apex to base in the frontal view, B (cm) is the maximum breadth in the same view, and T (cm) is the maximum depth in the lateral view (Figure 26). The borders of the heart are relatively sharp in the frontal picture, but on the lateral plate they are often indistinct, and the figure obtained for T is somewhat subjective.

The diffusing capacity of the lungs and the total blood volume can both be estimated by a bloodless technique that involves measuring the steady rate of absorption of carbon monoxide from a mixture containing a low and non-toxic concentration of this gas (0.1–0.2%). Errors of the method are discussed by T.W. Anderson and Shephard (1968a), and application to an arctic population is described by Rode and Shephard (1973a). The inspired and expired gas concentrations are measured by infra-red analysis, and the concentration of carbon monoxide in alveolar gas is either calculated (using an assumed value for the dead space of the airways) or is assumed to correspond with the concentration found in the last part of the expirate. The calculation of blood volume takes account of the volume of carbon monoxide absorbed, and relates this to the increased concentration of carbon monoxide in the blood stream, as estimated by a rebreathing procedure. The assumption is made that a percentage (different authors assume 6–15%) of the absorbed carbon monoxide leaves the blood stream to become fixed to the red pigment of the muscles (myoglobin).

The procedure for the estimation of haemoglobin should follow the internationally agreed protocol (International Committee, 1965; 1967; Lewis and Burgess, 1969; British Medical Journal, 1972a). Samples of capillary blood are treated with Drabkin's reagent, which converts the haemoglobin to cyanomethaemoglobin. The concentration of the latter is found from the absorption of visible light at a wavelength of 540 mμ; the spectrometer used in making these measurements is calibrated using a known solution of cyanomethaemoglobin provided by a reference laboratory.

Measurements of static and dynamic lung volumes, blood lactate, blood gas tensions, static and dynamic muscle strength, and endurance often form part of a detailed fitness survey, but techniques will not be discussed here. The examination of ECG records from static effort does not add to knowledge gained from rhythmic exercise tests (Haissly et al., 1974). Some authors regard flexibility measurements as an integral component of fitness assessment, although it is likely that if due regard is paid to endurance the flexibility needed by the average citizen will take care of itself. Many of the tests of static flexibility favour individuals with specific body builds; thus 'failure' of the Kraus-Weber test by many U.S. school children was due in part to their long legs, with associated difficulty in touching the floor while the knees were held straight. Tests of dynamic flexibility are difficult to administer, since the measuring instrument (goniometer) must be lined up precisely with the axis of rotation of the joint under investigation.

Certain anthropological observations, such as height, weight, and the thickness of selected skinfolds, should be obtained on all subjects; even for such simple items, reliable results require good instruments and well-standardized techniques (Weiner and Lourie, 1969; Durnin and Ramahan, 1967; Durnin and Womersley, 1971). More sophisticated estimates of body composition can be obtained from underwater weighing, the ingestion of tritiated water, and the measurement of radioactivity emitted by intramuscular potassium (the naturally present isotope ^{40}K); although the methods are quite involved, and use expensive equipment, all rely on the assumption that body composition throughout the world conforms to that determined on a small population of cadavers (Brozek, 1963; Symposium on Nutrition, Ageing and Longevity, 1965; Brozek, 1965).

5
Current levels of fitness

CHARACTERISTICS OF SPECIFIC POPULATIONS

How true is the current impression that people of the western nations in general, and of North America in particular, are unfit? Let us examine this question in terms of our prime criterion of endurance fitness, the maximum oxygen intake, deferring to a later section (Chapter 8) more general criteria of adaptation such as the incidence of fatigue, illness, and death.

Until fairly recently authors assumed that there was little published information on current levels of maximum oxygen intake. Thus Luft et al. (1963) commented that they had 'not been able to find any other studies on men 30–40 years of age of sedentary occupation with the exception of Robinson's.' Again, the only figures for maximum oxygen intake listed by the *Handbook of Respiration* (Dittmer and Grebe, 1958) were those of Robinson and of Åstrand. However, the available data have increased rapidly over the past decade. I assembled some 8500 observations about ten years ago (Shephard, 1966c), and in a more recent review noted over 770 references (Shephard, 1976e). Difficulties now arise not from the quantity of data but from uncertainties regarding its nature and quality. It is thus necessary to discuss the problems involved before presenting representative figures.

FACTORS INFLUENCING THE RESULTS REPORTED

Sampling
Few investigators have used randomly selected samples of the populations studied. Indeed, it is doubtful if a truly random sample can be obtained for other than the simplest of exercise experiments, if the free choice of the subjects is to be preserved with the rigour demanded by current standards of experimental ethics (Shephard, 1967e; 1972b). In one experiment involving school children

from the Toronto area, the percentage of the population prepared to participate in an investigation dropped from near 100% to as low as 35% when it was emphasized to both children and parents that they had a free choice in the matter, without prejudice to subsequent school records (Shephard, Allen, et al., 1968a). Likewise, only about a third of the adults randomly selected from the Saskatoon telephone directory attended the fitness testing laboratory.

In smaller communities, a better rapport can be established, with volunteer rates of 70–90% (Rode and Shephard, 1971a; Shephard, Lavallée, et al., 1976). Nevertheless, the general absence of a true random sample strikes at a keystone of traditional experimental design, and calls for new techniques. One approach has been to 'resynthesize' a representative population, taking data for one butcher, two bakers, and three candlestick makers as advised by the Dominion Bureau of Statistics; unfortunately, all of those who volunteer for exercise testing are then interested in fitness, and the average scores (Métivier and Orban, 1971) are unrealistically high. An alternative possibility is to recognize the bias in a sample and to measure its effects. If an experiment seems dangerous or offers a 'free' medical examination, it may attract an undue proportion of 'heurotic' volunteers. Thus in one study of volunteer servicemen at a Chemical Defence laboratory, the N (neuroticism) score on the Maudsley self-rating personality inventory (Eysenck, 1959) averaged 28, compared with 21 for an unbiased sample (Shephard and Kemp, unpublished data); fortunately, it was also possible to show that the influence of the high N score on the fitness of this sample was relatively slight (Shephard, 1966d).

Other sources of bias may be more serious. Many studies of primitive communities have used very small samples, with a tendency to examine the lazy and sick members of the tribe at the expense of the young and healthy (who are absent on long hunting expeditions). However, even if as many as 70% of the villagers are seen, significant sampling differences can arise between fitness and medically oriented research teams (Shephard, 1976e), the fitness experts attracting healthier specimens than the physicians. Many of the samples tested in western nations have been sought in or through schools of physical education, and such volunteers include an above-average proportion of fit individuals. Another popular recruiting site has been the YMCA. Here, the population has traditionally eschewed the use of tobacco, and has included an excess of men with a muscular 'mesomorphic' body build, many of them desperately fighting a bulging waistline. More general appeals for volunteers have attracted those concerned about specific health problems such as heart disease or obesity; even if neither is present, the subject's anxiety about the impending report on his health can lead to a high pulse rate, so that the response to submaximum exercise gives an erroneous underestimate of fitness (Shephard and Pelzer, 1966).

General health

The maximum oxygen intake is decreased by many medical conditions, particularly diseases affecting the cardio-respiratory system. In 'primitive' groups such as the arctic Eskimos, as many as 10% of a sample may show the after-effects of tuberculosis and other chronic chest ailments (Rode and Shephard, 1971a, 1973a); aerobic power is impaired in about a third of these (Shephard, 1976e). A preliminary medical examination thus contributes not only to the safety of an experiment, but also to its scientific validity. The dividing line between health and disease is sometimes fine. What of conditions such as mild anaemia and postural hypotension? Both should probably be regarded as falling at the 'poor' end of the normal health continuum, since an improvement in fitness often increases haemoglobin, while decreasing the tendency for the blood pressure to fall on standing. On the other hand, patients with conditions such as asthma and chronic bronchitis should probably be excluded from a normal sample even if they are in a quiescent phase, since a definite pathological process is involved.

Remarkably few authors discuss the medical status of their subjects. It is reasonable to assume that those with overt disease either did not volunteer or were excluded from testing. On the other hand, subjects having abnormalities compatible with normal life and employment may well have been examined particularly when sampling isolated communities that did not speak the language of the investigators. A substantial proportion of older subjects (up to 50% of those over the age of 65) have some minor medical abnormality, and it is perhaps unrealistic to exclude all such cases from a normal population. The ability to perform a full day's work seems a more useful criterion for separating the normal from the abnormal in an aging population.

Tobacco consumption

The haemoglobin of smokers shows a 5–10% saturation with carbon monoxide (page 252); this percentage of haemoglobin is not available for oxygen carriage, and the maximum oxygen intake is correspondingly reduced (Apthorp et al., 1958; Ekblom and Huof, 1972; Vogel and Gleser, 1972). About a half of the carbon monoxide stored in red cell pigment is lost from the body within four hours of stopping smoking. The specific effects of nicotine on the heart and airways are reversed even more rapidly, usually in an hour or less. It is thus a nice question how long cigarettes should be withheld prior to testing (Halicka-Ambroziak et al., 1975). If one is interested in normal levels of fitness, should not measurements on the smokers be made while they are in a nicotinized state? Few authors give details of either the immediate or the long-term tobacco consumption of their subjects. However, most subjects lack both the opportunity and the bravado to smoke during the initial period of waiting and preparation for a test, and a minimum of one hour's abstinence from tobacco can reasonably be assumed in most experiments.

Age

Most authors have reported results by decade (for example, the maximum oxygen intake of 50 men aged 40–50 years). This is a convenient abstraction, but with non-random sampling it leads to a slight bias in the data. Younger subjects volunteer more readily for testing than those who are older, and the mean age for the group cited would more likely be 43 than 45 years.

Test methods

The influence of test methods has already been considered (Chapter 4). The maximum oxygen intake is about 7% smaller when cycling than when running uphill on a treadmill; in an average population it may also be underestimated by 8–10% when it is predicted from the heart rate during submaximum work rather than measured directly.

Environment

Direct measurements of maximum oxygen intake are less susceptible to variations of environment than are predictions based upon the heart rate during submaximum work. A disproportionate increase of heart rate caused by anxiety or heat can lead to substantial underestimation of the maximum oxygen intake by prediction methods. Surprisingly, few investigators specify environmental conditions, and wide cultural differences in concepts of a 'comfortable' room temperature (24–27°C in North America, as low as 13–16°C in the homes of some hardy Britishers) contribute to apparent regional differences in the response to submaximum exercise.

An increase of altitude leads to a decrease of maximum heart rate (Figure 16), and this can influence predictions of maximum oxygen intake (page 129). However, the effect is slight below 7000 ft (2135 m), and this problem may therefore be discounted except in a few specific populations living at medium and high altitudes.

MAXIMUM OXYGEN INTAKE AROUND THE WORLD

For the most part, the published data must be taken at 'face value,' having due regard to the problems of measurement discussed above. However, a few simple corrections may be applied to facilitate comparisons: (a) Data presented as the PWC_{170} may be converted to a predicted maximum oxygen intake, using the formulae of the Åstrand and Ryhming nomogram (1954) with appropriate age

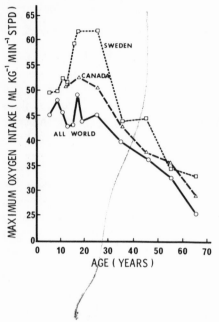

Figure 27 The maximum oxygen intake of 6633 non-athletic men from a wide range of developed countries compared with (a) data reported from Sweden and (b) author's data for 505 Torontonians. All observations have been adjusted for systematic errors listed on pages 145 et seq. For sources of data, see Shephard (1966c).

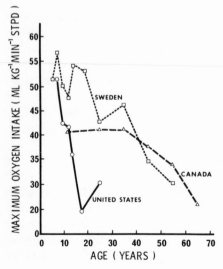

Figure 28 The maximum oxygen intake of women and children classified by region: (a) author's data for 156 Torontonians, (b) reported data for 286 Scandinavians, and (c) reported data for 211 U.S. citizens. For sources of information, see Shephard (1966c). The U.S. data include 58 subjects with very low maximum oxygen intakes reported by Rodahl et al. (1961).

TABLE 12

The maximum oxygen intake (ml kg^{-1} min^{-1} STPD) of 661 subjects from Toronto area (step test) and 1230 from Saskatoon (step and bicycle ergometer tests). Mean ±SD of results predicted from nomogram of P.O. Åstrand and Ryhming (1954) with appropriate age corrections

Age (yr)	Toronto, step test		Saskatoon, step test		Saskatoon, bicycle*	
	Male	Female	Male	Female	Male	Female
10–12**	46.9 ± 6.0 (n = 30)	37.3 ± 4.0 (n = 33)	–	–	–	–
15–19	48.8 ± 7.9 (n = 61)	–	47.2 (n = 102)	39.2 (n = 144)	42.5	33.7
20–29	47.0 ± 7.6 (n = 129)	38.2 ± 3.9 (n = 34)	40.1 (n = 104)	37.3 (n = 138)	36.3	30.6
30–39	39.5 ± 6.9 (n = 106)	38.6 ± 4.7 (n = 16)	37.1 (n = 163)	34.6 (n = 152)	32.4	28.1
40–49	34.7 ± 8.2 (n = 98)	35.1 ± 10.5 (n = 38)	33.8 (n = 84)	31.8 (n = 93)	27.0	24.4
50–59	33.0 ± 6.4 (n = 71)	31.6 ± 8.8 (n = 22)	32.3 (n = 68)	31.2 (n = 88)	25.7	21.9
60–69	26.8 ± 2.8 (n = 10)	24.1 ± 5.5 (n = 13)	30.7 (n = 33)	30.2 (n =56)	22.5	18.9

* n as for step test in Saskatoon.
** Submaximal treadmill test.

corrections. (b) Predictions of maximum oxygen intake based on submaximal test data may be increased by 8% to allow for the usual underestimation by extrapolation procedures. (c) Data obtained on the bicycle ergometer may be increased by a further 7% to make the figures comparable with those obtained on the treadmill. (d) Where the average age departs from the mean for a decade, a decline in maximum oxygen intake of 0.02 l. min^{-1} may be assumed per year of adult life. (e) Adults may be classified into three basic groups – normal sedentary subjects, trained subjects (including those performing heavy manual work), and athletes.

Results thus corrected for 6633 non-athletic male subjects and 653 female subjects are summarized in Figures 27 and 28. In these figures, the maximum oxygen intake has been expressed relative to body weight. The author's data for sedentary Canadians living in Toronto and in Saskatoon are presented in more detail in Table 12; this brings out the widening discrepancy between step and bicycle test data as subjects become older. With the exception of older men and women and children under the age of ten, the maximum oxygen intake of the

TABLE 13

The maximum oxygen intake, classified in terms of nationality and occupational category. Data for 12-year-old children and men aged 20–30 years, expressed relative to body weight (ml kg^{-1} min^{-1} STPD)

School children

	Male	Female
Sweden	57	50
Canada		
Anglophone	46,47	38,42
Francophone	55	46
Czechoslovakia	45,49	38
	51	
Germany	45	–
Holland	51	–
Israel		
Jews	53	45
Arabs	51	–
Italy	45,49	44
Japan	41,48	35,40
	49,53	42,45
Norway	49,56	–
Switzerland	49	–
United States	33,45	28,30
	47,49	49
All nations except Sweden	48.3	40.1

University students

	Phys. Ed.	Other faculties
Sweden	53,39	46,49
Belgium	39	57
Canada	54	40
Denmark	52	–
France	47	–
Norway	–	44[1]
South Africa	38	31
United States	48	30
All nations except Sweden	46.3	40.4

Soldiers

Sweden	64
Canada	44
Germany	33
U.K.	44
United States	49
	39
All nations except Sweden	41.8

Industrial workers

Sweden	53
Australia	44
Canada	44[2]
	49[3]
Holland	44
Norway	44[1]
All nations except Sweden	45.0

Note. For sources of information, see Shephard (1966c, 1976f), Shephard and Pimm (1976), Bottin et al. (1968), and references in notes 1–3.

1 K.L. Andersen (1964).   2 Cumming (1967).   3 Shephard, Jones, and Brown (1968).

Scandinavians seems large relative to that of subjects from other regions. The Swedish samples were non-random, and the majority of subjects concerned were associated in some way with schools of physical and health education. Many of the figures are also 25 or more years old. Nevertheless, the dominant position of Sweden persists when similar occupational groups are compared (Table 13). It is difficult to attribute such differences purely to technical factors, since regional variations in maximum oxygen intake are not found in young children or in trained subjects. The most reasonable explanation of the results is that the Scandinavian people are more active. This is borne out by the limited difference between 'trained' and 'untrained' subjects from Sweden. The attitude of the north European is illustrated by Engstrom's (1972) study of 2000 fourteen-year-old Swedish children. The boys in this sample were devoting an average of five hours per week to vigorous leisure activities and the girls an average of 3.5 hours. In contrast, a study from Quebec (Shephard, Lavallée, et al., 1975) found urban boys spending 30 hours and urban girls 22 hours per week watching television. Regional differences in the quantity and quality of food may also be involved. However, the obesity of North Americans is not the main explanation of their low maximum oxygen intakes, since both absolute and relative values are greater in the Swedes.

The possibility of a sampling bias has yet to be eliminated. Many of the Swedish data have been collected by the Central Gymnastic Institute in Stockholm, and it may be that the adults to whom they have access are of above-average fitness. Even when testing children, P.O. Åstrand (1952) did not draw a completely random sample; teachers were asked to select 'the best,' 'rather good,' and 'poor' members of their classes, and exceptionally fat children were excluded. However, his data are striking in showing that the maximum oxygen intake of teenage girls is well maintained, while that of the boys continues to increase into early adult life. In most other developed nations, fitness starts to deteriorate with the onset of adolescence. It is difficult to attribute the apparent advantage of the Swedes to a superior genetic endowment; if they were a 'master race' in terms of endurance fitness, this should be obvious in small children (where all nationalities are equally active), in athletes, and in old men (where all nationalities have become equally sedentary). The teenage deterioration of the North American seems rather an expression of lack of vigorous exercise. This is determined largely by the environment, a response to the current culture of the metropolis (although the purist could argue that inherited, constitutional factors predispose to overeating and lack of physical activity at this stage in life). There remains a need to test a Swedish population comparable with our 'telephone directory' sample of Saskatoon, but assuming that such an investigation were to confirm the suspicion of a difference in current fitness between the average

TABLE 14

Secular trend of maximum oxygen intake readings: (a) U.S. data for male Harvard students and faculty of 1938 compared with U.S. values for 1966; (b) Canadian data for 1966 and 1973

Age (yr)	(a) United States		(b) Canada	
	Robinson's data (1938) ($ml\ kg^{-1}\ min^{-1}$)	U.S. values as summarized by Shephard (1966c) ($ml\ kg^{-1}\ min^{-1}$)	Toronto 1966	Saskatoon 1973 ($ml\ kg^{-1}\ min^{-1}$)
20-30	48.7	37.6	47.0	40.1
30-40	43.1	36.2	39.5	37.1
40-50	39.2	35.7	34.7	33.8
50-60	37.6	35.7	33.0	32.3

young Swede and his North American counterpart, there is little doubt this would disappear if the North American were to undertake systematic physical training. In the Saskatoon sample, the average maximum oxygen intake of those taking little or no physical activity was 29.9 $ml\ kg^{-1}\ min^{-1}$ in the men and 26.1 $ml\ kg^{-1}\ min^{-1}$ in the women, but in those taking very frequent physical activity the corresponding figures were 39.3 and 31.2 $ml\ kg^{-1}\ min^{-1}$ (Bailey et al., 1974a).

Since the laziness of the North American may be a recent and developing phenomenon, it is interesting to make some historical comparisons (Table 14). S. Robinson (1938) tested 'non-athletic' university students, faculty, and office workers, and the values he reported were almost without exception higher than current figures for the United States. There also seems a small downward trend between step test data for Toronto (1966) and Saskatoon (1973).

Primitive and rural populations

It has commonly been suggested that the maximum oxygen intake of primitive and rural populations is greater than that of city-dwellers, since hunters and farmers live a relatively active life. Early collections of data (for example, Cumming, 1967) did not support such a hypthesis. The maximum oxygen intake of the primitive communities listed was unremarkable; indeed, values for certain samples of Bantu mining recruits and Eskimos were poorer than for sedentary western men of the same age. Even if a primitive man is more active than a city-dweller, he also faces more hardships. Often he must battle against disease, malnutrition, and thirst. After contact with the 'white' man, such problems may be compounded by alcoholism and a debilitating dependence upon 'welfare' (Shephard and Itoh, 1976). Detailed studies of Eskimos living at Igloolik in arctic Canada (Godin and Shephard, 1973a; Shephard and Rode, 1973) showed that only 29 of 147 adult men were actively engaged in hunting; the majority of the villagers remained within the settlement, living a relatively sedentary life. Wyndham, Strydom, et al. (1966) noted that when Bantus moved from their native 'reserves' to the mining 'compounds' of Johannesburg, the first few months of employment were marked by a substantial increase of lean body mass and a corresponding gain of maximum oxygen intake. This may reflect both the hard physical work required in the mines as well as improved standards of nutrition and medical care.

Primitive populations differ widely in activity. In general those living in a cold climate find the search for food and shelter hard, and they must engage in vigorous physical work if they are to survive by traditional means. Of the Canadian Eskimos at Igloolik, those that had accepted the 'white' life-style had an aerobic power of only 50 ml kg^{-1} min^{-1}, but the most active of the continuing hunters had an aerobic power of 65 ml kg^{-1} min^{-1} (Rode and Shephard, 1971a, 1973e). K.L. Andersen (1967a,b) compared nomadic Norwegian Lapps with Pascuans who lived in the idyllic surroundings of Easter Island; again, the maximum oxygen intake of the Easter Islanders was at least 10 ml kg^{-1} min^{-1} lower than that of the Lapps at all ages. It is tempting to attribute this difference to a lack of physical activity among the Pascuans. The Lapps are constantly on the move tending their reindeer, while the Pascuans are for the most part a sedentary people. Equally, in the tropics (Table 15), substantial differences can be seen between active and inactive tribespeople in both Nigeria and Tanzania. A further possible variable is the nature of the terrain. The highlanders of New Guinea and the Tarahumara of Mexico develop extremely high maximum oxygen intakes despite a poor diet and the need to conduct tests at altitudes of 1500–3000 metres. The prime explanation seems not the effect of altitude itself but rather the additional work involved in moving about a hilly countryside. In some of the tribes noted, a high aerobic power is encountered not only in adults but also in quite young children, where more uniform activity patterns might be anticipated between 'civilized' and 'primitive' groups. Infant mortality is high in most 'primitive' communities; for example, 200 of every 1000 children die in the first year of life among Eskimos who persist with their traditional hunting patterns (Godin and Shephard, 1973a). Natural selection, a 'survival of the fittest,' may thus contribute to the unusual aerobic power of some primitive groups.

Rural populations have also been presumed more active than their city-dwelling brethren. Morris (1967) organized a study of heart disease in farmers based on this assumption. Thirty years ago, farm-life often demanded physical activity. A man forming part of a human conveyor belt on the side of a hayrick, for instance, had a very strenuous 12-hour day, and the 24-hour energy expenditure of

TABLE 15

Aerobic power (ml kg^{-1} min^{-1} STPD) of young men aged 20–30 years
living in rugged or mountainous country, tropical regions, and arctic regions[*]

Rugged country and high altitude		Tropics		Arctic	
Canada		Congo		Canada	
Igloolik hunters	56.4	Hoto	42.7	Eskimo	52.3
Chile		Twa	47.5	Indians	49.1
Aymara	49.1[†]	East Africa		Greenland	
Ethiopia		Dorobo	46.0	Eskimo	40.7
Amhara	39.9[†]	Israel		Japan	
India		Kurds	48.4	Ainu	44.4
Tamil	40.3[†]		44.5	Skandinavia	
Mexico: Tarahumara		Yemenites	52.4	Lapps	49.0
'Civilized'	38.9[†]		46.9		53.0
Runners	63.0[†]	Jamaica	47.0	United States	
New Guinea		Malaya		Eskimo	42.3
Lufa	67.0[†]	Temiars	53.2		
Migrant highlanders	63.2	New Guinea			
Peru		Kaul	53.2		
Nunoa	40.1[†]	Nigeria: Yoruba			
		Active	55.5		
		Inactive	45.9		
		Pascua	42.0		
		South Africa			
		Bantu	41.1–47.8		
		Kalahari	47.1		
		Tanzania			
		Active	57.2		
		Inactive	47.2		
		Trinidad			
		Negroes	38.3		
		East Indians	39.4		
		United States			
		Navajo	44.0		
		Venezuela			
		Waras	47.9		

[*] For sources of data, see Cumming (1967) and Shephard (1976e).
[†] Test measurements made at altitudes of 1500–3000 m.

a goatherd climbing the Alpine peaks could be as much as 5000 kcal (20,950 kJ),
twice that of the city office-worker (Durnin and Passmore, 1967). However, a
farmer of the current generation, sitting in the air-conditioned comfort of his
combine-harvester, does little more physical activity than an office-worker.

Equally, Norwegian fisherman based on the islands of Vaerøy and Røst have an aerobic power of only 40.6 ml kg^{-1} min^{-1} at an average age of 40.6 years (Fugelli, 1974), while Italian subalpine farmers have no advantage of maximum oxygen intake over city-dwelling Milanese (Steplock et al., 1971).

Even among children, not all investigators have demonstrated an advantage to the rural groups. Green (1967) found that rural boys from Alberta had an aerobic power 0.3 l. min^{-1} greater than the city-dwellers, and girls from the country had a superiority of 0.13 l. min^{-1}. On the other hand, F.H. Adams et al. (1961) observed no significant difference of PWC$_{170}$ between children living in Stockholm and their counterparts from a farming district a few miles to the north, while studies from French Canada (Shephard, Lavallée, et al., 1974) and from Czechoslovakia (Seliger, 1970) have revealed slightly higher fitness levels in the urban communities. Explanations of this paradox include greater opportunities for organized sports in the towns, coupled with the provision of school buses for rural children. Daily activity diaries show that town children are more active, mainly because they walk as much as two miles to and from school each day.

REGIONAL DIFFERENCES IN PHYSICAL PERFORMANCE

The possible relationship between physical performance and endurance fitness poses two types of question. The first is raised by those selecting athletes for international competition and children for specialized training programs: If the maximum oxygen intake is measured, will it identify the best immediate performers or those with potential for top performance in a long distance race? The second question is the converse of the first, and is raised by those who do not have access to a physiology laboratory: If I measure the performance of my subjects, will it indicate their endurance fitness?

Unfortunately, it is not possible to give a simple affirmative answer to either question. One cannot deny the existence of a statistical relationship between performance and fitness. A sedentary and obese youth with a maximum oxygen intake of 35 ml kg^{-1} min^{-1} undoubtedly has a poorer time for a one-mile run than an athlete who can achieve an intake of 75 ml kg^{-1} min^{-1}. It is also quite possible to establish a significant correlation between maximum oxygen intake and the performance of individuals within an athletic team. Dahlström (1964) reported a correlation of 0.54 between the PWC$_{170}$ (page 280) and times in a cross-country skiing contest, and Costill (1967) found a coefficient of correlation of 0.83 between aerobic power and the times achieved by a team of cross-country runners. Our laboratory has shown equally good correlations between peer ratings of performance and physiological variables such as maximum oxygen intake and muscle strength in various groups of endurance sportsmen, including university class swimmers (Shephard, Godin, and Campbell, 1973), rowers (G.R.

Wright, Bompa, et al., 1975), whitewater paddlers (Sidney and Shephard, 1973), and dinghy sailors (Niinimaa et al., 1974); further, we have discussed techniques whereby the physiological scores can be combined to yield objective ratings as a guide to both selection and the regulation of training (Shephard, 1975c; 1976c). Nevertheless, the aerobic power of national level endurance athletes ranges quite widely from 70 to 85 ml kg^{-1} min^{-1} (Saltin and Åstrand, 1967), whereas times for performance of a distance event often differ by only a fraction of a second. Evidently other factors such as the skill of the performer, the efficiency of his movements, the extent of the oxygen debt incurred, the choice of an optimum pace, motivation, and reactions to the psychological pressures of top-level competition (Shephard, 1976c) are at least as important as the maximum oxygen intake in deciding the winner of an endurance event.

Performance tests at first inspection seem a rather attractive method of assessing the fitness of a large population when a minimum of equipment is available. Two 'batteries' of tests have been devised with this objective in view, one by the American Association of Health, Physical Education and Recreation (AAHPER, 1958), and the other by its Canadian counterpart (CAHPER, 1966). Similar test items are included:

AAHPER test battery	*CAHPER test battery*
Sit-ups (untimed)	One-minute speed sit-ups
Chin-ups	Flexed arm hang
Standing broad jump	Standing broad jump
Shuttle-run	Shuttle-run
50-yard (45.7 m) dash	50-yard (45.7 m) dash
600-yard (548 m) walk-run	300-yard (274 m) run
Soft-ball throw*	

Both test batteries have been applied to very large groups of children. One might object that neither includes a good measure of endurance. It is rumoured that a one- or two-mile (1.6-3.2 km) run was considered and rejected on the grounds that it was too exhausting and too dangerous for children. Certainly, in college-age adults, the correlation with direct treadmill measurements of maximum oxygen intake rises from -0.67 for half-mile times to -0.85 for two-mile (3.2 km) times (Ribisl and Kachadorian, 1969). In young children, a combination of poor pacing and limited enthusiasm for endurance effort give low coefficients of correlation over all distances (Lavallée et al., 1974); however, the best of a series of unsatisfactory correlations is seen over distances of 600 yards (0.5 km). Irrespective of the distance run, the correlation between test scores and maximum oxygen intake largely disappears once allowance has been made for the size of the

* This item will be omitted in a revised formulation of the test.

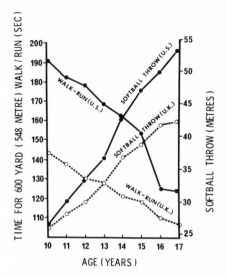

Figure 29 A comparison of the performance of U.S. and European children on two common fitness test items: the 600-yard (548-m) walk-run, and the softball throw (based on data of Campbell and Pohndorf, 1961).

subjects. Cumming and Keynes (1967) first demonstrated this point for children (where size varies greatly and maximum oxygen intake per unit weight varies relatively little), and subsequent work from this laboratory (Drake et al., 1968) has established that the same is true of adults. If due allowance is made for age and easily measured size variables (height, weight, and the thickness of subcutaneous fat), a battery of six or seven performance tests contributes no significant information on either the maximum oxygen intake or the strength of the subjects. Presumably it measures mainly skill and determination relative to the individual test items. Regional differences in the results of performance tests have been described, for instance between Danish and U.S. school children (Knuttgen, 1961) and between South African, U.K., and U.S. children (Sloan, 1963). Apparent racial differences in performance have also been noted among the several populations of Ceylon (Cullumbine, 1949–50) and South Africa (Cluver et al., 1942; Smit, 1961; Sloan, 1966; Sloan and Hansen, 1969). In the regional comparisons, U.S. children have shown the poorest scores, and it has been tempting to attribute their lack of performance to limitations of endurance and strength. However, skill, determination, simple familiarity with the tests, and even track conditions provide important explanations of differences in scores (Knuttgen and Steendahl, 1963). This point is brought out when the results for individual items are compared. Thus, the U.S. children fared particularly poorly on the 600-yard (548 m) walk-run, but did better than the Europeans and South Africans on what was for them a familiar task – the soft-ball throw (Figure 29).

TABLE 16

Changes in results of motor performance tests on 13-year-old
children in Oakland, California, U.S.A., between 1934 and 1958
(table based on data of Espenschade and Meleney, 1961)

	Boys	Girls
Height (cm)	+5.6	+2.3
Weight (kg)*	+4.7	+2.7
50 yard (45.7 m) dash (sec)	+0.2	+0.5
Ball throw (m)	+6.24	−0.62
Broad jump (cm)	−12.7	−12.7
Jump and reach (cm)	+5.1	+2.5
Grip strength (kg)†	+2.2	0.0

* By modern terminology, body mass.
† 1.00 kg = 9.8N.

Further proof of the effects of practice on test scores was forthcoming when the
U.S. national population was retested (AAHPER, 1965); although there was no
evidence that the fitness of the children had increased since 1958, results for all
performance tests were substantially improved because the test battery had been
used frequently in most participating schools.

Espenschade and Meleney (1961) compared the motor performance of Cali-
fornian school children over the longer period from 1934 to 1958 (Table 16).
Interpretation of their results is complicated not only by differences in test
learning but also by an advancement of maturation with a considerable increase
of average heights over the intervening years. The increase of height (Von
Döbeln, 1966; Asmussen and Christensen, 1967; Shephard, 1976e) favours performance in ball-throwing and the jump and reach test. It is difficult to predict
how opportunities for the practice of track and field items have changed over
the years. The deterioration in times for the 50-yard dash, for instance, might
reflect urban overcrowding rather than a true deterioration of fitness.

The question of performance test batteries should not be left without reference to the claim of Falls et al. (1966) that they could estimate the maximum
oxygen intake from the results of the AAHPER test with a 'standard error'
(standard deviation) of ±12%. This sounds impressive until it is realized that the
subjects tested were a rather homogenous group; the standard deviation of maximum oxygen intake for their population was only about 19% if no reference was
made to scores in the performance tests. The reduction of variance from 19% to
12% was due almost entirely to the influence of age, body size, and obesity upon
both performance test scores and aerobic power.

TABLE 17

The relationship between the distance covered in
12 minutes of all-out running and the maximum
oxygen intake (based on the data of Cooper, 1968)

Distance (km)	Maximum oxygen intake (ml kg^{-1} min^{-1} STPD)
<1.6	<28
1.6–2.0	28–34
2.0–2.4	34–42
2.4–2.8	42–52
>2.8	>52

In well-motivated adults, good predictions of aerobic power can be obtained by measuring the distance run in 15 minutes (Balke, 1954) or 12 minutes (Cooper, 1968). Correlations as high as 0.90 have been claimed when using this approach on young soldiers (Table 17), but results are much poorer in children, women, and older men (Maksud and Coutts, 1971; Wiley and Shaver 1972; Kearney and Byrnes, 1974). The various problems and dangers of such 'all-out' efforts are conveniently circumvented in the Canadian home fitness test. Although intended primarily for the home, it can be used in a field laboratory as well; given no more than a long double step and a gramophone turntable, groups of 16 or more subjects can be tested simultaneously (Bailey and Shephard, 1976).

CURRENT VALUES FOR OTHER MEASURES OF FITNESS

Obesity
Many authors have regarded obesity as a specific clinical condition, characterized by a certain minimum of excess weight. However, observation shows a continuum from the healthy to the obese, along which a substantial proportion of the adult population slide during their middle years. Two simple measures of the extent of obesity are the excess weight relative to actuarial height standards and the thickness of the skinfolds.

The 'ideal' weights proposed by the Society of Actuaries (1959) have a somewhat arbitrary derivation, but nevertheless describe the average young 'white' Canadian quite well. If a young athlete exceeds the 'ideal' weight, this may indicate an unusual development of the body muscles, but when excess weight first appears in middle age, it is usually due to an increase of body fat. In older subjects, accumulation of fat may occur even without an increase of body weight, since there is often an associated loss of lean tissue (Forbes and Reina, 1970).

There is reliable evidence that subjects who carry an excess weight have a poor life expectancy, although some authors have argued that this merely reflects the association of excess weight with a high blood pressure and abnormalities of blood lipids (Seltzer, 1966; Keys et al., 1972; British Medical Journal, 1973e). One might envisage the problem as an increased total body mass, supported and propelled by a shrunken cardiac and skeletal musculature. Is it more dangerous to accumulate an excess of fat than an excess of muscle? Surprisingly, this does not seem to be the case. There are few extremely obese victims among patients sustaining the commonest form of middle-aged death, a 'coronary' attack (Friedman and Rosenman, 1974). It may be hypothesized that manifest coronary disease has a predilection for a particular body type, the mesomorphic, aggressive, driving, 'Type A' individual; the really obese person is never sufficiently aroused, either emotionally or physically, to develop an overt 'coronary' incident! We may also ask whether there is any disadvantage in having a weight lower than the actuarial 'ideal.' In the past, low weights have been associated with 'wasting' diseases, such as tuberculosis and cancer, but at the present time it is quite possible for a healthy young person to have less than the 'ideal' weight. Canadian Eskimos (Rode and Shephard, 1971a) and other primitive groups (Shephard, 1976e) find no disadvantage in carrying much less body fat than the normal young 'white' Canadian who meets the actuarial standard. It is more debatable whether weight loss is desirable if it is attained at the expense of lean tissue (as can happen both in figure-conscious young ladies and endurance athletes who train extremely hard).

In the majority of city-dwellers, excess weight can be equated with fat, and this in turn reflects a low level of habitual activity (Durnin and Passmore, 1967). Thus, if the average weights for a population exceed the figures recommended by the life insurance companies, it is a reasonable first assumption that the population in question is unfit. In North America, men and women over the age of 40 commonly exceed the 'ideal' by 10 kg or more. The author's data for Canadians living in Toronto (Table 18) have been replicated by other surveys from many parts of this continent (Young et al., 1963; Wessel et al., 1963; Norris et al., 1963; U.S. Public Health Service, 1966; Sabry, 1973). There are indications that obesity is now becoming a problem in other affluent western nations. In wartime Britain (1943) the average weight of the 50-year-old man was 65.8 kg (Kemsley, 1952); by 1960, the 50-year-old Birmingham worker weighed 67.2 kg (Khosla and Lowe, 1967), while men seen by the British Institute of Directors (1964–68) averaged 69.1 kg (Richardson and Pincherle, 1969). At the corresponding height (177 cm in shoes), U.S. 'whites' weighed 72.5 kg and Bengalese men only 58.6 kg (Kemsley et al., 1962). 'White' South African miners aged 45–49 years had a similar average height (174.8 cm without shoes), but weighed 78.5 kg; part

TABLE 18

Average body weight relative to actuarial tables, and average thickness of eight skinfolds (author's data for Canadians living in the Toronto area [Shephard, Jones, et al., 1969])

Age (yr)	Men		Women	
	Excess weight* (kg)	Average skinfold (mm)	Excess weight* (kg)	Average skinfold (mm)
10-12	3.2[†]	8.0 ± 3.5 (n = 29)	2.1[†]	10.3 ± 3.5 (n = 33)
16-19	0.8 ± 9.4 (n = 68)	11.3 ± 5.9 (n = 68)	–	–
20-29	1.7 ± 8.7 (n = 78)	11.2 ± 5.3 (n = 78)	8.3 ± 5.3 (n = 6)	16.2 ± 3.8 (n = 6)
30-39	6.4 ± 8.5 (n = 66)	16.1 ± 10.6 (n = 65)	1.4 ± 5.3 (n = 18)	13.5 ± 5.2 (n = 18)
40-49	9.3 ± 9.5 (n = 75)	14.0 ± 5.8 (n = 76)	6.8 ± 8.4 (n = 37)	17.3 ± 5.4 (n = 38)
50-59	8.8 ± 7.7 (n = 60)	15.2 ± 6.7 (n = 63)	4.9 ± 7.2 (n = 22)	18.2 ± 5.1 (n = 23)
60-69	5.1 ± 7.3 (n = 9)	15.4 ± 2.7 (n = 10)	4.5 ± 9.5 (n = 14)	22.5 ± 7.9 (n = 11)

* The traditional term 'excess weight' has been retained. Actually, this is an excess body mass.
† Expressed relative to Holt's data for school children of equivalent height.

of their excess weight may have been muscle, although they had weighed 9 kg less in their late teens and were currently 6.3 kg heavier than British miners of the same age and height (Wyndham and Sluis-Cremer, 1968a; Wyndham, Watson, and Sluis-Cremer, 1970). Canadian Eskimos carry a substantial excess weight (average 5.7 kg for all adult males [Shephard, 1974c]), but this is due partly to a substantial muscle mass and partly to stocky limbs that make the normal weight for height tables inappropriate. In contrast, data from 17 'primitive' tropical tribes (Shephard, 1976e) shows an average weight 5 kg lower than the actuarial 'ideal.'

A double fold of skin and subcutaneous tissue has a thickness of 2-3 mm if the tissues immediately under the skin are free of fat (D.A.W. Edwards et al., 1955). In North American men, the average thickness is 11-15 mm, while in women it ranges from 14 to 22 mm, depending upon age (Table 18). Readings of 30 or 40 mm are not uncommon in the abdominal region of both sexes. Such massive deposits of fat serve no useful function unless a 20-mile swim in icy water is contemplated – they are merely evidence of an overnourished and unfit population. The body composition of the 'primitive' tribesman is very different (Shephard, Hatcher, and Rode, 1973); 6 groups living in mountainous areas had an average skinfold thickness of 6.3 mm, 11 tropical populations an average of 6.5 mm, and 13 arctic groups an average of 7.1 mm (Shephard, 1976e). The two exceptions to this pattern were groups acculturated to western 'civilization': the Eskimos of Point Barrow (11.0 mm) and the East Indians of Trinidad (10.6 mm). As with body weight, there is some evidence that skinfold readings are becoming progressively larger in the western world. Thus Colley (1974) noted that 14-year-old British schoolgirls were substantially fatter than their counterparts examined in 1959; by 1971, 3.6% of 14-year-old boys and 32.4% of the girls had triceps folds greater than 25 mm!

Haemoglobin
Despite general evidence of overnutrition, there are still pockets of undernutrition even in affluent western society; their influence on working capacity is revealed by measurements of the haemoglobin level. As noted in Chapter 3, the haemoglobin level determines the oxygen carrying potential of unit volume of blood and can be almost as important as the maximum cardiac output in determining an individual's maximum oxygen intake.

Several groups are particularly liable to a low haemoglobin level. In young children, the needs imposed by a combination of growth and high levels of physical activity may not be met by the diet (Durnin, 1967a). The deficiency of haemoglobin can be sufficient to reduce the child's activity and thus predispose to obesity. Some women are made anaemic by a heavy menstrual loss of blood (R.H. Davis et al., 1967; H.T. Andersen and Barkre, 1970). The elderly are also liable to anaemia; in this group, an impaired formation of red pigment may be compounded by the restricted diet possible for those living on a small pension. In some primitive tribes dietary anaemia is made worse by recurrent haemorrhage associated with parasitic infections such as bilharzia and hookworm (Davies and Van Haaren, 1973; Gardner, personal communication). One final group susceptible to anaemia is endurance athletes (page 95).

Despite these various exceptions, relatively few people in the western world are anaemic, and in most subjects the haemoglobin level is quite close to the mean normal value (Table 19).

Strength
Strength is related primarily to fitness for brief periods of activity. However, it can also be important in the context of endurance fitness, since the strength of the active muscles determines the influence of a given work load on local blood

TABLE 19

The haemoglobin content of the blood of male and female subjects living in the Toronto area (the internationally accepted 'normal' figures are 156 g l.$^{-1}$, 9.7 mmol l.$^{-1}$ for men, and 138 g l.$^{-1}$, 8.6 mmol l.$^{-1}$ for women). The mean and standard deviation of results are shown for each age group

Age (yr)	Haemoglobin level					
	Male subjects			Female subjects		
	g l.$^{-1}$	mmol l.$^{-1}$	n	g l.$^{-1}$	mmol l.$^{-1}$	n
10–12	141 ± 11	87 ± 7	26	141 ± 080	87 ± 5	32
16–19	157 ± 11	97 ± 7	68	–		
20–29	160 ± 14	99 ± 9	77	141 ± 12	87 ± 7	6
30–39	156 ± 14	97 ± 9	66	140 ± 13	87 ± 8	18
40–49	156 ± 12	97 ± 7	75	138 ± 13	86 ± 8	37
50–59	154 ± 10	95 ± 6	59	136 ± 10	84 ± 6	22
60–70	155 ± 08	96 ± 5	9	144 ± 9	89 ± 6	14

flow (page 245) and the resultant blood pressure response. A static (isometric) contraction or rhythmic contractions occupying more than 0.3 of the total performance time often cause some restriction of muscle blood flow, but this does not embarrass function until the intensity of the contraction reaches a fixed proportion of maximum voluntary force for the muscle concerned (Royce, 1959; Lind and McNicol, 1967). If a subject who is not accustomed to riding a bicycle performs maximum work on a bicycle ergometer, the intensity of contraction in the quadriceps muscles passes the point of embarrassment before the capacity of the heart has been fully taxed. The subject thus complains of local fatigue and weakness, and ceases cycling before his true centrally limited maximum oxygen intake has been reached.

An assessment of strength should include representative tests of force and endurance for arm, leg, and back muscles. However, most authors have been content to measure hand-grip force, using some form of hand dynamometer. Clarke (1966) has argued that the hand-grip readings show a correlation of 0.80 with more general measures of muscle strength, implying that the single reading will yield two-thirds of the information that could be obtained from a more-extensive battery of muscle strength tests. Hand-grip data provide an unsatisfactory basis of evaluation in individuals whose strength is localized to this specific region of the body, for example tennis players and some classes of manual labourer. Nevertheless, it is generally safe to assume that if an entire population has a low grip strength, their muscular development is poor.

TABLE 20

Grip strength of dominant hand (kg)* (data for various nations as shown)

Age (yr)	Males				Females		
	Toronto[1,2,3]	Denmark[4]	United States[5,6]	U.K.[7]	Toronto[1,3]	Denmark[4]	U.K.[7]
9–10	19.0 ± 2.6	–	21.4	–	15.5 ± 3.0	–	–
11	21.0 ± 4.7	–	24.1	–	18.7 ± 4.0	–	–
12–13	23.3 ± 3.3	–	26.4	–	23.1 ± 6.0	–	–
16–19	54.2 ± 9.2	51.0	50.0 45.0	–	–	33.8	–
20–29	54.0 ± 8.6	59.9	56.8 53.6	44.4	–	36.2	24.9
30–39	52.1 ± 8.7	58.5	50.7	–	–	35.7	–
40–49	55.2 ± 10.5	55.6	49.1	–	31.2 ± 5.7	33.5	–
50–59	47.0 ± 7.4	51.6	45.9	–	28.3 ± 5.6	32.5	–
60–69	44.1 ± 6.8	46.4	44.3	–	27.5 ± 4.5	30.7	–

* The traditional units have been used in this table. Strictly speaking, handgrip force should be expressed in N or kN (9.80 N = 1.00 kg).
1 Shephard, Allen, et al. (1968a).
2 Shephard, Jones, and Brown (1968).
3 Brown and Shephard (1967).
4 Asmussen and Heebøll-Nielsen (1961);   data for 175-cm men, 160-cm women.
5 Burke et al. (1953).
6 Bookwalter (1950).
7 Adamson and Cotes (1967).

The author's data for the grip strength of Torontonians are presented in Table 20. The results seem comparable with U.S. data, better than for one United Kingdom sample, but inferior to data obtained in Copenhagen. The earliest grip strength readings are those of Porter (St Louis, 1892) and Carmen (Saginaw, 1899); re-examination of the Saginaw children in 1964 (Montpetit et al., 1967) showed a 5-kg increase of grip strength in the girls and older boys. However, this was due entirely to the larger size of the current generation, and when grip strength was expressed as a ratio to body weight the Saginaw children of 1964 were inferior to the St Louis children of 1892.

Other variables
A complete survey of endurance fitness should include many other measurements, as discussed in Chapter 4. There have been few representative studies covering these other variables as yet. Indeed, in some instances agreed techniques have still to be devised. Complete surveys are costly in terms of staff, equipment, and the subject's time, and are best reserved for subsamples, particularly when the total population to be evaluated is large. Examples of more comprehensive studies of working capacity can be found in the appropriate synthesis volume of the Human Adaptability Project of the International Biological Programme (Shephard, 1976e).

THE EFFECTS OF GROWTH AND AGING
ON THE MAXIMUM OXYGEN INTAKE IN DIFFERENT COMMUNITIES

Activity patterns change as a person becomes older. The young child is naturally active, and becomes restive if restrained. The tempo lessens with adolescence, and continues to slow throughout adult life. Whether one is examining athletes who allege that they are continuing their training, or ordinary sedentary members of the population, it is difficult to distinguish the growth and aging of endurance fitness from responses to concomitant changes in physical activity.

In boys, a maximum oxygen intake of 50 ml kg^{-1} min^{-1} is typical of almost every nation where tests have been conducted (Shephard, 1971c; 1976e). Samples of Swedish children (Figure 27) and Canadian Eskimos (Rode and Shephard, 1971a) maintain or surpass this figure throughout adolescence and early manhood. This probably indicates what could be expected if a person with average physical endowment remained reasonably active; however, the usual finding in North America is a decline to 42–48 ml kg^{-1} min^{-1} in a young adult. In girls, puberty is associated with an increase in the percentage of body fat, and the maximum oxygen intake per unit of body weight inevitably shows some decline. However, there are again regional discrepancies. Swedish teenagers (Figure 28) and

Canadian Eskimos sustain an aerobic power close to 50 ml kg^{-1} min^{-1}, whereas in North American 'white' society adolescent girls show a rapid decline to figures of 40 ml kg^{-1} min^{-1} and less.

In adult life, both sexes suffer a further gradual loss of aerobic power; the influence of this loss on working capacity is usually enhanced by a progressive increase in the percentage of body fat. My data (Table 12) and other information from the world literature (Figures 27 and 28; Bink, 1962; Dehn and Bruce, 1972; Åstrand, 1973; Shephard, 1976e) show that the maximum oxygen intake of the average man decreases by 11-14 ml kg^{-1} min^{-1} between the ages of 25 and 55 years, with a steeper fall of 6-7 ml kg^{-1} min^{-1} between 55 and 65. Women retain a relatively constant aerobic power from 20 to 35 years of age, but lose 8-14 ml kg^{-1} min^{-1} from 35 to 55 years, and a further 7 ml kg^{-1} min^{-1} from 55 to 65 years. Regional comparisons suggest that the rate of aging is somewhat less in U.S. citizens (who are already inactive in their early twenties) and in circumpolar groups such as the Lapps and Eskimos (who may remain active until relatively late in adult life). Our enquiries (Godin and Shephard, 1973a) indicate a rapid decline in both the activity and the fitness of Eskimo hunters once they become grandparents and have the privilege of choosing the best cuts of meat from the caribou without the necessity of tracking it across the tundra.

Hollmann (1966) and Dehn and Bruce (1972) both claimed that the rate of aging was less in athletes than in sedentary subjects. However, these claims rest mainly on the atypical behaviour of the non-athletes. Thus Hollmann found that the maximum oxygen intake of a group of athletes decreased by 7 ml kg^{-1} min^{-1} between the ages of 44 and 59 years, with a loss of 14 ml kg^{-1} min^{-1} in 'non-sports persons.' Likewise, the rate of deterioration among the continuing athletes of Dehn and Bruce (1972), 0.56 ml kg^{-1} min^{-1} per year, was similar to that seen in most sedentary people over a comparable age span. Other figures for continuing athletes (Table 21) support this conclusion. Nevertheless, the athlete should not despise a continuation of his sport. Although he may lose aerobic power at the same absolute rate as a sedentary individual, he conserves his advantage over the inactive person and has a greater reserve to meet the problems of old age.

Any development of maximum oxygen intake, either in childhood or as a result of training, is associated with a roughly proportionate growth in the lean tissues of the body; indeed, the relationship of maximum oxygen intake to lean mass is sufficiently close that the ratio between the two variables has been suggested as an index of cardio-respiratory fitness (Buskirk and Taylor, 1957). The growth of lean body mass involves both the heart and the skeletal muscle, and is contingent upon the availability of an adequate diet. The case of the Bantu miners (page 151) has already been mentioned. It also seems possible for athletes to train to the point where lean tissue is being lost from the body (Kavanagh, Shep-

TABLE 21

Rate of aging in continuing athletes (data expressed as loss
of maximum oxygen intake [ml kg^{-1} min^{-1}] per year)

Subjects	Loss	Author
Physical Education teachers		
male	0.57	Asmussen and Mathiasen (1962)
female	0.70	
Sportsmen, male	0.70	Hollmann (1965, 1966)
Runners, male	0.67	Dill et al. (1967)
Orienteers, male	0.34	Saltin and Grimby (1968)
Athletes, male	0.56	Dehn and Bruce (1972)
Physical Education teachers		
male	0.69	I. Åstrand et al. (1973)
female	0.44	I. Åstrand et al. (1973)
Track athletes, male	0.56	Kavanagh and Shephard (1976b)

hard, et al., 1973; Shephard, Campbell, et al., 1974; Wright, Nicoletti, and Shephard, 1976), and there are rumours that some endurance competitors have exploited this phenomenon in attempts to better their performance.

The stunted growth of German school children during the latter part of World War II (Tanner, 1962) is probably attributable to poor nutrition (Figure 30). The converse may be equally true. If a population is well fed, it will grow larger, and this may in itself produce an increase of maximum oxygen intake. Over the last hundred years, the average height of western man has increased by about 10 cm. Although caused partly by better health, better environmental conditions, and a wider choice of marriage partners, the main basis for this 'secular trend' is thought to be improved nutrition (Suzuki, 1970). Currently, the rate of increase of stature is particularly fast in traditionally short populations such as the circumpolar tribes (Rode and Shephard, 1973d; Shephard, 1974c).

The past century has witnessed a vast improvement in athletic records (Frucht and Jokl, 1964; Jokl and Jokl, 1968; Ryan, 1974; Shephard, 1976c). The increase of standing height with associated developments of muscular strength and maximum oxygen intake (Bailey, Ross, et al., 1974) have undoubtedly contributed to this trend (Figure 31). It is less certain how the performance of the average man has fared. His absolute maximum oxygen intake has almost certainly increased with the general increase in body size, and some improvement of maximum oxygen intake per unit of body weight could have occurred, since a century ago many of the population were short of body-building proteins. However, it is likely that most sedentary adults have dissipated this potential gain through an

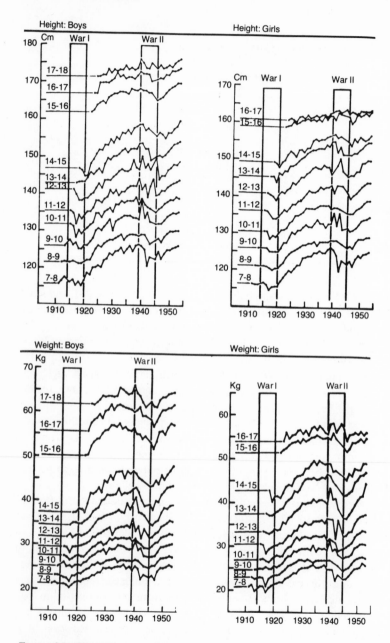

Figure 30 The influence of two world wars on the height and weight of German school children (Tanner, 1962).

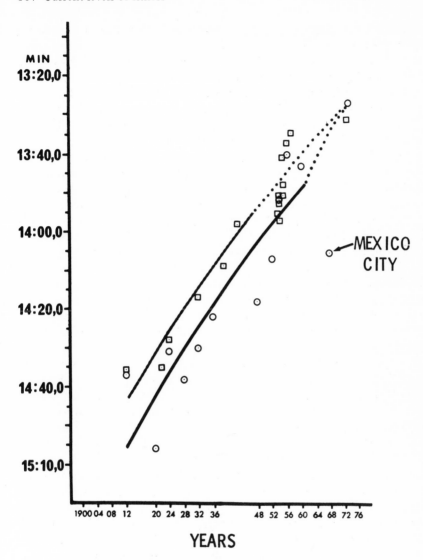

Figure 31 The improvement in athletic records for the 5000-m race from 1908 to 1975 (based in part on data of Frucht and Jokl, 1964): x, individual world records; o, Olympic performance.

increase in the percentage of body fat. The rate of maturation of children has also increased over the last century, further augmenting the average height at any given age. Paediatric work physiologists have thus given much thought to methods of comparing such variables as maximum oxygen intake and muscle strength in children that differ in size (Von Döbeln, 1966; Asmussen and Christensen, 1967; Shephard, 1976e). In theory, both aerobic power and strength should be proportional to the square of standing height, but in practice the height exponent is often 2.9–3.0.

Information on the biology of aging is tantalizingly limited. A number of studies, mainly cross-sectional in type, have shown that body weight reaches a maximum around the age of 45 years. Between the ages of 45 and 65 years, there is a constant or a decreasing body weight, but the thickness of the skinfolds does not change (Shephard, 1976e). We may thus presume that lean tissue is decreasing. A further factor influencing cross-sectional data, particularly in the oldest age categories, is an attrition of the sample through the death of overweight individuals. Readings for muscle force parallel predicted changes of lean tissue (Table 20); results are relatively constant in both sexes from 25 to 45 years, but thereafter decline by 20% to the age of 65 years. Anaerobic power shows a rather larger change, in men from an equivalent of 170 ml oxygen kg^{-1} min^{-1} at the age of 20 to 100 ml kg^{-1} min^{-1} at the age of 60, and in women from 145 to 80 ml kg^{-1} min^{-1} over the same age span (di Prampero and Cerretelli, 1969).

It is doubtful whether physical activity can slow these and other accompaniments of aging. Comfort (1964) concluded that human life could probably be prolonged, but he was unable to answer the question 'by what factor?' because so little was known of the processes determining human senescence. When Shock (1967) reviewed the influence of physical activity on aging, he was unable to produce concrete evidence that increased activity would slow the loss of physiological function or increase life expectancy. Careful 'longitudinal' experiments might answer both problems, but such investigations would be expensive and time-consuming. The experimenter would find it necessary to recruit a large population of older people and divide them randomly into two groups; one group would live a life of ease and inactivity, while the second would report for regular sessions of controlled exercise. At intervals of perhaps one or two years tests of physiological function such as the measurement of maximum oxygen intake would be carried out, and observations would continue until all of both groups were dead. Unfortunately, an investigator with the organizing ability, powers of mass persuasion, and patience needed for such an experiment has yet to be found; indeed, it is doubtful whether such a test is practicable in a free society.

6
Modifications of fitness

It is a matter of common experience that a period of prolonged bed rest is associated with substantial loss of fitness, and that a normal exercise tolerance is restored over several weeks of convalescence. However, until recently, there have been few quantitative studies of this phenomenon.

H.L. Taylor, Henschel, et al. (1949) confined a group of students to bed, and found that there was a 17% loss of maximum oxygen intake over a three-week period. Normal function was completely restored following 36 days of 'reconditioning.' Saltin et al. (1968) carried out a similar experiment, but persisted with training after the immediate period of convalescence was completed. Three sedentary subjects and two athletes showed a comparable (27%) loss of maximum oxygen intake during 20 days of bed rest; decreases of stroke volume during submaximal effort and maximum cardiac output were of similar magnitude. There was a 30% improvement of maximum oxygen intake in the first few weeks after getting out of bed, and the three sedentary subjects showed a further 33% gain over a total of 55 days of intensive conditioning. However, the two athletes did little more than restore their initial status despite continued training.

Immobilization following industrial injury can give rise to a similar picture. Fried and Shephard (1969) noted that many of the patients attending the Workmen's Compensation Board Hospital following leg injuries complained of weakness, fatigue, and dizziness. Two-thirds of the group had an aerobic power 5% or more below the anticipated figure for sedentary Torontonians, and skinfolds were 4 mm thicker than average. A four-week program of endurance training was sufficient to remove the excess fat and to increase aerobic power by 15%, without loss of lean tissue. In many instances, the subjects initially showed specific weakness of the immobilized muscles (Fried and Shephard, 1970). Appropriate isometric exercises increased limb strength by 13% over a four-week period, but there was only a 1% augmentation in muscle mass; the discrepancy between muscle force and size presumably reflects partly avoidance of pain through an initial voluntary limitation of force, and partly a development of skill with performance of the test task by an increased number of motor units. Davies and Sargeant (1974b) tested the two legs separately. Following injury, the aerobic power of the injured leg dropped by 26%, while the loss in the other leg was only 19%. These changes were proportional to the loss of leg volume. After rehabilitation, there were gains of aerobic power, 17% for the injured limb and 9% for the uninjured.

Further examples of detraining are provided by patients who have been hospitalized following elective surgery (Bassey and Fentem, 1974; Carswell, 1975) or a 'heart attack' (myocardial infarction). Our initial data for the latter group show an aerobic power about 70% of that anticipated for the sedentary population. Progress is quite slow during the initial few months of rehabilitation, but by the end of the first year there is typically a gain of some 20%. Younger patients without complications such as anginal pain or high blood pressure continue to improve, some to the point where they can complete a 42-km marathon in 3¼ to 3½ hours. At this stage, their maximum oxygen intake has increased to 110–115% of the age-related normal value (Kavanagh, Shephard, and Pandit, 1974; Kavanagh and Shephard, 1976a).

The physiological basis of the changes in endurance fitness with bed rest is not yet fully resolved. There is probably a loss of venous tone, so that an undue proportion of the total blood volume pools in the leg veins when the patient stands. The same phenomenon has attracted attention as a hazard of weightlessness during space travel (Müller, 1963; P.C. Johnson, Leach, and Rambant, 1973; Rummel et al., 1973, 1975). Prolonged immobilization is associated with wasting of muscles, decalcification of bones, and (unless food intake is curtailed) the development of obesity. The combination of muscle weakness and loss of functional connections ('coding') in the brain can also cause a debilitating deterioration of balance (Haines, 1974).

Acute illnesses in general make an individual disinclined to undertake vigorous exercise. Furthermore, in some diseases such as influenza, involvement of the heart muscle can make such activity dangerous. If effort is enforced, the ability to work for a few minutes may prove to be unchanged. However, this is not true if the disease process is affecting a link in the oxygen transport chain, as in pneumonia (where pulmonary gas exchange is impaired) or malaria (where there is an acute reduction of haemoglobin level [Henschel et al., 1950]). If the required activity is more prolonged, performance is impaired by most acute illnesses. Loss of blood volume due to sweating, impaired heat regulation, and a reduction of food stores secondary to a poor appetite all contribute to the reduced exercise tolerance.

Chronic illness also affects performance by attacking one or more links in the chain of oxygen conductances. Slight radiographic evidence of past tuberculosis has little effect on oxygen transport (Rode and Shephard, 1971a, 1973a; Shephard, 1974c, 1976e), but more advanced tuberculous disease and various other respiratory conditions such as chronic bronchitis and emphysema (Mertens et al., 1976; Shephard, 1976f), paralysis of the respiratory muscles, and diseases of the rib cage can all reduce ventilatory function to the point where this becomes the most important factor limiting oxygen intake. In some forms of asthma, exercise may actually contribute to a temporary impairment of ventilation ('exercise bronchospasm' [Fisher et al., 1970; Fitch and Morton, 1971; Lefcoe et al., 1971; S.D. Anderson et al., 1972]). Other respiratory diseases – sarcoidosis and many of the fungal infections of the lung, for instance – act mainly at the alveolar level (Dickie and Rankin, 1960; Bates, 1962; Holmgren and Svanberg, 1966; D.C. Morgan et al., 1975). In such pathologies, it may be that oxygen uptake is restricted by a mismatching of ventilation and blood flow in the finer structures of the lung rather than by a true impairment of diffusion across the lung membrane (Read and Williams, 1959). But irrespective of mechanisms, conditions of this type seriously restrict oxygen transport. Chronic cardiac disease is another major cause of reduced effort tolerance, as might be expected from the dominant role of the heart in the normal transport of oxygen. In some congenital anomalies, such as mild narrowing of the pulmonary valve, small ventricular septal defects, and surgically corrected tetralogies of Fallot, the disability may have a iatrogenic component, and with appropriate encouragement from a physician the range of possible activities can be greatly extended (Cumming, 1976; Mocellin and Bastanier, 1976). Most forms of cardiac disease are marked by a low cardiac output, and thus a low maximum oxygen intake and a poor effort tolerance. Specific additional symptoms are noted with disease of the heart valves. Regurgitation of blood at the mitral orifice leads to an increase of pressure in the left atrium and pulmonary veins, a breathlessness that is disproportionate to the intensity of effort, and a propensity for dangerous water-logging of the lungs (pulmonary oedema). Leakage at the tricuspid valve gives rise to an increase of pressure in the right atrium and systemic veins (often visible at the root of the neck when the patient is recumbent), tenderness along the lower edge of the chest wall due to enlargement of the liver, and progressive water-logging of the lower part of the body (peripheral oedema). Narrowing of any of the valves (stenosis) prevents the normal increase of cardiac output during exercise; the systemic blood pressure fails to rise in the expected manner, and a poor blood flow to the skin is reflected in a blueness of the extremities (peripheral cyanosis). Stenosis of the aortic valve may also lead to acute pulmonary oedema; failure of the blood pressure to rise or a sudden drop in blood pressure during an exercise test is an urgent indication to halt the procedure.

Many other chronic ailments can affect performance. Often there is an associated anaemia, and as we have seen this can be almost as effective as a poor cardiac output in reducing maximum oxygen intake. Even the apparently harmless condition of varicose veins can lead to a poor effort tolerance by permitting an excessive pooling of blood in the enlarged venous reservoirs of the legs (Carlsten, 1972).

The average sedentary subject who is free of overt disease can still improve his maximum oxygen intake through participation in a program of sustained endurance training. However, he is unlikely to make good more than a third of the discrepancy between himself and a superb athlete (Shephard, 1976e). Many training experiments have now been carried out (Pollock, 1973; Shephard, 1975e). Some have been based on voluntary participation in sports or gymnastics. A competitive atmosphere can then be arranged, and the motivation of the subjects is good, but it is difficult to ascertain the intensity, frequency, and duration of the exercise that is performed. In most of the more recent experiments, the laboratory bicycle or treadmill has been used for training. The 'dosage' of exercise is then better controlled, but something of the spontaneity of the voluntary program is lost.

Irrespective of procedure, the largest gain of maximum oxygen intake reported in the absence of preliminary bed rest seems about 20% (Shephard, 1965). In some cases, the improvement of maximum oxygen intake has been supplemented by a loss of fat, so that the increase of oxygen intake per unit of body weight (ml kg^{-1} min^{-1}) has been somewhat greater than 20%; however, in other experiments the fat has been replaced by lean tissue with little change of body weight. A few authors (for instance, Skinner et al., 1964) have reported the results of training experiments in terms of an augmented endurance for a specific heavy task such as uphill treadmill running. Changes in motivation and in tolerance of an oxygen debt then greatly influence a subject's score (Wright, Clarke, et al., 1976), and the increase of performance time may exceed the gain in oxygen intake by as much as an order of magnitude. Others have noted improvements of running speed (Mocellin and Wasmund, 1973); here factors of skill and pacing may contribute to observed scores. Many laboratories, not wishing to carry out maximal testing, have reported either the decrease in heart rate during performance of submaximal work, or the corresponding increase in predicted maximum oxygen intake. Again, the changes seen with training have sometimes exceeded 20%. However, interpretation of such data is complicated by the influence of learning and habituation on heart rate responses to submaximum exercise. Furthermore, there is evidence that some types of training have more effect on the performance of submaximum effort than on maximum working capacity, while for other more intensive patterns of training the reverse is true (Roskamm, 1967). Finally, when reviewing clinical data, it is necessary to look critically at reported gains in 'symptom-limited' maximum tests; lack of confidence on the part of the patient or the examining physician can cause a test to be halted prematurely at a first visit, leading to a large apparent gain of maximum oxygen intake when the same individual is retested after a brief period of training.

In addition to an increase in over-all maximum oxygen intake, training leads to development of individual links in the oxygen transport chain. The most noticeable response is an increase in the stroke volume of the heart, both at rest and in submaximum exercise (Simmons, 1969). The maximum output of the heart is increased in direct proportion to the gain of maximum oxygen intake (Ekblom et al., 1968; Simmons and Shephard, 1971b); if there is no rise of aerobic power because the program is not intense enough relative to the initial condition of the subjects, maximum cardiac output may also remain unaltered (Douglas and Becklake, 1968). Exploration of the basis for any increase of stroke volume has been limited to indirect procedures. Long-term training in the growing years increases the heart volume per kilogram of body weight (Cermak, 1973); however, more moderate stress (heart rate of 160 per minute for one hour daily) has no effect on the cardiac dimensions of 20–25 year old men (Roskamm, 1973). The mechanics of cardiac contraction have been studied by simultaneous recording of the carotid pulse wave, the phonocardiographic record of heart sounds, and the electrocardiogram. As training proceeds, the drive to the heart from the sympathetic nerve system diminishes both at rest and during exercise, and the isovolumetric phase of cardiac contraction is lengthened (Franks and Cureton, 1969; Wiley, 1971). Recent cardiac catheterization data (Roskamm, 1973) have confirmed the conclusions drawn by non-invasive techniques. At rest, indices of myocardial contractility such as the maximum rate of rise of intraventricular pressure are the same in sendentary and trained individuals, but in maximum effort both the heart rate and the rate of pressure rise decrease with training. Although stroke volume is increased, the relationship of stroke volume to heart size and the residual end-systolic blood volume of the heart are unchanged in the conditioned individual.

There is commonly (Saltin et al., 1969; Simmons and Shephard, 1971b; Roskamm, 1973) a widening of the maximum arterio-venous oxygen difference with training. This reflects a redistribution of blood flow away from the skin (Simmons and Shephard, 1971b) and the viscera (Rowell, 1974). During submaximum exercise the blood flow to the muscles may also be reduced (Treumann and Schroeder, 1968; Douglas and Becklake, 1968; Clausen et al., 1973), but in maximum effort muscle perfusion is increased (Rochelle et al., 1971; de Marées and Barbey, 1973).

Some authors have claimed that training induces a fall of resting blood pressure (Jokl et al., 1968), particularly in older subjects (Kilbom et al., 1969; de Vries, 1970) and those with hypertension (Choquette and Ferguson, 1973), but there are possibilities of artefacts from altered pulse-wave reflections and an improved fit of the measuring cuff. If there is an effect, it is small and of little practical significance (Ekblom et al., 1968; Frick et al., 1963; Tabakin et al., 1965).

Training usually augments the total blood volume, and there may be an increase in the haemoglobin content of unit volume of blood (although some forms of endurance training tend to cause anaemia, page 95). Some authors such as Holmgren et al. (1964) believe that working capacity is closely correlated with the total haemoglobin content of the body.

Many laboratories have found little effect of training upon respiratory variables such as vital capacity (Cureton, 1936), mean expiratory flow rate, and maximum voluntary ventilation (Cumming, 1971). Nevertheless, the maximum voluntary ventilation is larger in athletes than in non-athletes (Hollmann, 1966; 1972; Durusoy and Özgönül, 1971), and substantial coefficients of correlation can be established between vital capacity and performance measures such as times in a 5000-metre race, even if lung volumes are standardized for body weight (Ishiko, 1967). Especially large vital capacities are encountered in athletes using the thoracic musculature for their chosen sport (for example, rowers, paddlers, and swimmers); in such groups, both selection and specific training of the respiratory muscles (Delhez et al., 1967–68) seem contributing factors. The mechanical work of breathing at a given ventilation is unchanged by training, but there is some reduction in ventilation for a given oxygen consumption, so that the cost of breathing is effectively lower in a trained subject (Milic-Emili et al., 1962). This may be attributable in part to a reduction in sensitivity of the ventilatory chemoreceptors in the carotid body (Byrne-Quinn et al., 1971), and in part to a diminished production of lactate in near-maximal effort (Karlsson et al., 1972). The relationship of lung diffusing capacity to oxygen intake is unchanged by training, but since the maximum aerobic power is increased, a small increase in the maximum diffusing capacity may be presumed (Anderson and Shephard, 1968b).

At the tissue level, there are increases in the dimensions of individual muscle fibres, although such changes are less marked with endurance than with isometric training. Post-mortem examination shows a roughly parallel increase in the capillary bed of the muscles (Carrow et al., 1967; Tomanek, 1970; Hermansen and Wachtlová, 1971; Rakusan et al., 1971), so that, contrary to more optimistic predictions from early animal experiments (Vannotti and Magiday, 1934), the distance separating the typical mitrochondrion from its source of oxygen remains unchanged.

Changes in tissue enzyme concentrations have already been noted (page 99); their function is probably to facilitate the use of fat as a muscle fuel, thus sparing glycogen for bursts of anaerobic activity (Fitts et al., 1975). Some of the apparent gains of enzyme activity can also be attributed to methods of data expression. Thus concentrations are often stated per unit weight of 'muscle' (protein, fat, and connective tissue) rather than per unit weight of protein. Nevertheless, there is general agreement concerning an increase in the mitochondrial fraction of skeletal muscle (Kiesseling et al., 1973), with augmented activity of enzymes concerned in glycogen synthesis and breakdown (phosphorylase-a, synthetase I and D, glycogen branching and debranching enzymes [A.W. Taylor et al., 1974; A.W. Taylor, 1975]), glucose breakdown (phosphofructokinase), pyruvate oxidation (succinate dehydrogenase and cytochrome-c [Holloszy et al., 1971]), and the coupling of chemical energy to muscle proteins (mitochondrial ATP-ase activity [Holloszy et al., 1971]). Conversely, plaster immobilization of a limb leads to a diminution in the activity of key enzymes (Booth and Kelso, 1973). Possible mechanisms for the changes of enzyme activity include alterations in the proportions of 'inducer' and 'repressor' proteins and changes in regulatory and structural genes, all induced by muscle tension, and less inhibitory feedback because the products of the enzymic reactions are being consumed faster within the muscle fibres (Poortmans, 1975).

Training increases the myoglobin content of the muscle fibres (Holloszy et al., 1971) and their potential for glycogen storage (Saltin, 1974). It has been suggested that immobilization of a muscle leads to a progressive conversion of the aerobic white muscle fibres into anaerobic red fibres (Edgerton, 1975), with a potential for reversal of the process and even 'neuro-physiological doping' by an appropriate input of electrical stimuli to the motor nerves of the muscles concerned. However, other authors (Fitts et al., 1973; Holloszy, 1973) have found a rather equal development of the various muscle fibre types in animal training experiments.

Chemical changes are seen in bones and tendons, including an increased content of hydroxyproline and hexosamine (Kiiskinen and Heikkinen, 1975). Moderate training leads to a specific reinforcement of bone architecture in the exercised limbs, with a stimulation of bone growth in young subjects; more intense activity increases bone density but can have an inhibiting effect on growth (Booth and Gould, 1975). Other local effects of conditioning include a thickening of articular cartilages and an increase in the tensile strength of affected tendons (Tipton et al., 1975). Prolonged bed rest gives changes in the opposite sense. These are not averted by supine cycling, but can be checked by periodic weight-bearing.

With regard to mechanisms that regulate the development of fitness, Holmgren (1967c) has suggested that two types of training should be distinguished: 'regulatory' and 'structural.' The regulatory response is typified by the average pre-season training, where an improvement of function is sought in six weeks to three months. Over this period, the central blood volume is increased through an augmentation of tone in the leg veins. As with heat acclimatization, sweating is initiated at a progressively lower body temperature, and sweat production at a given percentage of aerobic power is increased. The skin temperature thus tends to be lower, and the same quantity of heat can be dissipated from the body with a smaller flow of blood to the skin. At the same time there is a shift from sympathetic to parasympathetic activity, both in the regulating centres of the hypothalamus (Raab and Krzywanek, 1966) and within the heart (increased local concentrations of acetylcholine and reduced levels of catecholamine [Herrlich et al., 1960; Tipton, 1965; de Schryver et al., 1969]).

The structural type of response is seen only with protracted training, measured in months and years rather than weeks. The weight of both the heart and the skeletal muscle may be increased, with parallel development of the capillary bed in these tissues. However, the likelihood of observing such a change is influenced by both age and the protein content of the diet. Oscai et al. (1971) found that male rats on an endurance exercise program gained weight more slowly than sedentary litter mates, and as an apparent consequence heart sizes were not increased relative to those for sedentary animals of equal weight.

Physical activity leads to changes in hormone secretion – an increased output of the growth hormone of the pituitary gland (L.H. Hartley, 1975; Shephard and Sidney, 1975) and of androgens (Lamb, 1975), with a decreased secretion of insulin (Vranic et al., 1975); all of these changes could influence protein formation. However, if they made a fundamental contribution to the structural changes seen in heart and skeletal muscle, one would anticipate that training would be more effective in children and adolescents than in older subjects (where growth had ceased and sexual functioning was waning). Certainly, the typical response to training is limited in the adult, but it is not noticeably less in elderly than in young adults; substantial gains of both maximum oxygen intake and performance have been obtained in middle-aged and elderly men and women when they have been persuaded to exercise with sufficient vigour and frequency (Skinner et al., 1964; Sidney, 1973, 1975). Furthermore, the responses of children to vigorous training are not exceptional (Shephard, 1976e). Current explanations of training phenomena thus look not at general hormonal effects, but rather at local influences of muscle tension upon protein synthesis within individual cells (Badeer, 1968; Schreiber et al., 1970, 1975; Hjalmarson and Isaksson, 1972; Zimmer et al., 1972). In the heart, the effect is seen as a sequel to 'after-load' (a rise of

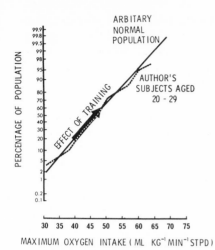

Figure 32 The distribution of maximum oxygen intake. A probit plot is used to compare the author's data for 58 men aged 20–29 years with an arbitrary population having a completely 'normal' distribution. The likely effect of training a subject with an initial oxygen intake of 39.4 ml kg^{-1} min^{-1} is indicated by the heavy arrow.

pressure) but not 'pre-load' (volume distension of the heart). During the first few hours of added after-loading, protein formation may diminish, but it becomes greater than normal within about a day. The increase in the force developed per unit cross-section of the fibres activates the nucleic acid DNA-RNA system, and this in turn stimulates protein synthesis. As the fibres increase in cross-section, they are able to develop a given pressure for a lesser force per cm^2; tension thus diminishes and the normal rate of protein synthesis is re-established.

GENETIC ENDOWMENT AND HABITUAL ACTIVITY

It is commonly held that heredity is more important than habitual activity in producing a person with a large maximum oxygen intake. P.O. Åstrand (1967a) writes: 'I am convinced that anyone interested in winning Olympic gold medals must select his or her parents very carefully.' His argument is based on the small effect of training relative to the much larger differences that separate most sedentary individuals from superb endurance athletes.

From Table 12, the coefficient of variation of maximum oxygen intake in Canadians is about 16%. A probit plot shows that individual subjects have aerobic powers distributed in a 'normal' pattern about the mean value for their age group (Figure 32). Thus, from the laws of statistics, 67% of subjects have a maximum oxygen intake within 16% of the mean value, 95% lie within 32% of the mean, and 99.9% within 48% of the mean. It follows that 67% of young men aged 20–29 years will have a maximum oxygen intake between 39.4 and 54.6 ml kg^{-1} min^{-1}. Let us now look sympathetically at a sedentary young man with a figure of 39.4 ml kg^{-1} min^{-1}. If he were submitted to rigorous training, he might increase his aerobic power by 20% (to about 47 ml kg^{-1} min^{-1}). However, despite valiant efforts, he would still be outclassed by 50% of the population, and would have no chance of reaching the values of 80–90 ml kg^{-1} min^{-1} found in some endurance athletes. At least two-thirds of the athletes' advantage is inherited (Shephard, 1976e).

More direct evidence regarding the influence of heredity is limited. Carter (1961) pointed out the association between the congenital stomach disorder of pyloric stenosis and a fine physique. Genetic factors are also known to contribute to high blood pressure (Cruz-Coke et al., 1973), diabetes, a high level of serum lipids, and a high risk of ischaemic heart disease (Gertler, 1967). Fortunately, many of these evils of parentage can be counteracted if the person at risk pays careful attention to diet and maintains a high level of habitual activity.

Specific information on genetic effects has traditionally been sought from comparisons of identical (monozygotic) and fraternal (dizygotic) twins. Gedda (1961) found that identical twins were more likely to have a similar interest in sports than were fraternal twins. Klissouras (1971) compared data for 15 pairs of monozygous and ten pairs of dizygous twins living in Montreal. His analysis apparently showed inheritance as accounting for 94% of the variance in maximum oxygen intake. However, the method of calculation that he used assumes the exposure of both groups of twins to a full potential range of environments, with adequate allowance for methodological error. The study can be faulted on both counts (Cotes, 1974; Shephard, 1976e), and in consequence it is likely that the genetic component of variance was overstated. The difficulty of interpreting twin data is illustrated by further experiments from Klissouras and his associates. Komi et al. (1973) reported that in most tests of physical performance variance was similar for monozygous and dizygous twins; however, the boys' scores on the Margaria test of anaerobic power, the patellar reflex time, and the reaction time appeared to be largely inherited. In 13-year-old boys, ten weeks of training led to a 12.5% gain of aerobic power, but supposedly untrained twins gained 16.0% over the same period (Klissouras and Weber, 1973). In contrast, trained 16-year-olds gained 20.8% and their untrained twins only 3.2%. Finally, a single well-trained 21-year-old twin had a 47.3% advantage of aerobic power, and a 61.0% advantage of maximum oxygen debt over his brother who had now adopted a relatively sedentary life-style (Klissouras, 1972). In summary, the various twin studies to date have indicated the genetic component of performance as ranging from almost zero to nearly 100%. The present need seems not for further experiments but rather for a more reliable method of analysing the data obtained from twin comparisons.

TYPES OF TRAINING REGIMEN

Several distinct patterns of athletic training have their own purpose and their particular advocates. These may be described briefly as follows:

1. *Continuous endurance training.* The subject exercises at a moderate and relatively steady intensity for quite long periods (ranging from 15 minutes to several hours, depending upon the enthusiasm of the trainee and the severity of the trainer).

2. *Brief interval training.* The subject undertakes short bursts of maximum anaerobic activity, interspersed with recovery periods of corresponding length when only light activity is allowed. For example, 200-metre sprints occupying 30 seconds may be alternated with 30-second periods of slow jogging.

3. *Prolonged interval training.* The pattern of exercise is as in 2, but the bursts of activity are prolonged to 2–3 minutes, with a corresponding extension of the recovery periods. The average subject thus alternates 600–800 metre runs with periods of slow jogging.

4. *Circuit training.* A typical circuit comprises ten varied gymnastic exercises – push-ups, running on the spot, and so on. The subject determines the maximum number of repetitions of each exercise that he can make. He is then required to move around the circuit three times. On each occasion, he performs 50% of his maximum number of repetitions at each of the ten stations. On subsequent days, he continues to make three complete circuits, but the number of repetitions is progressively increased (R.E. Morgan and Adamson, 1965).

5. *Other approaches.* We shall note shortly the role of individual and team sports, calisthenics, and the development of muscle strength and endurance through isotonic and isometric exercises.

In physiological terms, continuous training puts the heart and circulation under stress. Interval training also stimulates the heart, but there is the added factor that the oxygen debt is being taxed (R.H.T. Edwards, Ekelund, et al., 1973). With brief interval training, the alactate debt (page 56) is incurred, and some lactate is produced locally in the active muscles, but normal conditions are restored rapidly during recovery intervals (I. Åstrand, Åstrand, et al., 1960; Karlsson et al., 1967); brief interval work is particularly suited to improving the condition of patients who develop anginal pain during more sustained effort (Kavanagh and Shephard, 1975a). With more prolonged interval work, a maximum oxygen debt is developed, and lactate accumulates not only in the active muscles but also in the circulation as a whole. Aerobic power is developed more effectively by prolonged than by brief interval work (Knuttgen et al., 1973). Circuit training provides a substantial stimulus to the circulation, particularly if it is performed at speed, but it also exercises a wider range of muscles than continuous or interval training.

The effectiveness of the first four regimes has been compared in experiments on German army recruits. Hollmann et al. (1966) found that all procedures gave a 6–8% increase of heart volume (as measured from chest X-rays), with substantial improvements of maximum oxygen intake (16.1% for interval training, 15.3% for continuous training, and 13.2% for circuit training). A 9.1% gain of maximum oxygen intake was also registered by 'controls' who participated only in routine military sports. Circuit training, with a 12% gain of aerobic power, was the most effective procedure in terms of increasing muscle strength. Roskamm et al. (1966) found that the improvement in maximum working capacity following prolonged interval training was slightly superior to that seen following both short interval and continuous training. On the other hand, tolerance for prolonged activity developed best in those receiving continuous training.

We may conclude that long interval training has a place in the preparation of some classes of athlete, particularly contestants in short and medium distance events who must learn to tolerate a large oxygen debt. On the other hand, the oxygen debt mechanism of the average citizen is rarely stressed maximally. He must learn to tolerate fairly prolonged activity, and his training needs are served better (and with greater safety) by more moderate continuous exercise. Perhaps for this reason, although there have been some studies of optimum patterns of interval work (Knuttgen et al., 1973; E.L. Fox, Bartels, et al., 1975), most authors have concentrated on defining optimum patterns of continuous training.

OPTIMUM PATTERN OF CONTINUOUS TRAINING

There are good reasons for seeking information on the minimum dose of exercise needed to develop and maintain cardio-respiratory health. Perhaps the most obvious is the laziness of many enquirers! However, the time of those who are not lazy may be limited, and excessive exercise has possible dangers for the middle-aged, particularly if it is performed irregularly in those with latent or manifest disease of the coronary vessels. Finally, the athlete may pose the question of overtraining. Often, this is a psychological rather than a physiological problem, a reaction to diminishing returns as peak condition is approached. However, if it can be avoided by appropriate regulation of the extent of training, this would seem advisable.

Certain inferences can be drawn from general physiological principles. Training is but one example of the more general process of stress adaptation. Adolph (1964) suggested that most processes of adaptation could be characterized by a threshold of stimulation, a maximum potential rate of adaptation, and a maximum final response. Both the rate of adaptation and the total amount of response depended upon the intensity of stimulation. Assuming that his generalizations are applicable to the training process, we would not expect to find any training until a certain minimum of activity was attained. We would also anticipate that the extent of the training response would depend more upon the intensity of effort above this threshold than upon the frequency and duration of activity.

Karvonen et al. (1957) were the first to provide evidence of a training threshold. They exercised medical students on a treadmill for half an hour, four or five times per week. In some of the students the speed of running was adjusted to give a terminal pulse rate of 135 min^{-1}, and in these subjects no training occurred. In the remainder, the terminal pulse rate was 160-180 min^{-1}; training in this group was such that it was necessary to increase the speed of the treadmill by 25-30% over a four-week period in order to maintain the chosen pulse rate. Subsequent authors have interpreted these experiments with regrettable carelessness, assuming that the findings were applicable to subjects of all ages, regardless of physical condition. The critical pulse rate has also been stated as 60% of maximum oxygen intake (135 min^{-1}), 60% of the difference between resting and maximum pulse rate (145 min^{-1}) and even 60% of maximum heart rate (117 min^{-1})!

Some investigators have found a lower training threshold than that suggested by the data of Karvonen et al. (1957), perhaps because they have used more sedentary subjects. Durnin et al. (1960) found substantial improvement in the endurance fitness of soldiers who were required to march 10 to 30 km per day. Presumably, their speed of marching was no more than 4.8-5.6 km h^{-1}, and it is unlikely that their pulse rate exceeded 120 min^{-1}. Bouchard et al. (1966) produced some training by having their subjects carry out no more than ten minutes of cycling per day at a heart rate of 130 min^{-1}.

At high work loads, quite short periods of activity seem adequate to induce training. Thus I found that when soldiers were exercised at a load of 140 watts (about 75-80% of their aerobic power), the improvements in response to the first of three 15-minute rides per day actually exceeded those seen during the first of three 30-minute rides per day. On the other hand, Petersen (1962) reported that when the total work performed was held constant, greater training resulted from 30 minutes of cycling than from shorter rides.

A series of treadmill experiments where subjects were allocated to training regimes differing in intensity, frequency, and duration of exercise (Shephard, 1968f) emphasized that the improvement in performance depended mainly upon the intensity of effort and the initial fitness of the subjects (Figure 33); with the number of individuals tested, the components of residual variance due to frequency and duration of effort were statistically insignificant. There have been

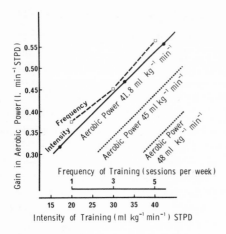

Figure 33 The influence of intensity of exercise (expressed as oxygen consumption, ml kg^{-1} min^{-1} STPD), initial fitness (expressed as aerobic power, ml kg^{-1} min^{-1} STPD), and frequency of exercise upon the gain in aerobic power during training (from Shephard, 1968f).

many repetitions of these experiments, almost all with young university men (Pollock, 1973; Shephard, 1975e). Reports have claimed an effect of intensity (Faria, 1970), of intensity but not initial fitness (Gledhill and Eynon, 1972), of fitness and intensity (Sharkey and Holleman, 1967) with the latter variable insignificant after equating work loads (Sharkey, 1970), of intensity despite equation of initial fitness and total work performed (Wenger and MacNab, 1972), of intensity and duration (Davies and Knibbs, 1971), and in some (Pollock et al., 1969; Sidney et al., 1972) but not all (Bartels et al., 1968) investigations an effect of frequency of sessions, seen only if differing total amounts of work were performed (J.S. Hill et al., 1971). Conflicting results may reflect the use of small samples of subjects differing in initial fitness; in some samples, part of the apparent gain of aerobic power (ml kg^{-1} min^{-1}) has also reflected a reduction of obesity proportional to total caloric expenditure rather than the intensity of effort. The loadings have ranged from around 50% to almost 100% of aerobic power, and in some instances the lower intensities have barely exceeded the effort encountered in daily life. Often the period of study has been quite short; Durnin et al. (1960), for example, exercised their soldiers for only ten days. However, Pollock et al. (1969) claimed that the difference in response to two and four sessions of exercise did not emerge clearly until 20 weeks of activity had elapsed. 'Regulatory' adaptations may well be completed within ten days, but if 'dimensional' or structural changes are sought, observation must continue over months or even years of training.

Another source of confusion has been the training criterion. Although the majority of recent authors have used the maximum oxygen intake, several early reports studied changes in the endurance of just submaximal work, and others examined alterations of the heart rate during submaximal effort or the aerobic power predicted therefrom. Not surprisingly, these various approaches have yielded differing answers (Roskamm, 1967; Hill et al., 1971). The endurance time for near maximal effort is important to the athlete, but is of less concern to the average citizen; the scores obtained are influenced by motivation, habituation, muscle strength, lactate accumulation, and above all by changes in the margin between the required effort and the maximum oxygen intake. It is less clear why training responses should be observed in submaximum but not in maximum effort, and why three sessions per week should sometimes be more effective than five (Hill et al., 1971). Habituation to the test procedure could cause difficulty if training and testing are performed on the same equipment (Sharkey, 1970), but this problem is largely overcome by one or two practice sessions (Shephard, 1969b). It is possible that when unfit subjects perform five training sessions per week, they fail to recover completely before testing, and that because of persistent fatigue and/or dehydration the normal habituation to strenuous exercise is replaced by an increase of anxiety or arousal. Some of the changes in response to submaximum effort may also reflect locally induced changes in sympathetic drive (Clausen et al., 1970, 1971) such as a decrease in afferent impulses from well-trained limbs, a decrease in the cortical discharge to hypertrophied muscle fibres, and a lesser accumulation of anaerobic metabolites due to learning of the task, muscle hypertrophy, and the development of tissue enzyme systems.

Several recent authors (Sharkey and Holleman, 1967; Hill et al., 1971; Sidney et al., 1972; Wenger and MacNab, 1972) have had all of their subjects perform the same total amount of work while training. However, from the practical point of view, it seems more urgent to decide whether to spend 30 minutes on vigorous activity five times per week (I. Åstrand, 1967) or whether five minutes of jogging per day will suffice (Cooper, 1968). Current evidence suggests that the former is needed to train a subject who is already in moderate condition, but that the milder Cooper prescription can benefit a very sedentary individual.

Some investigators believe that children can be trained more readily than adults (Andrew et al., 1972; Ekblom, 1969a, 1971; Eriksson, 1972), particularly with respect to gains of organ size. However, a complicated dimensional analysis is needed to separate the effects of training and growth (Von Döbeln, 1966; Shephard, 1976e), and it is by no means clearly established that training increases the ultimate size of a growing child. In addition, differences of aerobic power between the child athlete and his average classmate are by no means remarkable; Cunningham and Eynon (1973), for example, found a maximum oxygen intake of only 56.6 ml kg^{-1} min^{-1} in male swimmers who were Ontario provincial-class champions. Finally, there is no evidence that training is particularly effective at the time of the pubertal growth spurt (Cumming et al., 1967; Klissouras and

Weber, 1973); indeed, many (Cumming et al., 1969; Seliger et al., 1973; Mocellin and Wasmund, 1973; Bar-Or and Zwiren, 1973; Kemper et al., 1974) but not all (Ekblom, 1971; Rutenfranz et al., 1973; Shephard, Lavallée, et al., 1976) authors have found that children benefit little from additional physical education classes.

If training were age-dependent, we might anticipate a lesser response in the elderly, but in practice subjects over the age of 60 years react surprisingly vigorously to a conditioning program (Reville, 1970; Sidney, 1975). Naturally, even a small absolute gain at this stage represents a large percentage improvement, and it may have considerable functional significance. One factor predisposing towards positive changes in the elderly is their poor initial condition. The hormone balance seems unlikely to favour rapid anabolism, and there is thus interest in the possibility of facilitating structural gains through an appropriate combination of a high protein diet and carefully graded doses of anabolic steroids (page 266). Zuhlke et al. (1966) have described the inhibition of dimensional changes by the use of a low-protein diet and treatment with actomyocin D or puromycin, and it is tempting to suppose we are on the threshold of discovering converse procedures that may enhance tissue protein synthesis during training.

There have been few formal studies of training in young (Yeager and Bryntson, 1970; Knibbs, 1971) or older female subjects (Kilbom, 1971a,b; Drinkwater, 1973). Typically, the aerobic power of the city-dwelling girl ceases to develop beyond about 13 years of age. However, this is partly a cultural phenomenon, and is less marked in the Eskimo girl who must work relatively hard during her adolescent years (Rode and Shephard, 1971a). The responses of the sedentary adult woman to a short-term training program seem much as in a man with comparable initial physical condition.

Many authors have shown a rapid reversal of training gains with cessation of conditioning (Fardy, 1969; Siegel et al., 1970; Kilbom, 1971a,b; Kendrick et al., 1971; M.H. Williams and Edwards, 1971; Drinkwater and Horvath, 1972). At least two and possibly three days per week of training seem necessary to maintain endurance fitness (Roskamm, 1967; Saltin et al., 1969), and if the chosen method of exercise is jogging, a total weekly mileage of as much as 8 miles may be required (Kendrick et al., 1971).

EXERCISE PRESCRIPTION FOR THE MIDDLE-AGED

The sedentary middle-aged male, in a fit of sudden remorse, commonly confronts his physician or physical education director with a request for an exercise program. The physical educator may have had some instruction in the principles underlying an exercise prescription, but unfortunately few medical schools provide even rudimentary tuition in this important area. There is thus a danger that the doctor will treat a request for exercise with more levity than a complaint calling for the administration of potent drugs. It is not unknown for 'more exercise' to be proposed in such vague terms that the patient is either stimulated to an excess of zeal or (perhaps more commonly) makes no alteration in his exercise habits.

A sudden return to an active life has potential hazards for the tendons and the cardiovascular system, as discussed in subsequent sections, while physical deterioration of the patient will continue unless the increase of activity is adequate. A nice judgment must thus be exercised in selecting both the initial intensity of training and the subsequent rate of progression for any given patient. Many patients need repeated stimulation and encouragement in order to attain their training objectives, but the highly competitive ('Type A') coronary-prone business man (Friedman and Rosenman, 1974) may have to be restrained from an attempt to undo ten years of indolence in two days! The main emphasis for the sedentary person should be on continuous isotonic exercise (for instance, fast walking progressing to brisk running). Patients should be taught to count their pulse by light carotid palpation (Banister and Taunton, 1971), and in 'post-coronary' patients it is often useful to describe the symptoms of anginal pain and ventricular extrasystoles. A safe training heart rate is defined by a preliminary progressive exercise test; the value chosen is age-related and is insufficient to cause frequent extrasystoles or marked depression of the ST segment of the electrocardiogram. In a patient seen immediately after hospitalization for a myocardial infarction, it may be necessary to commence with a pulse ceiling corresponding to 50% of aerobic power (about 120 beats per minute), but the hope will be to progress first to 60 and then 70% of aerobic power as this is shown to be safe by clinical observation of gymnasium performance and repetition of laboratory exercise tests (Shephard and Kavanagh, 1975b). A given daily session should include a progressive warm-up (light calisthenics and flexibility exercises, with a pulse rate of less than 110 per min), and a final five minutes of 'warmdown' such as slow walking. The main part of the exercise comprises fast walking and/or jogging. In addition to the pulse ceiling, the patient is given a target distance and time, for example two miles to be covered in 30 minutes. Appropriate speeds can be gauged from the predicted maximum oxygen intake of the patient and graphs relating the oxygen cost of walking and running to speed (for example, Figure 20).

If seen immediately after a period of bed rest, a patient may not have the strength to carry out 30 minutes of exercise at one session. It is thus desirable to split the daily prescription into two segments of perhaps 15 minutes each until a modicum of condition has been restored. Symptoms such as frequent extrasys-

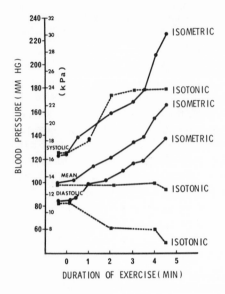

Figure 34 A comparison of the changes in systolic, mean, and diastolic arterial pressure during rhythmic (isotonic) and sustained (isometric) exercise. The isotonic exercise was treadmill walking for 3 minutes at a speed producing an oxygen consumption of 28.5 ml kg^{-1} min^{-1} and thereafter for 2 minutes at an oxygen consumption of 43.8 ml kg^{-1} min^{-1}. The isometric exercise was a hand grip sustained at 30% of the maximum voluntary contraction. (Based on data of Lind and McNicol, 1967)

toles or anginal pain and minor musculo-skeletal problems are an indication for a temporary slowing of the rate of progression. The exercise prescription may also need a transient adjustment for such things as a period of unusually hot weather and 'pressure' from domestic or business worries.

Given these simple principles, it is not difficult to recommend a suitable exercise program to a middle-aged patient. Individual preferences should be humoured as far as possible, since the availability of facilities and equipment and the enjoyment of training provide substantial motivation for its continuance. While the 'loner' likes the solitude of a jogging program, an extrovert often prefers to follow his program in a communal gymnasium such as the YMCA or a commercial 'fitness studio' (Massie and Shephard, 1971). The patient who visits a gymnasium should be cautioned that many forms of calisthenics do little to develop cardiorespiratory health (Seliger, 1967). He should also be warned that exercises with a substantial isometric component, such as the lifting of heavy weights, are undesirable in the middle-aged individual. If an isometric contraction is sustained, there is a large increase of systemic blood pressure (Lind and McNicol, 1967); this throws a heavy strain on the aging heart (Figure 34), since a rise of ventricular pressure has much more effect on the work-load of the heart than does an increase of muscle blood flow (Shephard, 1972b). Regular isometric training has the further disadvantage of causing a substantial increase in the bulk of specific muscles such as the biceps, without a parallel gain of cardiac power (Van Uytranck and Vrijens, 1971). An Atlas figure looks impressive on the beach, but the mass to be supported and moved during daily life is greatly increased; furthermore, the body gains no mechanical advantage from such 'top-heavy' development except on the rare occasions that great efforts are required of the arms. There is also a danger that the patient will conclude his training requirements have been satisfied once he has spent some time on 'muscle-building.' Despite our general condemnation of the narcissistic 'muscle cult,' it is reasonable to undertake exercises designed to strengthen the spinal and abdominal muscles; back injuries (J.R. Brown, 1972) and herniae are common causes of disability in middle age. The worker who uses his hands above his head (for example, a house-painter, I. Åstrand, Gahary, and Wahren, 1968) may also need arm exercises. As the arm muscles are strengthened, local blood flow is facilitated; this reduces the likelihood of an excessive rise of blood pressure and complications such as anginal pain when working.

Gymnasium time is best devoted to track work, the use of bicycles and rowing machines, and vigorous swimming if there is a pool. Feats of jumping, balance, and agility contribute little to the health of a middle-aged man, and may result in tendon and bone injuries.

Some subjects find it more convenient to carry out the well-documented 5BX and 10BX programs (Royal Canadian Air Force, 1962) in their homes. These exercises contain a substantial element of running, and would thus be expected to improve endurance. However, the gains of aerobic power demonstrated by formal tests have sometimes been disappointing (Malhotra et al., 1973). If unsupervised, the subjects may become bored and fail to persist with their exercises; indeed, the tedium of the required daily routine is one important criticism of the 5BX system. In some patients more serious problems have arisen from exacerbation of back injuries. Twisting exercises should be recommended with discretion for any middle-aged patient who has a history of back pain.

Many patients prefer the less regimented approach of participation in games and sports. These activities provide pleasant relaxation, but unfortunately the stimulus to the cardio-respiratory system is often inadequate. The energy cost of various common pastimes is given in Table 22. An expenditure of 33 kJ min^{-1} (8 kcal min^{-1}) produces a pulse rate of about 130 min^{-1} in a sedentary young man. The popular sports of the suburbs – golf, bowling, sailing, leisurely horse-riding, hunting, archery, and gentle walking often give a heart rate of no more than 100 beats per minute. If the speed of walking is increased to 7-8 km h^{-1}, a heart rate of at least 120-130 min^{-1} is achieved, and very rapid walking provides an effective initial procedure for the training of elderly subjects (Sidney, 1973). However, few people walk faster than 5 km h^{-1}, and for many 3-4 km h^{-1} is a more normal pace. Other popular weekend activities such as swimming and downhill skiing have quite a high potential metabolic cost; however, when pur-

TABLE 22

The reported gross energy cost of participation in various sports (Durnin and Passmore, 1967). Most figures are for small numbers of male subjects, and do not take account of rest pauses

Light activity

	kcal min^{-1}	kJ min^{-1}
Archery	3.2-5.7	13.4-23.8
Billiards	2.7	11.3
Bowls	4.1	17.1
Cricket	5.0-8.0	20.9-33.4
Golf	4.7	19.6
Table tennis	3.6-5.2	15.0-21.7
Volleyball	3.5	14.6

Moderate activity

	kcal min^{-1}	kJ min^{-1}
Badminton	6.3	26.3
Canoeing	3.0-7.0	12.5-29.3
Cycling	4-20	16.7-83.6
Dancing	4-8	16.7-33.4
Gardening	3-5	12.5-20.9
Gymnastics	2.5-12.0	10.5-50.2
Field hockey	8.7	36.4
Horse riding	3-10	12.5-41.8
Cross-country skiing	9.9-18.6	41.4-77.7
Downhill skiing	Up to 10	31.8
Swimming	5-15	20.9-62.7
Tennis	5.7-8.5	23.8-35.5

Heavy activity

	kcal min^{-1}	kJ min^{-1}
Athletics	Up to 20	83.6
Basketball	9.0	37.6
Boxing	9.0-14.4	37.6-60.2
Climbing	7.0-10.0	29.3-41.8
Cross-country running	10-11	41.8-46.0
English football	5-12	20.9-50.2
Rowing	4.1-11.2	17.1-46.8
Squash-rackets	10.1-18.2	42.2-76.1

sued as recreations, the speed of movement is slow and the training effect is often slight. The individual concerned spends much of his time changing, talking, and watching other participants. These pitfalls can be avoided in the competitive racquet sports, particularly if the pace is set by a fitter or a more experienced opponent.

One problem that arises when pursuing assorted forms of recreation is to equate the diverse activities and ensure that an adequate 'dose' of training is received each week. Cooper (1968) made a useful contribution to this question by proposing a simple 'points' scheme; this enabled the general public to make approximate comparisons of the training derived from such items as a game of tennis, a quarter-mile swim, and a brisk jog. Details of the scheme can be criticized from a scientific point of view (Massie et al., 1970). For example, some activities earn more poins than others for an equivalent energy expenditure. Furthermore, we lack the necessary information to make a precise comparison of the merits of brief intense and slower but more prolonged exercise. Nevertheless, Cooper has rendered a useful service to the lay reader in suggesting how training can be gauged and programs adapted to immediate local opportunities.

The merits of incorporating exercise into the daily routine deserve emphasis. A two-mile walk to the subway station allows little scope for procrastination, and with suitable timing of the departure from home, there is a strong motivation to walk at 8 rather than 4 km h^{-1}! If a briefcase containing 10–15 kg of books is carried alternately in the left and right hands, useful stimulation is also applied to the muscles in the upper half of the body. Staircases are another useful source of activity, immediately available to every apartment dweller and office-worker. A sedentary executive who climbs a flight of 20–23 cm steps at a rate of 30–40 steps per minute is achieving about 50% of his maximum oxygen intake. A useful, if brief 'work-out' is thus obtained whenever he climbs three floors (30–40 steps). As the ankle and leg muscles become stronger, the speed of ascent can be increased, and the stairs taken two at a time. The three floors should then be climbed in 30 seconds or less, and the executive has progressed to the brief form of interval training. The average demands of office life call for at least 10 journeys to other floors in the course of a day. The executive who uses the staircase is saved at least 10 minutes previously spent in waiting for elevators, in addition to gaining a source of healthy exercise. In many buildings, he will discover that he can outpace the elevator over journeys of 10–15 floors. A study by Fardy and Ilmarinen (1975) showed that aerobic power could be increased in as little as 12 weeks by the deliberate use of 25 or more flights of stairs per day. The London bus-conductors (page 222) climb about 60 flights per day (Morris, personal communication), and perhaps partly as a consequence of this experience less ischaemic heart disease than the drivers. It is disappointing that in many modern buildings the staircase is hard to find, unattractive, and ends in a fire-door to be opened 'only in an emergency.' The cause of fitness would be well served if the staircase were restored to the central place it occupied in Regency and Colonial buildings, while the elevator was banished to the tradesmen's entrance or some similar obscure corner.

The response to training should be assessed regularly, irrespective of the mode of exercise that is being followed. Gains of test scores are important to the motivation of the subject. Simple 'feedback' can be obtained from regular performance of the Canadian home fitness test (Bailey, Shephard, and Mirwald, 1976), although there are naturally advantages to personal contact with a physician or coach; an exercise counsellor can decide whether adequate exercise is being taken without the development of untoward symptoms, and can also advise on the next steps in a systematic program to develop fitness and improve general lifestyle. If the heart rate is 170 min^{-1} at the first assessment, but two weeks later it is 162 min^{-1} at the same work-load, the patient is convinced he is making progress, and is encouraged to continue with his efforts. On the other hand, if the heart rate remains 170 min^{-1}, it is likely that the exercise is not being pursued with sufficient vigour, and the subject may require further stimulation from his advisor.

SAFETY OF TRAINING REGIMES

The dangers of top-level competition are well recognized. Howell and Howell (1969) cited an early catastrophe involving world champion oarsmen from St John, N.B., and Newcastle-upon-Tyne, England; the race of 1871 had to be abandoned because James Renforth, the Tyne stroke, suffered a heart attack. Five years later, there was a similar disaster in the ten-mile foot race at Ogdenburg: 'Fleetwood ... burst a blood vessel at the end of the fifth mile, and Brown therefore had the field to himself.' The popular press still chronicle similar events occurring in recreational pursuits. A twenty-year-old student dies of a coronary attack while carrying out warm-up exercises on the horizontal bars in a university gymnasium. A busy housewife suffers a back injury while tobogganing, and is immobilized for three months. Such cases are recalled more readily than the countless thousands of successful graduates of training programs. They have a strongly negative influence on the motivation of the public. But are such fears warranted? How safe is exercise?

In terms of fatalities, the answer is moderately reassuring. Dogs have died of heart failure following prolonged treadmill exercise, but in man exercise is usually limited by psychological rather than physiological factors. Occasional deaths have occurred during football games in the southern part of the United States, but these have been due to heat stress rather than overexertion (Murphy and

Ashe, 1965; Buskirk, 1968; Goodman, 1968; Spickard, 1968; Shephard, 1976a,c). Nylon clothing looks pretty on the football field and is easily laundered, but it is also fatally impermeable to sweat. Fox (personal communication) commented that over a one-year period, eight deaths of men wearing jogging clothes were reported from Orange County, California; however, there was no means of determining whether this was a larger number than would have been anticipated by the chance that kills two or three of every thousand middle-aged men per year. Åstrand (personal communication) noted that the two major cross-country skiing events in Sweden have together attracted about 10,000 entrants per year for the last 50 years. Many of the participants are middle-aged, yet only two fatalities have been recorded, both in 1971. Vuori (1974) found reports of ten deaths during some 12 million man-hours of cross-country skiing in Finland. Between half and three-quarters of the Finnish villagers join in these events, and the calculated death rate is about four times that for a comparable population under resting conditions. It is further arguable that the acute bout of exercise has merely precipitated death in a vulnerable person who would have succumbed in the near future; viewed over a time frame of months or years, the exercise habit could have improved rather than worsened life expectancy for an average member of the population.

Jokl (1958) argued that if sudden death occurred during exercise in a temperate climate, post-mortem examination invariably revealed some abnormality of the heart or circulation. Hinckle et al. (1969) also suggested that if abnormalities of ventricular rhythm were provoked by ordinary physical activity, then there was usually underlying coronary arterial disease. This is probably true, but not particularly helpful, since some atherosclerosis can usually be found in the hearts of those dying as children or young adults (Jaffé and Manning, 1971; Enos et al., 1955). Jokl (1958) collected reports on 76 cases of sudden death during exercise; three main conditions were described: (a) narrowing or occlusion of the coronary vessels supplying the heart muscle (34 cases), (b) rupture of the heart or major artery (22 cases – aortic, 11; cerebral, 5; cardiac, 4; pulmonary vascular, 2), and (c) central cardiac failure (17 cases – chronic infection or degeneration of the heart muscle, 8 cases; acute infection, 5 cases; congenital or degenerative lesions of the heart valves, 4 cases).

Such figures substantiate the popular impression that the main hazard of overexertion is a coronary attack. It is thus of interest to question those recovering from an infarct as to their activity at the time of the acute episode. A study of 203 primary and 30 secondary attacks in patients attending an exercise-rehabilitation program (Shephard, 1974k) showed that 30 were engaged in various types of sport and a further 21 were doing heavy physical work around the home at the moment of infarction, both figures being larger proportions of the sample than would be anticipated for a sedentary group of Toronto business men. In contrast, there were significant deficits of attacks during sleep and during normal office work. Almost all types of activity were cited, including walking (13 episodes), running (8 episodes), snow-shovelling (9 episodes), and (with diminishing frequency) curling, tennis, baseball, hockey, soccer, basketball, squash, dancing, showering after calisthenics, and sexual intercourse. Often the activity was of unaccustomed severity, such as the portage of a canoe from a summer cottage, or the driving of two-inch screws into a concrete basement wall. Sometimes there was also associated emotional stress, such as participation in the final competition of a curling championship. Nevertheless, there seems little question that the immediate chances of a coronary attack were increased by a factor of six to twelve while the group were exercising. A formal exercise test in a doctor's office, with the stress of an anticipated report on medical condition, is even more hazardous. Several of the patients in our series had their attacks while attending a hospital or a doctor's office for treatment of an unrelated condition. McDonough and Bruce (1969) reported one attack of ventricular fibrillation for every 3000 maximum exercise tests, and one attack for every 15,000 submaximum tests; however, a high proportion of their patients had known or suspected heart disease. Rochmis and Blackburn (1971) noted 16 deaths in 170,000 exercise tests, with a further 40 patients admitted to hospital for severe chest pain or dysrhythmias; the majority of those affected were again suspected or proven cases of ischaemic heart disease, and in this study there was no difference in the incidence of cardiac emergencies between maximum and submaximum stress tests. Such statistics show the need for caution, but they do not imply that the coronary-prone individual should be prohibited from exercise. As discussed in Chapter 8, it is probable that the long-term chances of avoiding a coronary episode are reduced by a graded increase of activity. Nor are occasional 'coronary' deaths a firm argument for rigid supervision of mass testing and exercise programs. It can be calculated that if a population of five million middle-aged Canadians each carried out a six-minute exercise test once per year, it would be necessary to wait 16–33 years for there to be one fatality attributable to the test (Shephard, 1976a). Further, the cost for physician supervision of such tests would be about $12 billion per successful resuscitation! Plainly, the real need is for a wider distribution of primary care equipment to paramedical groups such as ambulance drivers and firemen (White et al., 1973), coupled with the development of simple, self-administered questionnaires that will distinguish the majority of individuals needing closer medical supervision.

It is probable that several types of pathology are associated with 'heart attacks.' In some patients there is complete blockage of a coronary vessel by a thrombus; such a lesion seems at least as likely to develop during sleep as during exercise or anger. In other instances, a detached thrombus has lodged at a more peripheral site, or there has been haemorrhage into a plaque that had previously partially obstructed a vessel (Burton, 1965); such lesions could well be precipitated by an increase of cardiac work, whether from emotion or physical activity. Sometimes, a typical 'coronary death' is reported, but at post-mortem examination none of the coronary vessels are completely blocked. It may then be suspected that an increase in the work of the heart has caused relative oxygen lack beyond a site of vessel narrowing. The irritability of the heart may also have been augmented by such factors as an increase in circulating adrenaline, an alteration in the mineral content of the heart muscle (T.W. Anderson, 1973), or an acute infection (viral myocarditis). Ventricular fibrillation is triggered by the combination of oxygen lack and other stimulants, and a continuous writhing contraction of the heart muscle makes normal function of the cardiac pump impossible. Unconsciousness develops rapidly, and unless fibrillation is checked within about four minutes, the patient dies. In such a situation, early first aid by a well-trained paramedical worker is inevitably more effective than delayed care from a physician or a hospital. The city of Seattle is currently conducting the interesting experiment of teaching techniques of cardiac resuscitation to all of its 80,000 high-school students.

Rupture of a major blood vessel only occurs when there is some pre-existing structural weakness, either congenital or infective in type. An aneurysmal swelling of the vessel may have been present for some time, but the final rupture is usually precipitated by a sustained rise of blood pressure. Vigorous isotonic exercise leads to some rise of systolic blood pressure, particularly if exercise is prolonged (Figure 34), but the increase is much larger and of more rapid onset when muscles undergo isometric contraction (Lind and McNicol, 1967). It is thus not surprising that there is a history of isometric work in about a third of the exercise fatalities collected by Jokl (1958). Prolonged isometric effort is undesirable at any age. If the strength of individual muscle groups is to be developed through a program of isometric training, then the duration of individual contractions should be short (less than 10 seconds), and the intervening rest pauses should be long enough (more than 30 seconds) to permit repayment of the accumulated oxygen debt.

Heart failure occurs when the venous input to the heart exceeds the output for more than a few beats. A momentary increase of ventricular filling usually leads to an increase in the output of the heart, but further filling soon brings the heart to the point where the muscle is overstretched and cannot contract efficiently. Cardiac output then decreases and failure develops rapidly. There is no fundamental reason why a normal heart could not fail during sustained maximum exercise. Indeed, as already noted, some varieties of dogs have been run to their death. However, other factors such as breathlessness, pain or weakness in the limbs, and even loss of the vertical posture usually cause a man to abandon exercise before this point is reached. Thus, heart failure does not occur unless there is some predisposing factor such as narrowing or leakage at one of the heart valves, or disease of the heart muscle. A particularly ominous sign, and a warning to stop exercise urgently, is a sudden fall in the systemic blood pressure.

The ideal arrangement would be for everyone to receive a full medical examination prior to entering a training program. This should detect most potentially fatal abnormalities of the cardiovascular system, with the exception of congenital weakness of the arteries at the base of the brain and certain forms of degeneration of the heart muscle. A full examination should include electrocardiograms taken at rest and during graded intensities of exercise and a chest radiograph; unfortunately, this makes the procedure rather expensive to consider within the framework of mass participation in exercise and the universal pre-paid delivery of health care. Many features of a normal clinical examination are helpful in identifying the 'coronary prone' individual. He is tense, ambitious, and aggressive in his attempts to climb the social scale, and has an urgent sense of the passage of time. There is often a family history of sudden death. The individual may be overweight, he smokes an excessive number of cigarettes, and has little time for exercise. The systemic blood pressure is high. Biochemical investigations show a poor glucose tolerance, high serum cholesterol and triglyceride readings, and sometimes a high serum uric acid level. The exercise electrocardiogram typically shows a horizontal or downward-sloping ST segment, and there may be other abnormalities such as frequent multifocal ventricular extrasystoles and blockage of atrio-ventricular conduction during effort (Figure 25). Anuerysms of the great vessels, points of weakness where rupture may occur, should be visible on the chest radiograph. Doubtful cases should be referred for radiographic screening; the pulsatile nature of the swelling can then be clearly established. Diseases of the heart musculature and valves are indicated by a heart shadow that is large relative to working capacity, and by specific abnormalities of the resting electrocardiogram. Details of the latter are given in standard texts of cardiology, and will not be discussed here. Particular care must be taken in recommending sports to patients with single organs. While the present toll of eye injuries continues in hockey, a boy with but a single eye would be well advised to avoid this game. Similarly, a person with but a single kidney would do well to avoid violent contact sports.

With a few obvious exceptions, it is rarely necessary to restrict the planned activities of a patient. The physician must guard against a caution that would keep the majority of his patients from realizing their physical potential, while condemning a proportion to a life of unnecessary invalidism. Particular care is necessary in the evaluation of functional ('innocent') murmurs of the heart. These are found in as many as 75% of normal children (Olley, personal communication; Iliev and Velev, 1976). The majority disappear before adolescence, and it seems better to risk missing an occasional significant pathology than to create an enormous population of neurotics.

There are severe practical problems in finding funds and personnel for a preliminary medical examination of all potential exercise enthusiasts. Many investigators in the United States still think in terms of providing a clinical examination with stress electrocardiogram not only for cases with identifiable heart disease, but also for all other patients over the age of 35 who express an interest in exercise (Cooper, 1970; Erb, 1970; Kattus, 1972). A close look at economic realities has convinced Canadians this is an impractical solution (Cumming, 1973; Orban, 1972). The proposed alternative is a physical activity readiness questionnaire, to be completed by the individual who is contemplating entering a training program (Chisholm, personal communication). This advises telephone contact with a physician if a positive response is made to any one of four questions: (1) over the age of 65 and unaccustomed to vigorous exertion? (2) told previously of heart trouble, a high blood pressure, or a bone and joint problem made worse by exercise? (3) a history of fainting or severe dizziness? or (4) any good physical reason not to follow a program of vigorous activity? Assuming all four answers are negative, and the individual does not have a temporary minor illness such as a common cold, he is allowed to undertake the Canadian home fitness test, and on the results of this evaluation to commence a gently graded exercise program.

Surgical problems can arise from an increase of physical activity, and indeed death from injury is not unknown in sports involving body contact. About two-thirds of such fatalities are due to injuries of the head and neck, and many of the remainder reflect severe damage to abdominal organs, particularly the liver, kidney, and spleen. Whether caused by trauma or heart failure, deaths provide headline material for the mass media. Fortunately, such incidents are relatively uncommon. Lesser accidents are a more significant practical preventive problem. They occur with annoying frequency; they may cause considerable inconvenience and expense to participants in a sport or training program, and they have a powerful deterrent effect on those with a marginal interest in fitness. Thorndike (1942) found that over a nine-year period 32.8% of all participants in organized sport at Harvard University suffered injuries of sufficient severity to cause them to miss at least one day's practice or play; when relatively 'safe' sports such as swimming or rowing were excluded, the proportion was even higher. Assuming an average of four years in university, the injury per participant-year would be 8.2%. A study from Toronto (MacIntosh et al., 1972) found an almost identical figure of 8.4% per participant-year, with a big discrepancy between the hazards

TABLE 23

The relative safety of different sports, tabulated according to the
average number of days' play that elapse before an injury is sustained
(based on data of Thorndike [1942] and MacIntosh et al. [1972])

	Harvard University (days)	University of Toronto (days)
American football		
Fall season	42	51
Spring season	100	–
Association football	116	140
Field hockey	147	–
Ice hockey	–	190
Cross-country running	222	–
Squash	–	253
Baseball	486	–
Lacrosse	486	–
Rugby football	552	54
Track and field (winter season)	568	–
Basketball	765	107
Track and field (spring season)	917	–
Rowing	3344	7865
Swimming	5844	1399

of intramural sport (5.7%) and intercollegiate competition (50.9%). Individual
sports can be rated in terms of the number of days' play before an injury occurs
(Table 23). In the college setting, injuries are particularly frequent for American
football, wrestling, soccer, and field hockey. The influence of local ground conditions is reflected in the relative figures for American football during fall and
winter seasons, for track and field sports during winter and spring seasons, and
for basketball at Harvard and Toronto (ankle injuries occur rather frequently in
Toronto due to a cramped gymnasium). The adverse influence of severe competition is illustrated by the tenfold difference of rates between intramural and intercollegiate competition, and by local differences in the risks of swimming (a
Toronto specialty) and rowing (a Harvard emphasis). The injury can take many
forms (Table 24). At both Harvard and Toronto, the commonest problem was a
sprain or a strain (Table 24). However, the pattern of injury depends to some
extent upon the type of activity and the age of the participants. Among Edmonton school children, where the main emphasis was on gymnastics, fractures were
more common than tendon injuries at the elementary level of education, although

TABLE 24

The types of injury sustained by 12,429 participants in sports programs
at Harvard University (8.2% of participants injured per year) and 8020
participants at the University of Toronto (5.7% of intramural and 50.9%
of intercollegiate participants injured per year), based on data of Thorndike (1942) and MacIntosh et al. (1972)

Injury	Harvard (%)	Toronto (%)
Sprains	22.6	40.2
Strains	14.3	4.7
Simple contusions ('bruises')	8.8	} 23.8
Muscle contusions	21.3	
Fractures of bones	12.2	6.0
Dislocations of joints	–	3.5
Lacerations and abrasions	9.5	7.3
Concussion	–	1.9
Conditions involving infection or inflammation	11.3	4.4
Other injuries	–	8.2

TABLE 25

Proportions of fractures/dislocations and sprains/strains among injuries incurred
at different ages (based on data of Mendryk and Dickau [1968] for school children
in Edmonton, Alberta)

Student classification	Sprains/strains	Fractures/dislocations
Elementary school (age 6–11)	69/247 (27.9%)	73/247 (29.6%)
Junior high school (age 12–14)	251/584 (42.9%)	170/584 (29.1%)
Senior high school (age 15–18)	156/360 (43.3%)	79/360 (21.9%)

at high school sprains and strains were again the commonest types of injury
(Table 25; Mendryk and Dickau, 1968).

Many factors can contribute to an undue incidence of injuries, and all should
be considered in a thorough preventive program. The influence of adverse
weather conditions has already been noted; injuries are increased by play on
either frozen or wet and slippery grounds. Poor facilities such as a cramped
basketball court, an overcrowded swimming pool, worn artificial turf (Bowers
and Martin, 1975), or an excessively hard gymnasium floor (such as polyvinyl

tile laid on concrete [Yarr, 1968]) can have a similar disastrous effect. Lack of familiarity with the ground, track, or equipment, inadequate refereeing when a game becomes rough, and poor matching of the contestants in terms of ability and physique are other external factors that increase the chances of injury (Ryan, 1974). Failure to wear proper protective helmets, shoes, and other equipment is a common individual problem (Stoddard, 1974; Bowers and Martin, 1975; Boustingl et al., 1975). The point is accepted for contact sports, but is also true of seemingly more innocuous activities. Painful tendon injuries of the lower leg and ankle are caused by running and jumping in shoes that give inadequate lateral support or permit undue stretching of the calf muscles. Poorly designed protective equipment may itself cause injury to the wearer or an opponent (Stoddard, 1974). Other personal factors that increase the risk of an accident are lack of sleep, fatigue, anger, and attempts to rush the training process. Both old and recent injuries leave a sportsman more vulnerable, some regions such as the shoulder having a particularly high incidence of recurrent lesions (MacIntosh et al., 1972). A few subjects seem particularly accident-prone.

An initial medical examination can direct attention to the condition of joints, tendons, and ligaments likely to be stressed by the proposed regimen. Defects of posture and muscle balance can be noted, and corrective exercises prescribed where necessary (Klein and Allman, 1969). Joint mobility can be explored, and the presence of old injuries and arthritic conditions excluded. However, the single most important factor in any program of injury prevention is an appropriate regulation of the rate of training. Many hazards cannot be avoided, but if the subject is allowed time to develop strength and agility, he can overcome with safety and confidence situations that would result in certain injury for the noviarte.

7
Current activity patterns
and attitudes

In previous chapters it has been suggested that the best current criterion of endurance fitness is the direct measurement of maximum oxygen intake. However, it has also been pointed out that this criterion has limited practical value in assessing the immediate status of the individual, since the test result is influenced more by genetic background than by the state of training. There is thus an urgent need for a new and imaginative method of assessing personal fitness.

In view of the relationship between activity and fitness, one possible alternative approach is to measure activity patterns rather than any changes of physiological status that they may produce. There are several practical problems in implementing such a philosophy. Fitness represents the summated response to weeks if not months of activity. Activity patterns on one specific day may differ widely from the norm for the individual and it is difficult to make representative measurements without studying a subject very closely over a long period. The expense of the investigation can become prohibitive, and problems may also arise from invasions of personal privacy (Shephard, 1972b). Furthermore, the form of the relationship between activity and fitness has yet to be resolved. Do we want to know the average level of activity for a typical day, or are we interested in that period of the day during which activity exceeds a certain threshold? If we believe in a threshold, is this the same for all individuals, or does it vary with their initial level of fitness? Is it enough to measure a physiological response to activity (such as the increase of heart rate), or must the nature of the activity also be considered?

Despite these unanswered practical questions, the direct study of human activity holds substantial promise for the future. Not only may it yield the key to a new procedure for assessing fitness, but it also has important applications in the field of community health. If sociological and psychological studies are carried out in conjunction with observations of activity, much may be learned about current attitudes to physical exercise, and the 'hidden persuaders' can be armed with new techniques to manipulate human behaviour in the interests of an improved life-style.

METHODS OF MEASURING HUMAN ACTIVITY

A wide variety of methods for the measurement of human activity have been suggested at various times. Detailed reviews are available elsewhere (Edholm, 1966, 1970; Monod, 1967; Shephard, 1967b, 1968d, 1976e), but the usefulness and limitations of some of the more common procedures will now be considered.

Diary-keeping
Typically, the subject is required to keep a detailed diary of his activities. Note-keeping is facilitated by a sheet ruled in minutes and hours. Standard abbreviations are suggested for all common activities (S for sleeping, Si for sitting, St for standing, W for walking, and so on). The subject enters the appropriate abbreviation in his diary when he alters his activity, and then marks successive minutes with a line until he begins to do something else.

The success of this type of diary-keeping depends very much upon the enthusiasm and intelligence of the subject. The author once studied a group of elderly people for 12 weeks. At first, they were quite keen to co-operate, but after three or four weeks variations in the diary entries became almost non-existent. In this particular experiment, the subjects were encouraged by thrice-weekly visits from a physician. It is likely that the quality of the diary records would have deteriorated even faster without such reinforcement of their motivation.

A second problem in keeping a detailed prospective diary is that the process of annotation can alter habitual activity. Many people have a rather short 'attention span.' They work only 5 or 10 minutes at their appointed task before standing to talk, smoke, drink coffee, or otherwise waste time. However, a diary that will be inspected by even a 'neutral' observer acts as a powerful conscience. A lazy subject may also prefer to remain seated rather than make an extra entry in his notebook.

While a full 24-hour record is important when determining daily caloric expenditures, from the viewpoint of endurance training much simpler information may suffice. In our studies of post-coronary patients, we have found it quite practicable to issue subjects with weekly diary sheets (Figure 35) on which they record brief details of up to three vigorous activities per day. Others have used simple diaries quite successfully in large-scale community-type investigations of

Day	Main activities		Time actually active (min)	Points (Cooper system)
Sunday	(1) Skiing (downhill)		30	3
	(2) Jogging	1.6 km	12	2
	(3) –		–	–
Monday	(1) Walking	2.4 km	30	0
	(2) Jogging	1.6 km	12	2
	(3) –		–	–
Tuesday	(1) Walking	5.0 km	60	1½
	(2) Squash		10	1½
	(3) Jogging	1.6 km	12	2
Wednesday	(1) Squash		10	1½
	(2) Walking	1.6 km	20	0
	(3) –		–	–
Thursday	(1) Jogging	1.8 km	12	3
	(2) Skating		30	2
	(3) Walking	5.0 km	60	1½
Friday	(1) Jogging	1.7 km	12	3
	(2) Squash		10	1½
	(3) –		–	–
Saturday	(1) Golf		9 holes	1½
	(2) Walking	1.6 km	20 min	0
	(3) –		--	0
Total points per week				26

Figure 35 Example of a simplified weekly activity diary, used to regulate the personal training of 'post-coronary' patients (Kavanagh, Shephard, et al., 1970; Shephard, 1972b).

coronary arterial disease (for instance, the Framingham study [Kannel, 1967] and a study of English civil servants completed by Morris, Chave, et al., [1973]).

Observation
A technician can be trained to keep records similar to those proposed for personal diary-keeping. If the observer has a quiet and unobtrusive manner, activity

patterns are altered relatively little by his note-taking, and the accuracy of the data is greater than when a diary is kept by the subject himself.

The main objection to continuous observation is that the technician can often shadow only a single subject at any one time. The expense of studying a population is thus high. The method is best suited to groups such as army recruits (Edholm et al., 1970; O'Hara et al., 1976) or a ship's company (Southgate and Shirling, 1970), where men are living and working in close proximity to each other. A party of 20 or more soldiers often follow a stereotyped routine, and one technician can then observe several subjects simultaneously. Nevertheless, the method has also been applied successfully to the study of primitive tribespeople such as Eskimos hunting across the arctic tundra (Godin and Shephard, 1973a).

Retrospective questionnaires

An experienced observer may question subjects about their recent activities, or they may themselves complete a multiple-choice questionnaire (Montoye, 1971, 1975). Some questionnaires run to twenty or more pages. The quality of the information obtained then becomes highly suspect, particularly if the procedure is self-administered to entire populations covering a wide spectrum of intelligence and motivation. Subjects commonly exaggerate their activity when completing questionnaires. This is not necessarily a matter of bragging, or a wanton disregard of the truth; often it reflects the limitations of the questionnaire. The average tennis player, for example, may find no alternative but to classify the time occupied in changing, conversation, and searching for lost balls as 'playing tennis.'

The retrospective questionnaire is thus one of the less accurate methods of obtaining information on activity. More accurate information can sometimes be obtained if a bulky form is replaced by a simple classification of activity. In one group of soldiers (Shephard and McClure, 1965) answers to three leading questions ('do you play sport regularly?' 'do you undertake specific training for this sport?' and 'do you train more than once per week?') accounted for almost 40% of the variation in physiological responses to exercise. A sample of 1500 adults living in Saskatoon (Bailey, Shephard, et al., 1974) rated their physical activity on a five-point scale, ranging from 'none' or 'infrequent' through 'regular' (2-3 sessions per week of moderate activity such as jogging, tennis, squash, and swimming four lengths or more) to 'very frequent' (4-5 sessions of moderate activity per week, or regular training 3-5 times per week for a specific sport). Again, there was a clear gradation of aerobic power with activity category (Table 26).

Pedometers and accelerometers

A pedometer is a simple pendulum-like device fixed to the subject's belt. The mechanism is based on a pocket watch, and the intention is that each leg pace

TABLE 26

Relationship between habitual physical activity
and aerobic power. Data for sample of 1500 adults
living in Saskatoon (Bailey, Shephard, et al., 1974)

Activity level	Aerobic power $(ml \, kg^{-1} \, min^{-1} \, STPD)$	
	Men	Women
None or infrequent	29.9	26.1
Regular	33.3	28.7
Very frequent	39.3	31.2

will trigger a unit movement of the gear wheels connected to the clock face. The scale of most pedometers is calibrated in miles or kilometres rather than in paces, so that the individual's average pace length must be judged; the accuracy of the distance recorded depends on this estimate. The information yielded by a pedometer is plainly of limited value if a subject spends much of his day doing hard physical work with his hands rather than his legs. It might be thought more useful for the sedentary city-dweller whose most vigorous pursuit is walking. However, critical analysis has shown that the common designs of pedometer fail to respond to moderate walking, while if the subject runs faster than 10 km h^{-1} two or more paces are recorded for every step (Kemper and Verschuur, 1976). More accurate recordings of movement patterns might be obtained if accelerometers were strapped to various parts of the body and the resulting electrical signals were transmitted to a central receiver by a radio-telemetry system. However, the simplicity of the pedometer approach would then be lost, and a meaningful synthesis of extensive movement records would create practical problems of data reduction.

Oxygen uptake measurements
The most accurate method of assessing the intensity of physical activity is the direct measurement of the individual's oxygen uptake. There are two portable devices that can be used for this purpose: the Kofranyi-Michaelis respirometer (Müller and Franz, 1952; Kofranyi and Michaelis, 1949) and the Wolff IMP (Wolff, 1958). The Kofranyi-Michaelis respirometer (Figure 36) is a rugged mechanical gasmeter that can be strapped to the subject's back. The volume breathed is indicated directly in litres, and a reciprocating pump diverts a known fraction (0.3 or 0.6%) of the expired volume into a neoprene bag for subsequent gas analysis. The apparatus works well for all normal activities, although it is a

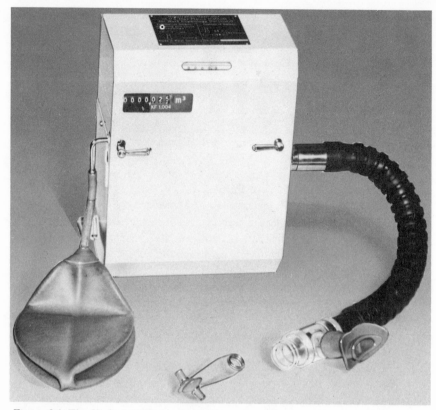

Figure 36 The Kofranyi-Michaelis respirometer. The apparatus is strapped on the subject's back. A counter records the respiratory minute volume, and a small percentage of the expired gas volume (0.3 or 0.6%) is collected in a rubber bag for subsequent chemical analysis.

little cumbersome for wear during sport, and its capacity is exceeded by the ventilatory volumes of maximum effort. Little maintenance is necessary other than periodic calibration against a suitable pump; in our hands, the calibration factor is remarkably stable, providing the apparatus is not badly mistreated. The main disadvantages are that (i) the activity of the subject is somewhat restricted by the mouthpiece, noseclip, and respirometer, (ii) skilled technicians are needed to determine the oxygen and carbon dioxide content of the gas samples, and (iii) individual observations cover a fixed time-span of a few minutes. Neither very brief nor very prolonged activities can be examined, and on this account the respirometer is often used in conjunction with a diary technique.

The Wolff IMP is an electrical form of gasmeter. A sliding contact is driven along a potentiometer by each expiration; an electrical signal is produced thereby, and this drives a small motor and counting unit. The system is rather complicated for field use, and it requires more frequent and more careful maintenance than the Kofranyi-Michaelis respirometer. The calibration of the IMP changes quite quickly, and if the subject takes a deep breath it is possible for the contact to jam at one end of the potentiometer. A further objection to the usual commercial form of the Wolff apparatus is that the expired gas is collected by an inadequate facemask; this was originally designed to supply oxygen to sedentary aviators, and it was rejected even for this purpose some years ago. The bulk, weight, and airflow characteristics of the IMP are similar to those of the Kofranyi-Michaelis apparatus; however, a modular design allows the individual components of the electrical integrator to be distributed along a waist band if desired. Another advantage that can be claimed for Wolff's machine is the aspiration of a smaller gas sample. Brief activities are studied less readily, but it becomes possible to follow steady activities over periods of up to an hour.

Indices of oxygen uptake
In view of the practical problems inherent in large-scale measurements of oxygen uptake, many investigators with an interest in human activity have sought to predict oxygen uptake from simpler and more readily recorded physiological indices such as heart rate, ventilation rate, and deep body temperature.

The heart rate may be recorded using a radio-telemeter and receiver. This approach is particularly appropriate in the study of sports, since most telemeters have a range of no more than a few hundred yards. Alternatively, the electrocardiograph signal may be stored on a small tape-recorder carried by the subject (Holter, 1961), with subsequent play-back of tapes into a suitable counting and printing unit (Figure 37). Commercial recorders carry twelve-hour tapes, and minute-by-minute counts of heart rate can be obtained over this period. If the subjects are freely moving, the main practical difficulties are to maintain good electrode contact and constant tape speed. The machines operate well when new, but the bearings deteriorate rapidly with repeated vibration. A third heart-rate recording system, pioneered by Wolff (1966), uses the electrical impulse from the heart beat to carry out an electrochemical reaction. In the initial format, iodide solution was reduced to iodine, and in more recent models silver has been deposited on a gold electrode. A small recording cell is brought to a standard initial state, is worn for a specified time, and is then restored to its initial condition by passage of a measured electrical current. The average number of heart beats during use can be deduced from the quantity of current needed to restore the initial state (Baker et al., 1967). The Wolff system is relatively cheap, and easily

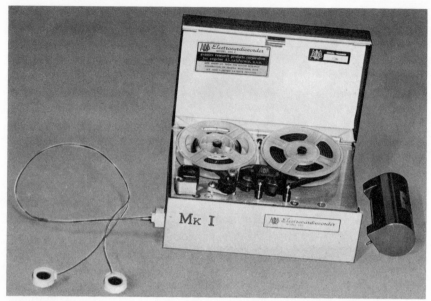

Figure 37 Portable tape-recorder used in obtaining 12-hour records of patient's heart rate.

portable, but in practice the results have been disappointing, owing to problems in determining whether the count has been increased or diminished by electrode artefacts. Edholm et al. (1973) were reduced to deciding whether results were trustworthy on the basis that the night heart rate fell within the range 40-90 beats per minute, and the daytime rate lay between 55 and 110 min^{-1}; on this criterion, only about three-quarters of their measurements were acceptable. Sidney (1975) carried out simultaneous measurements by tape-recorder and electrochemical integrator, and he also found large disparities between the two sets of data in many subjects. The electrochemical device may yet be rendered functional by using a series of integraters, with categorization of the cumulative heart rates. If individual cells only accepted data within certain ranges, it should be possible to direct most of the artefactual signals to units recording rates of less than 50 min^{-1} and more than 200 min^{-1}. Subjects with high readings in either of these units could then be eliminated from data analyses. A fourth possible method of counting the pulse rate is to apply a photo-cell to the ear lobe. The change of optical density with each pulse wave drives a counting device (Müller and Himmelmann, 1957). This technique has been used in some industrial studies, but is not particularly suitable for vigorous activity since double counts and other false signals can be generated by movement of the earpiece. Wrist-watch type counters have been used occasionally to accumulate signals derived from the electrocardiogram (Glagov et al., 1970; Masironi, 1971, 1974); such devices are mechanically sound, but suffer from all the problems of hidden artefacts discussed above.

The volume of gas respired per minute can be measured by the Kofranyi-Michaelis respirometer or the Wolff IMP. As when these machines are used to measure oxygen consumption, it is necessary for an observer to travel with the subjects, recording the counter readings at fixed intervals. However, the number of measurements is no longer restricted by the need to collect and analyse gas samples. Telemetry of the respiratory signal is usually limited to transmission of the breathing rate. This provides an uncertain indication of oxygen consumption. Nevertheless, there is no fundamental reason why the volume output of the Wolff IMP should not be transmitted by radio-telemetry or stored on a small tape-recorder.

The heart rate and ventilation are used quite extensively as indices of human oxygen consumption under field conditions. With both approaches, the assumption is made that the chosen index is linearly related to oxygen consumption. This is true of the heart rate from about 50% of maximum oxygen consumption to near maximum effort. However, at the lower intensities of activity encountered in normal life, the increased oxygen needs of the tissues are met in part by an increase in the stroke volume of the heart and in part by a greater extraction of oxygen from the circulating blood, so that the increase of heart rate for a given increase of work load is relatively less. The influence of work on heart rate also depends on the form of activity. Leg work produces a smaller increase of heart rate than a corresponding amount of arm work, particularly if the subject is standing (Asmussen and Christensen, 1939; Bevegard et al., 1960) or using his arms above his head (I. Åstrand, 1971b). Isometric work leads to a much greater increase of heart rate than does rhythmic work (Lind and McNicol, 1967). A man carrying a suitcase will not have a much higher oxygen consumption than his friend who is walking beside him, but his pulse rate may be increased from the normal pedestrian value of 105 beats min^{-1} to 150 beats min^{-1}. The relationship between heart rate and oxygen consumption also varies somewhat with age and sex, and it is distorted by anxiety, high environmental temperatures, recent meals, exhaustion, and many other factors. Ventilation is linearly related to oxygen consumption at low work loads, but it also is subject to various disturbing influences. It is more closely linked to carbon dioxide output than to oxygen intake, and at higher intensities of effort lactic acid formation leads to the washing out of carbon dioxide from the body, with a disproportionate increase of ventilation.

Under favourable conditions, the error of individual predictions of oxygen consumption using either heart rate or ventilation measurements is about 10% (Shephard, 1968d). This is adequate to estimate activity levels in a population, but is rather marginal when following the behaviour of individual subjects.

Other physiological indices of activity include measurements of deep body temperature and the rate of excretion of the breakdown products of adrenaline and noradrenaline (the catecholamines). As yet, such techniques are in the developmental stage.

Studies of food intake

Because of difficulties in obtaining accurate indices of energy expenditure, some authors have approached the problem from the opposite standpoint, measuring the intake of energy in the form of food. Over short periods, there are substantial differences between energy expenditure and intake of food, but the two estimates usually show substantial agreement over a week or more (Durnin and Passmore, 1967; O'Hara et al., 1976). The main disadvantage of the dietary approach is that it can give only an average activity figure for a long period, covering both work and recreation; unfortunately, the shorter periods of more intense activity are more important in the context of endurance fitness, and perhaps also in the prevention of ischaemic heart disease (Kavanagh, Shephard, et al., 1973; Morris, Chave, et al., 1973).

CURRENT LEVELS OF ACTIVITY

Most observers are convinced that the average adult city-dweller engages in very little physical activity, but until recently documentation of this belief has generally been limited to the use of questionnaires. Morris et al. (1973) found that 18.5% of a large sample of executive-class British civil servants aged 40–64 years were taking 15 or more minutes of vigorous activity (>7.5 kcal min^{-1}, 31.4 kJ min^{-1}) per day. The U.S. President's Council on Fitness (1973) distributed activity questionnaires to a random sample of 3875 adults. Some 45% of respondents, whether men or women, took no deliberate exercise. The two commonest forms of voluntary activity were walking and bicycle riding, both being slightly more prevalent in metropolitan than in non-metropolitan areas. Voluntary activity was also more common in the young, better educated, and more affluent segment of the American population. Some 22% of the sample claimed to be walking almost every day, often for 20 minutes or longer. An analogous study of Canadians living in Saskatoon (Bailey, Ross, et al. 1974) found 14% of the adult men and 9% of the women taking vigorous exercise (walking a mile or more, jogging, tennis, squash, or swimming four or more lengths) four or five times per

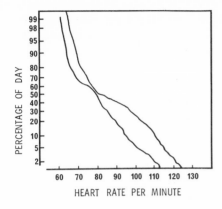

Figure 38 Twenty-four-hour heart-rate records of a sedentary subject living in Metropolitan Toronto. The record to the left is taken from a normal working day; that to the right is from a week-end period of more vigorous activity (Shephard, 1968b).

week. A further 26% of the men and 27% of the women were taking such exercise two or three times per week. By way of comparison, a survey of 2000 fourteen-year-old Swedish children (L-M. Engström, 1972) showed that the boys were devoting an average of 5 hours per week to active leisure pursuits such as soccer, ice-hockey, and swimming, while girls were spending 3½ hours per week on swimming, cycling, and walking. Only 5% of the boys and 10% of the girls in Sweden had no active leisure pursuits.

K.L. Andersen (1967b) collected tape-recordings of heart rates in a number of subjects. In lumberjacks, he found that the mean heart rate during a working day was 135 min^{-1}, and values of 150 min^{-1} were not uncommon. In manual industrial workers, occasional peaks of 130–150 min^{-1} were encountered, but the mean rate was only 110 min^{-1}, while in Oslo office workers, heart rates greater than 100 min^{-1} were uncommon. Similar findings have been reported from Toronto (Shephard, 1967c; Sidney, 1975). Young adults were studied for 24-hour periods both on weekdays and at the weekend, and the evidence of the tape-recordings was supplemented by a diary record. The only sources of activity for many individuals were occasional walks and stair climbing. Since many North Americans are rather careful to avoid both walking and stairs, it must be concluded that the level of activity of a modern young metropolitan man is often even lower than that shown in Figure 38. In 65-year-old subjects, we found average heart rates of 90 min^{-1} in the men and 80 min^{-1} in the women, with little difference between afternoon work and evening leisure. Other observers have noted similar findings. Boas and Goldschmidt (1932) quoted rates of 78 for young men and 84 for young women performing their daily work. Friedman et al. (1963) found figures of 86 for 'Type A' workers, and 85 for 'Type B,' their two groups separating aggressive, competitive individuals from those who were non-aggressive and easy going. Goldsmith and Hale (1971) reported readings of

TABLE 27

Daily energy expenditures of Scottish workers (Durnin and Passmore, 1967), Guatemalan farmers (Viteri et al., 1971), Jamaican farmers (G.J. Miller et al., 1972), Kurdish and Yemenite farmers (Edholm et al., 1973), !Kung bushmen (Lee, 1969), and Canadian Eskimos (Godin and Shephard, 1973a)

	kcal day^{-1}	kJ day^{-1}		kcal day^{-1}	kJ day^{-1}
Scotland			Jamaica		
Office staff	2520	10,600	Farmers	3250	13,600
Construction	3000	12,500	Israel		
Steelworkers	3280	13,700	Kurdish men	3080	12,900
Farmers	3550	14,800	women	2320	9,700
Coal miners	3660	15,300	Yemenite men	3025	12,600
Forestry	3670	15,300	women	2340	9,780
Guatemala			Africa		
Peasants	3873	16,200	!Kung bushmen	2140	8,950
Horsemen	4271	17,900	Canada		
Carpenters/masons	3530	14,800	Eskimo hunters	3670	15,300
Dairymen/herdsmen	3145	13,100	Employed villagers	3350	14,000
Foremen	2778	11,600	Married women	2400	10,000
			Single women	2300	9,610

86-94 for working policemen, the counts dropping to 83-85 during their leisure hours. Lastly, two studies of young housewives found heart rates of 95 and 108 min^{-1} during daytime activities (Brunner, 1969; I. Åstrand, 1971a).

Is it possible to exclude workers in 'heavy' industry from the general indictment of insufficient daily activity? Is it reasonable to assume that the occupational activity of 'heavy' workers allows them to maintain an adequate level of fitness? The heart rate recordings of Andersen (1967b) might suggest that this is the case, but the high recorded values could also reflect heat exposure or isometric work. Other information on the energy expenditures of heavy manual workers comes partly from wartime dietary surveys, and partly from the observations of industrial physicians and their assistants (Table 27). At first glance, a miner who burns 3660 kcal (15,300 kJ) of food per day seems much more active than the office worker who consumes 2500 kcal (10,500 kJ). But if the additional 1160 kcal (4850 kJ) is spread over a possible six hours at the coal face, it amounts to an average of only 3.2 kcal min^{-1} (13.4 kJ min^{-1}). Neglecting the complication of weekends (when the office worker may be as active as the miner), the 3.2 kcal may be added to the office-worker's consumption of 1.7 kcal min^{-1} (7.1 kJ min^{-1}) to yield a total consumption of 4.9 kcal min^{-1} (20.6 kJ min^{-1}), about a third of the maximum energy expenditure of a young man. The industrial physician rates an expenditure of 3.3-5.4 kcal min^{-1} (13.9-22.7 kJ min^{-1}) as 'moderate' work, 5.4-9.0 kcal min^{-1} (22.7-37.8 kJ min^{-1}) as 'heavy' work, and more than 9.0 kcal min^{-1} (37.8 kJ min^{-1}) as 'very heavy' work (J.R. Brown and Crowden, 1963). In a typical worker, the corresponding heart rates would be 90-105, 105-140, and over 140 min^{-1} respectively. Thus only 'very heavy' work does much to improve endurance fitness. In the highly automated factories of North America, it is rare to reach even the category of 'heavy' work. As factories are progressively modernized, the same is becoming true of other parts of the world. Thus, in a study from Australia, Allen (1966) was able to show little difference of endurance fitness between office workers and those employed in 'heavy' industry. It seems clear that the factory worker, like the clerk, must look to his leisure if he wishes to develop his fitness (Montoye, 1971).

In some primitive tribes, the active members of the community have substantial energy expenditures, particularly if account is taken of the small size of the individuals concerned (Table 27). However, even in the remote areas of the Canadian arctic and the Kalahari desert, the weekly averages tend to be reduced by the fact that vigorous effort is necessary on only two or three days per week. Lammert (1972) recorded the heart rates of Eskimos living on the west coast of Greenland. When on board their fishing launches, heart rates approximated normal resting levels, but when tracking seals in their kayaks, heart rates of 120-140 min^{-1} were recorded. Godin and Shephard (1973a) noted vigorous activities not only in the hunting Eskimos but also in employed villagers; readings on the latter group included garbage collection (6.5-7.8 kcal min^{-1}, 27.3-32.8 kJ min^{-1}), unloading of the supply ship and aircraft (5 kcal min^{-1}, 21 kJ min^{-1}), and ice delivery (5.0-5.3 kcal min^{-1}, 21-22.2 kJ min^{-1}). The women of the village also had fairly vigorous tasks such as preparing skins and carrying babies on their backs in the traditional amauti. In contrast, Ekblom and Gjessing (1968) showed that the Pascuans of semi-tropical Easter Island were relatively inactive. Two outdoor labourers had average working heart rates of 102 and 86 min^{-1} respectively, a fisherman averaged 90 beats min^{-1}, and three housewives 87, 91, and 101 beats min^{-1}.

The opinion is sometimes expressed that sexual activity still provides both the laziest of desert islanders and metropolitan men with at least one vigorous pursuit! Most scientists consider detailed physiological study of the sexual act an unwarranted invasion of personal privacy. However, occasional heart rate recordings have been obtained during intercourse (Boas and Goldschmidt, 1932; Masters and Johnson, 1966). Some of these studies have used prostitutes and mechanical masturbation, and it is uncertain how far such findings can be extrapolated to normal individuals in more normal circumstances; heart rates of 140-

150 min^{-1} have been seen during orgasm, with values of 120 min^{-1} for some 20 minutes before and after reaching a climax. These figures do not necessarily reflect high rates of energy expenditure, since the muscles involved are relatively small. The increase of heart rate is partly an emotional reaction, and partly a response to isometric work. The sexual act probably has little significance as a means of improving fitness. On the other hand, the increased work load imposed upon the heart during coitus could cause the problems associated with isometric exercise in general (page 245). An extended account of a coronary attack brought on by climbing four flights of stairs and anticipation of sexual intercourse is given by Winifred Holtby in the novel *South Riding* (Collins). Many family physicians also are familiar with individual cases. In a series of some 200 coronary events, we found two were associated with intercourse, whereas chance would have yielded less than one attack in a population which was sexually active only one night in five (Shephard, 1976a). If evidence accumulates that sexual prowess depends upon the state of the coronary vessels, a new basis of motivation for the improvement of personal fitness may well result! However, Hellerstein and Friedman (1969) have argued that both the dramatic cardiac response to sexual activity and the associated risks are an expression of promiscuity; in their experiments, normal marital relationships produced heart rates no higher than 120 min^{-1}, an effort that Hellerstein compared with the ascent of two flights of stairs.

Sexual intercourse is not the only situation where the heart rate can give a misleading impression of the intensity of activity. If a subject is sitting and reading a not too lurid novel, his pulse rate may be 65 beats min^{-1}. If he concentrates upon a mathematical calculation, it rises to 80 or 85 beats min^{-1}. If he drives his car, a pulse rate of 80–100 beats min^{-1} is normal (Shephard, 1967c; Littler et al., 1973), and values of 140–150 min^{-1} may be encountered when joining an urban expressway in heavy traffic. Passengers, particularly 'back-seat drivers,' can have pulse rates of 120–130 min^{-1}, and figures of 180–200 min^{-1} have been reported in racing drivers prior to a race (Lonne et al., 1968). Again, aircraft pilots may develop heart rates of 140–160 min^{-1} when landing at a crowded or unfamiliar airport (Howitt et al., 1966; British Medical Journal, 1973b; Mulder and Van der Meulen, 1973). Under all of these conditions, the metabolic activity is light, amounting to no more than 1.6–2.0 kcal min^{-1} (6.7–8.4 kJ min^{-1}). The pulse rate can also remain elevated for as long as seven hours following strenuous activity such as distance cycling (Brooke and Firth, 1972). Thus, if minute-by-minute pulse records are to be interpreted in terms of activity, it is vital that the pulse information be supplemented by some form of diary. Periods when the subject is performing isometric work or is under emotional tension can then be disregarded, and due allowance made for long-term disturbances of fluid balance caused by previous activity.

Activity patterns tend to be modified by age, sex, obesity, and climate. However, in the sedentary populations of North America, the baseline of activity is so low that changes are hard to detect. In general, not only are the young more active than the elderly, but the rate of performance of any given self-paced task also decreases with age. Klimt (1966) found heart rates of 160-180 min^{-1} during the spontaneous play of pre-school children. Older children sustained heart rates of 150-160 min^{-1} for long periods of play, and laboratory studies showed ten to twelve year old boys capable of sustaining 70-80% of their maximum oxygen intake for an hour or longer without exhaustion (Oseid et al., 1969). Average heart rates for the waking day were higher (~90 min^{-1}) in 12-year-old boys than in 16-year-olds (~80 min^{-1}), with the latter group spending significantly more time sitting (Seliger et al., 1974).

Figures collected by Durnin and Passmore (1967) further illustrate the influence of age on the energy cost of walking. Boys aged 9-11 years had an average energy expenditure of 3.0 kcal min^{-1} (12.5 kJ min^{-1}) while 'walking.' The equivalent rate of progression in a man of the same weight would be more than 6.4 km h^{-1} (4 mph); this is hardly a typical speed for an adult! Durnin and Passmore put the total activity of their Scottish boys on a par with that of colliery workers. It is not surprising that boys of this age have a reasonable standard of endurance fitness. Young girls are as active as boys. However, with the onset of puberty, most girls learn to move more slowly. In the age range 9-11 years, Durnin and Passmore found that the average energy expenditure of their female subjects during walking was only 2.0 kcal min^{-1} (8.4 kJ min^{-1}), two-thirds of the figure for the boys. At the age of 14 years, energy expenditures at the customary rate of walking again showed a sex difference of 0.7 kcal min^{-1} (2.9 kJ min^{-1}). The total daily energy consumption of the older girls was 2300 kcal (9600 kJ), 500 kcal (2100 kJ) less than for boys of the same age. This is in keeping with the deterioration of endurance fitness shown by urban girls during the 'teen years' (page 149).

Some studies of childhood activity patterns are becoming dated, and it is questionable how far they represent the current generation of young people. In most developed countries children now spend a large part of their leisure time watching television. One study from Quebec (Shephard, Lavallée, et al., 1975) showed urban boys spending 30 hours, rural boys 20 hours, urban girls 22 hours, and rural girls 16 hours per week in front of their television sets. In consequence, there was a wide discrepancy between expressed interests in sports and active participation. Almost all of the boys and most of the girls said they were interested in ice hockey and baseball, for example, but of 40 boys only 18 played ice hockey regularly and only 12 played baseball, while among the 40 girls only 2 were playing ice hockey and 3 baseball.

Obesity increases the energy cost of a given task. On the other hand, the obese are less active than an average person (Chapter 9).

Extremes of climate reduce activity by confining people to their homes. Thus, we found a significant increase of subcutaneous fat in Eskimo hunters during the coldest winter months (Rode and Shephard, 1973c). On the other hand, outdoor activity may cost more in a cold climate, partly because resting metabolism is increased, partly because more clothing is worn, and partly because the average person prefers to move more briskly in an attempt to keep warm. In a hot climate, the reverse is true; the resting metabolism falls, less clothing is worn, and the newcomer to the tropics soon learns the wisdom of the leisured movements that characterize the permanent resident.

ATTITUDES TOWARDS ACTIVITY

Little is known of the reasons why some people are active and others are lazy. Personality differences can be demonstrated between athletes and non-athletes, but it may well be that they are caused by athletic success rather than that they contribute to it. Thus, Werner and Gottheil (1966) found the athletes of a military academy to be sociable, dominant, enthusiastic, adventurous, tough, group-dependent, sophisticated, and conservative relative to cadets with no previous sports experience. However, all students were required to participate in sports while at the academy, and at the end of four years the personality of the initial non-athletes was no closer to that of the athletes than was the case during the first investigation. Tillman (1965) had a similar experience when he applied a vigorous physical fitness program to the poorest 15 per cent of a high school gymnasium class. R.C. Brown (1967) suggested that in both English and American children activity was influenced more by social factors than by personality.

The attitude of a subject to a proposed program of activity may depend in part upon its apparent relevance to his health. Thus, in one study of cardiac patients and controls (Paivio, 1967), the cardiac patients all showed positive changes of mood, feelings of happiness, pleasantness, confidence, success, cheerfulness, and the like, but these changes could not be demonstrated in normal subjects who performed the same amount of exercise. The only personality change found in both normal subjects and cardiac patients was a decrease of manifest anxiety. A major factor contributing to the positive response of cardiac patients is the severe depression engendered by the acute episode (Friedman and Hellerstein, 1973; Kavanagh, Shephard, and Tuck, 1975; Coustry-Degré et al., 1975). This apparently regresses as the patient undergoes successful rehabilitation.

In several studies, improvements of mood have been most marked in those members of the group with an initial psychological disturbance. W.P. Morgan et al. (1970) noted a reduction in depression scores over a six-week training period, but changes were confined to those subjects who were depressed at the beginning of the study. Likewise, de Vries (1968) saw a 25% decrease in resting muscle action potentials in response to chronic activity, but this was due largely to greater relaxation on the part of subjects who were initially tense. Popejoy (1967) and Folkins et al. (1973) reported decreases of manifest anxiety in young women undergoing training; although average changes were significant relative to groups being given instruction in golf and archery, a response was seen only in those with high initial anxiety scores.

When asked about the effects of an increase in physical activity, normal subjects typically claim that they 'feel better' (Massie and Shephard, 1971). Heinzelmann and Bagley (1970) studied 381 coronary-prone men. Half were assigned to a program of one hour's exercise three times per week, while the remainder served as a control. Those who exercised regularly reported positive feelings of sound health, more stamina and energy, and a greater ability to deal with stress. In addition the extent of gains was related to both program adherence and increases of cardio-respiratory performance.

The apparent gains of affect are not usually accompanied by changes in scores on formal psychological tests. Folkins et al. (1973) found no alteration in anxiety, depression, self-confidence, or adjustment when men underwent a training program. W.P. Morgan et al. (1971) noted that a group of young men and women 'felt better' after walking, but there were no associated improvements of psychological state. Massie and Shephard (1971) saw no psychological changes when middle-aged men followed an individual jogging program; in a second group allocated to gymnasium-centred activities, the only psychological effect was a small increase in extraversion score. Sidney (1975) evaluated exercise responses in 65-year-old men and women. His group again felt much improved after training, but they showed no changes in the 'life satisfaction index,' and only a small reduction of manifest anxiety scores.

Some studies have demonstrated an improvement of body image with training (Hammett, 1967). This has been reflected in the results of various 'projective' tests, such as interpretation of the Rorschach 'ink-blots' and drawing on a blank sheet of paper. Unfortunately, several of the groups examined had a poor initial body image, since they suffered from either neuromuscular disorders or mental retardation. It is thus less certain that increased activity is beneficial to the body image of normal subjects. Kreitler and Kreitler (1970) hypothesized that inactivity causes distorted perceptions – the body seems heavier and broader than it really is, movements feel clumsy and insecure, and activity is seen as excessively strenuous; a vicious circle of progressively diminishing activity is thus established. Massie and Shephard (1971) found no change in the body image of middle-aged businessmen in response to training. Sidney (1975) also saw no change in the group scores for his elderly subjects over the period of conditioning, but when he separated out those who trained the hardest, he found that this subgroup narrowed the margin between their presently perceived and ideal body images. Heinzelmann and Bagley (1970) also reported that their exercised subjects developed a more positive self-image. Many people who exercise regularly undoubtedly are seeking an improvement of body image – they hope that exercise will make them 'feel good' or 'look good.' However, if this is their main motivation to increased activity, then by implication the initial image of such subjects is poor – they 'feel bad' or believe they 'look bad.' Such studies provide no guarantee that a person with an average self-image will improve further through a program of graded activity.

Physical training may have a beneficial influence on job performance. Several studies from eastern Europe have extolled the virtues of a physical training break in place of a coffee break, and we were surprised to find that as many as a quarter of a sample of working men in Toronto favoured such an idea (Shephard, Jones, and Brown, 1968). In one group of radio-telegraph operators, four hours of exercise per week improved both working performance and scores on objective tests of attention and concentration. These changes were attributed by the authors to a lessening of anxiety. However, it seems fair to ask whether telegraph operators are an anxious breed, even in eastern Europe. The improvement of performance could equally reflect relief of boredom, and a greater arousal of the cerebral cortex initiated by a fresh type of activity could explain the gains of attention and concentration (Shephard, 1974h). Certainly, many people value physical activity for the arousal that it gives, particularly if their work calls for concentration and vigilance.

Other psychological inducements to exercise are familiar from personal experience. The aggressive instincts of a good 'organization' man must frequently be curbed at work, and it has been argued that sport provides an opportunity to release repressed emotions, through both the thrill of contest and the activity itself (particularly if body contact is involved). The success of this 'catharctic' role depends greatly upon the attitude of the sportsman, and in some instances aggressive play may enhance rather than diminish the aggressive tendencies of the individual concerned (Scott, 1970; Layman, 1970; Shephard, 1976c). Kenyon (1965) found that many teenagers valued the sensation of giddiness (vertigo), and would pursue any sport that involved rapid motion and fast turns. We have applied the same questionnaire to middle-aged men (Massie and Shephard, 1971) and older men and women (Sidney, 1975). As one might anticipate, the pursuit of vertigo and sport as a game of chance diminishes with aging, while there is an increase of interest in physical activity as a means of attaining health and fitness and as a social and aesthetic experience. Older people often value exercise for the companionship it brings; the ritual of the nineteenth hole may be as important to them as the activity itself (Stiles, 1967). Sometimes they are also driven by fear. A man is afraid of becoming old or of having a heart attack, while a woman fears her figure is deteriorating. With younger children, there are some practical difficulties in translating the rather abstract concepts of Kenyon's questionnaire into examples that are understandable. Nevertheless, we have attempted this with a group of 11-year-old French Canadian children (Shephard, Lavallée, et al., 1975). Our results suggest that relative to Anglophone teenagers there is less interest in vertigo and more appreciation of the elements of chance, health, and the ascetic and aesthetic value of sports participation.

Sociological factors influence attitudes towards activity. The habits of the growing child are moulded by his parents and his teachers. Some schools are fortunate enough to have extensive playing fields, and all pupils have the opportunity to exercise five afternoons per week. Such institutions seem more likely to develop a positive attitude towards sport than the average school, where a single dust bowl allows half an hour of play per week for each of 500 or 1000 students. Adults also are influenced by community attitudes and facilities. In Europe, the week-end cyclist or football player is accepted as a normal, sensible member of the community. On the other hand, in North America a man who professes an active interest in any exercise with the possible exception of skiing is classed as something of a 'nut,' while if a woman enjoys vigorous activity, even her gender becomes suspect. The lazy commonly blame their inactivity on a lack of physical facilities (Shephard, Jones, and Brown, 1968), but a careful inventory of most large cities shows a substantial unused potential for physical recreation. A number of government and private offices in Canada have installed exercise rooms in their basements, but the typical users are the 10–20% of workers who have least need of an improvement in their physical condition.

While psychological and sociological factors determine in large measure whether a person is active or inactive, physiological factors may also be involved. Some authors (Anend, 1961; Horvath, 1967) have postulated that a regulatory centre in the mid-brain influences the level of habitual activity. The main evidence for this suggestion is that when stimulating electrodes are placed in the hypothalamus, experimental animals can be induced to run to exhaustion and even death. Suggested mechanisms for the feedback of information to the hypothalamus in normal life include food sensors in the gastro-intestinal tract, receptors that report on the availability of glucose to the hypothalamic cells, temperature sensors, and possibly some as yet unexplained long-term control from body fat depots (Mayer, 1972). Obesity is usually associated with low levels of activity (page 240), and the body hormones may also play a significant role in mobilizing both glucose and fat (thus influencing activity patterns via the hypothalamic glucose detectors). The fat and lazy teenage boy often shows delayed sexual development. An excess of thyroid hormone, as in certain forms of goitre, is associated with hyperactivity, while a deficiency of the same hormone leads to both obesity and inactivity. There may also be differences in the inherent need for cerebral arousal – an extrovert needs the stimulation of vigorous physical activity, while the introvert is already highly aroused and prefers periods of quiet contemplation. Perhaps for this reason hyperactive children can be treated successfully by arousing drugs such as caffeine and the amphetamines (Schnackenberg, 1973).

Hunger, thirst, and disease predispose to less vigorous movement patterns. It is easy for a well-fed western man to accuse the peasants of an underdeveloped country of apathy and laziness, but their low productivity may be due at least in part to poor health and malnutrition.

MOTIVATION TO INCREASED ACTIVITY

Many people concerned with fitness and physical education consider the benefits of physical activity self-evident; they thus feel justified in preaching their conviction with missionary fervour. Let us suppose that, after due review of the available evidence (Chapter 8), we are inclined to agree that greater activity would be of benefit to many sedentary people. Are we justified in trying to manipulate public attitudes, and if so, how should we set about this task?

There can be little argument that the adult population is currently sedentary. Among a group of 181 working Canadian men, 88 claimed to be taking at least 120 kcal (29 kJ) of deliberate activity per day (Shephard et al., 1968c); however, only 21 reached the expenditure of 480 kcal (116 kJ) that epidemiological studies have suggested is necessary for protection against ischaemic heart disease (Shephard and Kavanagh, 1975a). In women aged 40–70, only one in six claimed to be taking even mild deliberate activity (J.R. Brown and Shephard, 1967). A much larger survey by Statistics Canada recently confirmed these findings. According to their data, about a half of Canadians under the age of 25 were taking no sport or regular activity, and after the age of 35 less than 20% were deliberately active.

Motivation towards an increase of physical activity can be based on positive conditioning (rewards such as fun and good facilities) or negative conditioning (fear of adverse consequences such as a heart attack). Commercial clubs use both tactics. To date, the main thrusts of policy by the Canadian government have been a modest advertising campaign by a crown corporation (Sports Participation Canada), a system of fitness performance awards to children, and an increase of spending on such items as national parks, hiking trails, and other public facilities. Such measures have not been particularly effective, and the time may be approaching when government will use negative reinforcement, saying that the health insurance premiums of otherwise healthy individuals will rise unless they meet certain minimum standards of fitness.

In some respects, the problem of increasing physical activity is analogous to that of decreasing cigarette consumption. Most people agree that more exercise would be beneficial, but they are not prepared to act on this belief. Fortunately, there are no massive vested interests committed to a maintenance of laziness by false propaganda, but there are still many popular misconceptions to be corrected by persistent education. As with smoking, the missionary approach can be successful with certain types of personality, particularly if it is accompanied by personal testimony and example. However, a larger percentage of lasting 'conversions' is likely to result from an educational approach, aimed at a progressive change in attitudes towards exercise. Regardless of the technique adopted, the percentage of converts is unlikely to be high. The habits of the adult are rigidly formed, and a cataclysm is necessary to induce significant change.

Since converts are few, their nurture is important. The newly found enthusiasm for activity must be maintained. The provision of adequate facilities, including showers and locker rooms, is critical, and it is encouraging to see that some government departments are giving such items high priority in the design of new office blocks. In some people, the payment of a substantial fee (as at commercial 'fitness studios') can add useful motivation.

Converts are more easily won among the young than the elderly. Appropriate interests should thus be fostered in the school child. Sports and pastimes that can be followed in adult life should be encouraged in preference to either games requiring thirty players or gymnastic feats needing elaborate apparatus. Particular attention should be paid to cross-country running, long-distance cycling, swimming, cross-country skiing, and the racquet sports. All of the class should be taught, irrespective of individual basic abilities. If the prospects of an increase in salary depend upon the defeat of a rival school, it is natural for the coach or trainer to concentrate upon his star pupils; however, as with any process of education, the true standard of judgment is not the success of the stars but the ultimate attitudes and attainments of average students.

8
Fitness and health

In this chapter, we shall examine objectively whether an improved level of endurance fitness can contribute to health. Areas of interest include not only the prevention of organic disease, but also the promotion of positive health in terms of better academic performance and increased industrial productivity.

The last fifty years have seen a remarkable increase in the number of deaths attributed to cardiovascular disease. As early as 1948 an analysis of the U.K. registrar-general's death certificates (Morris, 1951) showed a progressive increase of cardiac deaths, more marked in men than in women, with most of the increase attributable to acute cardiac deaths. Subsequent studies from the U.S. (U.S. Dept. HEW, 1969) and Canada (T.W. Anderson and Le Riche, 1970) have shown a comparable phenomenon. Further, it is difficult to dismiss such statistics as the result of more accurate diagnosis, with the abandonment of the picturesque descriptions of death favoured by previous generations of physicians (Morgan, 1968), since a detailed analysis of death certificates shows that the main increase has been in 'sudden deaths,' particularly events that are unequivocal 'coronary attacks' (Anderson and Le Riche, 1970).

Within Europe, trends have been variable. Norway and West Germany, for example, have shown a rapid increase in the mortality from arteriosclerotic and degenerative heart disease, the rates for men aged 55–64 years climbing from 398 and 450 per 100,000 to 599 and 540 per 100,000 between 1956 and 1966. In Czechoslovakia, on the other hand, the corresponding figures have remained relatively constant, being 413 per 100,000 in 1956 and 458 per 100,000 in 1966 (Rose, 1970). Traditional living groups such as Eskimos and indigenous Africans (Luijomba-Sengero, 1963) have as yet escaped the general increase in myocardial infarctions, but among the highly acculturated Eskimos of the north Alaskan coast, the prevalence of coronary heart disease is only a little less than in 'white' men of similar age (Maynard, 1976).

Many changes of life-style have occurred over the last half century, and each has been blamed in turn for the increase in cardiac deaths. One contributory factor is undoubtedly longevity. Pneumonia was once known as the 'old man's friend,' because it gave the aged a speedy release from the burden of life. Now, the antibiotics have conquered pneumonia and many other bacterial diseases, and an older man has little alternative but to die of a degenerative condition. However, this is not the entire explanation, since many cardiac deaths occur in early middle age. Other commonly blamed features of modern life are the stresses and strains of urban society, over-nutrition, lack of exercise, and a penchant for highly processed foods and soft water. Anxiety may play a direct role in causing coronary attacks, since it increases the work of the heart and makes it more irritable. T.W. Anderson (1973) has argued that processed foods and soft water may also lay the groundwork for a heart-attack by depleting the cardiac muscle of calcium and magnesium ions.

Over-nutrition and lack of exercise bear closely on endurance fitness, and their relation to cardiovascular disease will thus be considered in some detail. The contribution of an excessive body weight to premature death, particularly cardiovascular death, has been recognized by the life insurance companies for many years (Society of Actuaries, 1959). The chance of a cardiovascular death is 185% of normal in men who are 60 pounds overweight and 217% of normal in women with a similar excess weight. Over-nutrition is an increasing problem of affluent western society, and this could be one important reason why life-expectancy in the United States is poorer than in many materially less privileged nations (Jokl, 1967). However, some authors have argued that excess weight due to muscle is also bad for health. Certainly, the work-load of the heart depends on the total weight to be carried rather than the relative proportions of muscle and fat. Further, in terms of personality, an aggressive and muscular 'meso-morph' is more likely to undertake a sudden and dangerous burst of activity than a fat and somnolent 'endomorph.' Keys et al. (1972) have suggested that obesity is no longer a hazard if due allowance is made for associated risk factors such as a high systemic blood pressure and a high serum cholesterol level. Nevertheless, there is good evidence that a loss of excess weight will modify these other risk factors and thus diminish the chances of a subsequent heart attack (Ashley and Kannel, 1974).

Much of the evidence linking voluntary activity and the prevention of cardio-vascular disease has been obtained in retrospect, through comparisons of sup-posedly active and inactive populations. Some workers have studied longevity (see Chapter 2). Positive findings were reported by Karvonen (1959), who showed that skiers lived seven years longer than non-skiers. In Finland, cross-country skiing is a sport that is continued into old age, and Karvonen suggested that the vigorous activity entailed contributed to the greater life-expectancy of the skiers. However, the sportsmen were inevitably a self-selected group, and it is likely that the sick members of the community (including those with overt heart disease) did not participate in the skiing events. Other authors have examined the incidence of heart disease in selected occupational groups. Morris and his associates (1953) compared the coronary experiences of London Transport bus drivers with those of the conductors. It was presumed (and later shown by use of SAMI heart rate counters) that the conductor of a double-deck London bus had a more active life than the driver. A group of 31,000 men aged 35–64 were studied; after allowing for differences of age, the incidence of the first episode of coronary heart disease was higher in the drivers (2.7 per 1000 man-years) than in the conductors (1.9 per 1000 man-years). The mortality rate for coronary disease was also greater in the drivers than in the conductors; on the other hand, the symptom of cardiac pain, angina pectoris (a reflection of lack of oxygen in the heart muscle), was more common in the conductors. Similar comparisons have been carried out on several other occupational groups – postmen and sedentary civil servants, active and sedentary workers in the Jewish communal settlements (kibbutzim), switch-men and booking clerks on a United States railroad, blue- and white-collar workers in a Chicago utility company, farm owners and workers, lumberjacks and their sedentary colleagues, and various grades of longshoremen (S.M. Fox and Skinner, 1964; Epstein, 1968; Paffenbarger and Hale, 1975). Some of the 'active' occupations involved relatively low energy expenditures (400–900 kcal, 95–214 kJ per day), yet all except one of the studies (on Los Angeles civil servants) substantiated the findings of Morris et al., the sedentary groups usually having about twice the incidence of coronary events seen in their active counterparts. Unfortunately, the association between inactivity and heart disease cannot be proved conclusively by such retrospective investigations. This is partly because a certain type of job attracts a certain type of man. Morris, Heady, and Raffle (1956) soon found that bus drivers were fatter than conductors when their uniforms were first issued; the drivers thus started their careers with a greater risk of coronary disease. In some of the studies cited, there were other differences of pay, social status and aspirations, diet and initial health between active and inactive groups. Furthermore, there was inevitably a tendency for men with disabilities to move from active to sedentary employment.

Many of these confounding factors can be eliminated by means of a prospective study. Morris, Kagan, et al. (1966) took 667 bus crew members without initial evidence of heart disease and followed their health over a five-year period.

During this time, 7% developed clinical or electrocardiographic signs of coronary disease. Incidents were more common in the obese than in the slim, and drivers were also at a disadvantage relative to conductors. However, the two factors that contributed most to a coronary attack were a high systolic blood pressure and a high level of serum cholesterol. Those readers who have never visited London may wonder what intensity of activity is involved in collecting fares. The maximum work load would be two ascents of the staircase in every mile, or 24 ascents per hour. Over an eight-hour shift, a conductor would then perform 20–25,000 kgm (200–250 kJ) of work on the stairs, equivalent to four or five Harvard step tests. Dr Morris has spent time observing the conductors, and he tells me that eight ascents per hour is a more usual performance. Nevertheless, the intensity of these brief bursts of activity is quite high, and the conductor seems a good industrial model of a person undertaking deliberate interval training. Certainly, the cumulative effort should be sufficient to reveal the possible beneficial effects of exercise. The other unsolved problem of the London Transport studies relates to basic constitutional differences between drivers and conductors. The same difficulty has plagued examinations of leisure activities. Morris, Chave, et al., (1973) recorded the leisure pursuits of 16,882 executive-class civil servants on a specific Friday and Saturday. They were then followed prospectively for several years. Among those developing signs of coronary disease, only 11% recorded vigorous leisure activities (>7.5 kcal min^{-1}, 1.8 kJ min^{-1}) such as swimming, keep-fit exercises, digging, or getting about quickly; in contrast, 26% of controls gave such a history. However, Morris was quick to admit that his data did not indicate how much of the observed differences was due to the nature of the men (inheritance and experience), how much to what they currently did, and how much inheritance, experience, and environment interacted with current activity.

One possible method of circumventing these difficulties would be to allocate subjects randomly to 'exercise' and 'control' groups. The United States Public Health Service carried out feasibility trials for such a study a few years ago. In order to obtain a definitive result in a reasonable time, it was suggested that all of the subjects chosen should have a substantially increased risk of coronary disease (caused by high blood pressure, obesity, and so on). The 'exercise' group were to report for regular sessions of physical training, while it was hoped that the life-style of the 'control' group would remain unchanged. At the end of each year, the incidence of vascular disease between the two groups would be compared. The pilot trials quickly revealed two obstacles to completion of such a study – the vast cost (about $31 million in 1967) and a high rate of defections from both exercise and control groups (as much as 50% over the first six months). Largely for these reasons, the project is currently 'shelved.'

The group with the highest incidence of myocardial infarctions is composed of patients who have already sustained one or more coronary attacks. For this reason, such patients allow the cheapest and most effective study of the value of vigorous exercise in halting the ravages of ischaemic heart disease. Several 'tertiary preventive' trials of this type are currently underway in Europe, the United States, and Canada (Rechnitzer et al., 1975). We hope that within five years we shall know the benefit of added activity to such patients, and will have a more logical basis for discussing the cost-effectiveness of similar studies on individuals who have not yet sustained a heart attack.

There has been much discussion of potential mechanisms whereby exercise could modify the course of ischaemic heart disease. Some authors have argued that by middle age the pathological changes are irreversible. Certainly, post-mortem studies suggest that normal amounts of exercise do not reduce the number of fatty, atherosclerotic plaques in the walls of the coronary blood vessels. On the other hand, fibrous scarring of the heart muscle is less in active subjects (Morris and Crawford, 1958). How does exercise help the individual to live with his damaged coronary vessels? Eckstein (1957) suggested on the basis of animal experiments that exercise encouraged the development of an alternative ('collateral') vascular supply to areas of heart muscle beyond narrowed or blocked arteries. Burt and Jackson (1965) carried out similar animal experiments, with constriction of the coronary arteries after completion of training; they found no enhancement of collateral circulation in the exercised group. The human coronary vessels have been visualized by injection of radio-opaque dyes. Such studies have shown no special development of collateral vessels in individuals who have carried out moderate exercise after myocardial infarction (Kattus and Grollman, 1972), but it is still conceivable that more sustained and intensive effort might produce such a response.

Exercise may also be helpful in burning excess fat and establishing a better caloric balance, with reduction of serum cholesterol and triglyceride levels. The type of activity needed for such an effect has no threshold – excess calories can be burned equally by a brief run or by a longer walk, and indeed deliberate exercise can be avoided if the initial intake of food is sufficiently reduced. In some animal experiments, exercise has reduced the extent of atheroma, but the contrast of activity (between forced exercise and caging) has been extreme (Montoye, 1960). Conversely, plaque formation is accentuated if animals are fed a high cholesterol diet.

There are several other ways in which an improvement of endurance fitness could be beneficial to the potential coronary victim (Fox, 1974). Activity decreases the clotting tendency of the blood (McDonald and Fullerton, 1958). Gains of aerobic power and strength with a decrease of body weight reduce the stress imposed on the heart muscle for a given external effort (in terms of both the rise of blood pressure and the secretion of adrenaline) and such training responses may be supplemented by an increase of myocardial contractility. Pleasurable relaxation, camaraderie, and 'joie de vivre' are provided by quite low levels of recreational activity, while more vigorous contact sports may provide an outlet for aggressions generated in the board-room (Scott, 1970; Layman, 1970).

These various explanations must be held in abeyance until it has been demonstrated conclusively that exercise lowers the incidence of coronary disease. In the meantime, many may decide to find enjoyment from participation in their favourite sports, regarding the probable benefit to their hearts as a bonus yet to be declared. This is particularly true of the substantial group who have already suffered a coronary attack. Traditionally, physicians have prescribed rest and yet more rest for such patients, and they have created many chronic invalids by their advice. Yet invalidism seems unnecessary. There is good evidence that most coronary patients can be restored to full productivity through a graded program of activity (Hellerstein et al., 1967). In our Toronto series, 71% returned to full time work in their old job, 12% found a new full-time job, 6% accepted a part-time job, and 10% were unemployed. A proportion of the sample reached a higher level of fitness than before their heart attack, some to the point of running a 42-km marathon race in 3¼ to 5 hours (Kavanagh, Shephard, and Pandit, 1974). Many of those concerned with rehabilitation programs have been so impressed with their therapeutic value that they have not compared the experience of their patients with that of 'controls'; relative to data from other centres, a two- or three-fold reduction in subsequent coronary attacks has been suggested (Rechnitzer et al., 1971; Shephard and Kavanagh, 1975a), but this could be a by-product of the program rather than a direct effect of the activity itself. The subjects get advice on diet and smoking, their fears regarding a recurrence of the 'heart attack' are lessened by the support of a group with a positive outlook (Friedman and Hellerstein, 1973; Kavanagh, Shephard, and Tuck, 1975), and they may benefit because they escape from home or office several nights per week. Whatever their physiological basis, rehabilitation programs play an important role in modern society. If properly administered, they can restore to full efficiency the majority of men stricken by 'heart attacks' in the prime of life, including many who are leaders in their communities.

With experience, the timing of rehabilitation is being progressively advanced. At one time it was thought wise to wait six months, until scarring of the damaged heart tissue was complete. However, with such a delay, there is already a substantial burden of 'detraining' to reverse, and the potential interest in physical activity kindled by the critical incident is waning. Unless the patient shows signs of heart failure, shock, intractable pain, or uncontrolled abnormalities of heart rhythm, exercise should begin within 24 hours of infarction. Activities should be confined at first to light movements performed by individual muscle groups (total cost <2.5 kcal min^{-1}, 10.5 kJ min^{-1}). At the end of the first week, the patient should be sitting in a chair for up to three hours per day, and by the fourth week he should be walking up to half a mile at a stretch. Given such a preliminary program, formal rehabilitation can commence as early as eight weeks after infarction. Subsequent progression of the exercise prescription is carried out as rapidly as is judged safe from regular laboratory exercise tests and physician observation of the exercise sessions.

Which patients should be excluded from the formal program of vigorous training? Certainly, those with heart failure or ominous aneurysmal bulging of the heart shadow are not good candidates for rehabilitation. Most physicians are also agreed that cardiac pain (angina) at rest and abnormalities of rhythm not controlled by medication are contraindications to an aggressive conditioning program. There is less certainty whether angina should be provoked during exercise. Angina is a symptom of oxygen lack, and such oxygen lack may help in opening up new blood vessels to the heart muscle. On the other hand, a frequent recurrence of rather unpleasant pain may make the patient anxious, and there is also some risk that failure of the left side of the heart may develop during an anginal attack (Parker et al., 1966). Our current practice is to teach patients about the manifestations of angina, and to advise them to reduce their activity to a slow walk if any form of anginal pain is encountered. Where patients have a history of effort angina, the exercise is set at a level just below that likely to cause symptoms. Nevertheless, we have found difficulty in advancing such patients through a standard program requiring continuous effort; much larger gains can be accomplished through the use of an interval training regimen (Kavanagh and Shephard, 1975a).

A group program is generally more beneficial than individual exercise therapy, since the patient is encouraged by others who have already progressed in their rehabilitation. A group approach also permits personal supervision of the activity by a physician, and appropriate advice and treatment can be given to any of the group who develop cardiac pain. However, in view of the potential number of coronary patients needing rehabilitation, it is less certain that there are a sufficient number of physicians with the time and interest to provide such supervision. If group treatment is arranged, it is vital that activities be tailored to the capacity of individual participants. Patients must be warned specifically against indulging the competitive element that tends to develop in pursuits involving men with Type 'A' personalities. Hellerstein and his colleagues involve their patients in three forms of activity – calisthenics, a run-walk sequence, and recreation; attendance is for one hour, three times per week, and the intensity of activity is increased progressively until the patient is spending about 400 kcal (1670 kJ) of energy per session. The Toronto program is somewhat similar. It comprises 10 minutes of calisthenics for a 'warm-up,' 10 minutes of walking and jogging, 15 minutes of a game such as volleyball, 25 minutes of individually prescribed jogging and running, and a final brief warm down. In the early phases of training, our patients attend the rehabilitation centre twice per week, but once we are convinced that they understand the principles of training, they are transferred to a once-weekly attendance, with 'homework' to be carried out on at least four other days of the week. The prescription specifies the distance to be covered each day, the time to be taken, the permitted pulse-rate ceiling, and any special indications for stopping exercise (such as the development of anginal pain or the appearance of an abnormal pulse rhythm). Adherence to the prescription is checked by having the patient complete a weekly diary sheet (page 20) and observing his progress in the supervised exercise sessions. Adjustment of the prescription follows the typical plan of long-distance training. First the time specified for a given distance is reduced; once the patient is accomplishing the faster speed without problem, the distance is lengthened and the process is repeated. Some of our patients have advanced from an aerobic power 70% of the sedentary normal immediately post-infarction to as much as 112% of normal one to four years later (Shephard and Kavanagh, 1975a). The associated renewal of personal confidence is both remarkable and praiseworthy. Many office workers who have not yet had a coronary attack would hesitate to keep pace with our marathon team!

PHYSICAL ACTIVITY AND OTHER FORMS OF DISEASE

Does exercise help in the prevention and treatment of other forms of disease? In a few specific conditions, it has the opposite effect. The hot and sweaty skin of the athlete is susceptible to fungi ('athlete's foot') and bacteria (boils and other superficial infections). The swimmer has an increased chance of gastro-intestinal infection, since few pools and bathing beaches are completely free of intestinal pathogens (Crone and Tee, 1974); the sodden, macerated skin of the swimmer's external ear is also a favourite target of bacteria, and if the ear drum is damaged, infection may spread to the middle ear and the mastoid bone.

Exercise alters the number of circulating white blood corpuscles, and some change of immune reactions might be anticipated. However, there have been few studies of interactions between activity and more general forms of disease. Many infections enter the body by the respiratory route, and whether the microorganism is bacterial or viral in type, a certain critical number of organisms must be both inhaled and retained in order to overcome the body defences. While there is no evidence that the critical dose is altered by a change of fitness, the mere fact of taking exercise may modify the dose. A person who spends the evening in a crowded bar or theatre is more likely to inhale microorganisms than a man who is out running on the track. On the other hand, the removal of both particles and microorganisms from the trachea and bronchi depends largely upon the action of the hair-like cilia lining the airway. If the athlete inhales a large quantity of cold, dry, or polluted air while running, this can weaken the action of the cilia, increasing his liability to subsequent infection (Rylander, 1968). Further, the sportsman who returns to a crowded changing room while still breathing hard can draw an enormous number of microorganisms into his lungs.

Activity may also modify the manifestation of an acute infection. If a person exercises while he has a sinus infection, mucus may be aspirated into the chest, spreading the infection to the bronchi. Vigorous activity in the presence of a viral infection such as influenza can occasionally culminate in cardiac arrest or fibrillation. If one part of the body is exercised hard during the early stages of poliomyelitis, the virus responsible for this condition tends to localize itself to motor cells in the corresponding part of the spinal cord. The course of severe diseases also depends upon the initial fitness of the individual. If the reserve capacity of the heart or lungs is limited prior to infection, then the patient is particularly likely to succumb to the disease process. The bed rest needed in countering an acute infection leads to a substantial loss of cardio-respiratory power (page 169). A graded program of physical activity should thus be initiated to restore condition once the body temperature has returned to normal. As with other forms of rehabilitation, the training should emphasize vigorous isotonic exercise.

In a simple experimental study of the health effects of repeated exercise, Massie and Shephard (1971) compared the employment records of two groups of middle-aged men employed by a public utility company; in the control group, absences from work were noted over two successive seven-month winter periods; the test subjects were studied over the same two winters, but in the second season undertook a progressive exercise training program. Absences of the control subjects averaged 1.6 and 2.2 days for the two winters, while averages for the test group were 3.1 and 2.4 days; although suggesting a slight benefit from exercise, these differences were not statistically significant. Lindén (1969) also found some evidence that industrial absenteeism was inversely related to aerobic power. Cheraskin and Ringsdorf (1971) found an inverse relationship between habitual physical activity and scores on the Cornell Medical Index; however, it was unclear whether lack of activity was the cause or an effect of poor health. The same problem has plagued the frequently demonstrated association between habitual activity and good health practices (Palmore, 1970; Belloc and Breslow,

1972). Sidney (1975) had his group of elderly subjects complete the Cornell Medical Index before and after participation in a training program. Over-all scores showed no change, but conditioning led to a statistically significant decrease in positive responses to a section of the questionnaire (k), dealing with the frequency of illnesses.

Relatively little is known regarding activity and chronic diseases. High blood pressure, diabetes, and chronic infections of the gall bladder are more common in the obese, and such conditions may thus be related indirectly to a lack of physical activity. The direct effect of increased exercise upon a high blood pressure is minimal. There is some evidence that moderate activity controls peaks of blood glucose, and thus reduces the need of the mild diabetic for insulin. An exercise-induced decrease of serum cholesterol (page 237) could reduce the tendency to gall stone formation, and thus the liability to infections of the biliary tract.

Although chronic obstructive lung disease was once regarded as a progressive and incurable condition, a number of authors have now shown that progressive exercise is surprisingly effective in its treatment (W.F. Miller, 1967; Paez et al., 1967; Christie, 1968; Bass et al., 1970; Petty et al., 1970; Vyas et al., 1971; Alpert et al., 1974; Mertens et al., 1976; Shephard, 1976f). Some of the reported gains could have a psychological basis, reflecting the immediate response to a new form of treatment and the support of an interested medical team. However, many investigations also show an improved objective response to submaximal effort, with a diminution of heart rate, cardiac output, and respiratory minute volume; one may presume that without the stimulus of a regular prescribed program many patients fall into a vicious circle of breathlessness, diminished activity, loss of condition, further breathlessness, and further restriction of activity. In the less severe cases, renewed exercise not only improves aerobic power, but also leads to a strengthening of the muscles; there are increases of muscular endurance (Mertens et al., 1976) and a diminished accumulation of lactic acid in submaximum effort, the latter possibly being specific to the tasks that have been practised (Paez et al., 1967). The oxygen cost of activity may also diminish with training. This reflects partly an improvement of posture as the subject becomes less tense, and partly the adoption of a more efficient pattern of breathing. While patients feel much better as the result of exercise, it is less certain that the ultimate course of the disease process is changed; severely disabled patients show a continuing loss of lean tissue with an associated decrease of muscular strength (Mertens et al., 1976). On the other hand, there is no suggestion that exercise worsens long-term prognosis. Nor are there reports of exercise precipitating right-sided heart failure, even when individuals with a diagnosis of 'right ventricular strain' have been exercised (Bass et al., 1970). The main problem is implementation of the training program, compliance being poor relative to that observed in 'post-coronary' patients (Mertens et al., 1976). One reason is that the patients have experienced no critical incident to arouse their concern. Those with mild dyspnoea consider this as normal for their age, while those who are more severely disabled have great difficulty in carrying out any exercise unless supplemental oxygen is provided (Woolf and Suero, 1969).

The course of many chronic ailments is strongly influenced by the patient's state of mind. In any disease with a large psychosomatic element, exercise thus plays a useful role in directing the patient's thoughts away from his troubles. There is much unnecessary invalidism among chronically diseased patients, and a substantial proportion of those concerned could be restored to a useful place in society through an appropriate rehabilitation program.

EXERCISE AND ACADEMIC PERFORMANCE

Many physical educators apparently have felt a measure of guilt at taking time from a heavily loaded curriculum in order to teach students a non-academic topic. In an attempt to justify their discipline, they have sought a linkage between academic achievement and participation in athletics. One review noted that 70 studies of this type had been conducted in 434 high schools between 1907 and 1940 (Shaw and Cordts, 1960). Unfortunately, the authors cited were almost equally divided in their opinions regarding the academic prowess of athletes. Failure to resolve the problem seems due in part to inadequate definition of an athlete, and in part to inadequate measures of academic achievement. Clarke (1975) carried out a 12-year longitudinal study of U.S. boys; this showed that when junior high school athletes were matched with non-athletes for age, academic achievements in the sixth grade, and socio-economic status, the athletes had significantly greater academic success at the junior high school, the highest grades being seen for those playing upper-class sports such as golf, tennis, and crew, with poor performances from football and track athletes. Despite these studies, it can still be argued that the final differences of academic achievement between the athletes and the non-athletes reflect initial differences of class and constitution rather than a response to activity as such. Furthermore, even if the differences of achievement could ultimately be attributed to athletics, it would still by no means prove that some alternative form of ego-rewarding relaxation might not do just as much for intellectual achievement. In short, there seems no great future in the equation of exercise and intelligence. If we feel a need to justify physical activity, better ammunition will be obtained from studies of obesity, cardiovascular disease, and mood.

EXERCISE AND PRODUCTIVITY

A course of exercise could theoretically improve productivity in several ways. It might improve physical working capacity directly, and thus reduce fatigue. It might also act indirectly, increasing arousal (Shephard, 1974h), providing an outlet for aggression (Layman, 1970; Scott, 1970), and relieving boredom. Finally, it might reduce the amount of time lost through illness, industrial injuries, and other forms of absenteeism.

Working capacity and fatigue
Most mechanics are reluctant to permit the steady operation of a machine at more than 50% of its rated power. A similar margin of safety seems desirable for the worker. If such considerations are ignored, physical fatigue develops (Burger, 1964). There is a progressive increase of pulse rate, ventilation rate, respiratory gas exchange ratio (CO_2 output/oxygen intake), and deep body temperature, while lactic acid accumulates in the blood stream (Sadoul et al., 1966). Movements become poorly coordinated, and the quantity and quality of the work performed deteriorates.

Åstrand (1960) initially suggested that employees should be allowed to reach a 50% loading, but more recently she has favoured the restriction of work rates to 40% of aerobic power (P.O. Åstrand, 1967c). Bonjer (1968) recommended even lower limits, 63% for one hour, 53% for two hours, 47% for four hours, and 33% for eight hours of work. Where heavy work is self-paced, staff commonly operate at about 40% of aerobic power (Hughes and Goldman, 1970). There can be no question that the 50% limit is physiologically possible under favourable conditions, and indeed even in the hot and humid environment of the South African mines, the Bantu manage to work at 50-60% of maximum oxygen intake over one year or longer contracts. Nevertheless, a more conservative figure is preferable, particularly if working conditions are poor. In order to compute the percentage loading of an individual, it is usual to take the average figure for the energy expenditure during an eight-hour shift, adjust this for body weight (page 242), and relate the resultant cost to the subject's maximum oxygen intake. The latter may be measured directly or predicted from the response to a brief period of submaximum exercise (Chapter 4). A full evaluation of the industrial operation should also take account of the intensity and duration of more brief periods of activity, since these may exceed the reasonable capacity of the worker. It is further necessary to specify the nature of the task and the physique of the individual. A 50% load is acceptable in activities such as running, where a steady energy expenditure is distributed over much of the body musculature.

However, the same load becomes more of an imposition if the task is performed by a few specific muscle groups, particularly if the arms are used above heart level (I. Åstrand, Gahary, and Wahren, 1968; Åstrand, 1971b). Obesity increases the energy cost of most tasks (Chapter 9), partly because of gravitational work imposed by the heavy body mass and partly because fat impedes movement of the limbs; it is thus unreasonable to apply to the very obese worker the cost per shift averaged over the total labour force.

The conditions of employment have a substantial effect on the load that is tolerated. A high environmental temperature reduces the safety margin, since much of the potential increase of cardiac output is then diverted from the working muscles and the viscera to the blood vessels of the skin. Prolonged standing also reduces work tolerance, since fluid is progressively pooled in the blood vessels and tissues of the legs. Awkward postures such as reaching or stooping are even more disadvantageous; a substantial effort is involved in sustaining the ungainly posture, and it is impossible to bring many of the muscles that are normally used to bear on the task. The rhythm of work also influences the safety margin; a load much closer to the theoretical limit can be tolerated if the worker is allowed periodic rest pauses to oxidize any lactic acid that may have accumulated (Müller, 1953). Finally, the journey to and from work must be considered; if this is long and tiring (as in some sub-oceanic coal mines), it must be taken into account when reckoning the energy expenditure per shift.

How closely does the average worker approach his eight-hour limit? A young man with a maximum oxygen intake of 3 l. min^{-1} should be able to perform at an average daily rate of 7.5 kcal min^{-1} (31.4 kJ min^{-1}). As discussed previously (page 209), effort of this intensity is rarely required in modern industry. Many older men have a maximum oxygen intake of 2 l. min^{-1} or less (Table 12). Their potential for an eight-hour shift (5 kcal min^{-1}, 20.9 kJ min^{-1}) is thus marginal for heavy industries. It takes only a slight mechanical problem (such as failure to grease the wheels of a miner's tub [Williams et al., 1966]) or the onset of chronic disease to bring the worker within the range where fatigue will occur. In older women, the capacity is even more limited; a maximum oxygen intake of 1.5 l. min^{-1} is common, and activities for a working day may need restricting to an average of 3.5 kcal min^{-1} (14.6 kJ min^{-1}).

While a worker is operating well within his safety margin, it is unlikely that physical training will have a direct influence on productivity. However, many older men and women operate close to or over the safety limit. A conditioning program might well have a favourable influence on such workers with respect to both fatigue and work output; a 20% gain of aerobic power could be anticipated from an appropriate training regimen, with possible additional benefits from cessation of smoking (Chapter 11) and correction of any anaemia (Chapter 3). Lindén (1969) found that fitness levels influenced absenteeism in customs workers, but not in firemen or office-workers; 5 of the 10 customs men with frequent absences had high heart rates while they were working. Kilbom (1971a,b) instituted a seven-week physical training program for middle-aged female shop assistants; emotional well-being was unchanged by the program, but the subjects noted greater physical well-being at the end of the day, with less swelling of the feet and calves after long periods of standing.

It is surprising that complaints of fatigue are not more common among older employees who perform heavy physical work. One possible explanation is that as the safety margin is approached, the worker slows his pace of movement to a more acceptable level; in some instances, younger individuals may consciously or unconsciously help the older person who cannot bear an average share of the daily load. Experience may also enable an older worker to carry out a given task with less than the average energy expenditure. Finally, a proportion of employees gain promotion which takes them away from the shop floor.

Psychological benefits
In some European factories, it is customary to have regular breaks for organized calisthenics (Galevskaya, 1970). The factory managers concerned are presumably convinced that production is raised thereby. There is also some scientific evidence that active, gymnastic pauses are more effective in relieving fatigue than passive pauses, particularly in light or sedentary work (Geissler, 1960; Manguroff et al., 1960; Laporte, 1966). The Russian physiologists, still strongly influenced by the theories of Pavlov, interpret the improvement of performance as a form of 'disinhibition.' They apparently mean a release from anxiety. Exercise can certainly serve this function, and the performance of the busy executive may well be improved if his anxiety level is lowered. However, it is less probable that anxiety is limiting productivity in the simpler tasks of the factory floor. Another form of 'inhibition' is boredom, and it is very likely that this could be reversed by a few minutes of vigorous exercise. Regular gymnastics may also be beneficial in promoting an 'espirit de corps,' although the factory manager must be careful that an excess of energy is not diverted from productive work to the organization of recreational events (Shephard, 1974l).

Illness and injury
The influence of acute and chronic illnesses upon physical performance has been reviewed in a preceding section. If experienced workers are restored to full employment following a serious illness, progressive rehabilitation is making a useful contribution to the total productivity of the community. In industry, as in sport, injuries are most common when the body is overstressed and fatigued. A training

regimen can thus help the industrial safety officer by reducing the incidence of physical fatigue. Time is frequently lost through back injuries and the development of herniae (J.R. Brown, 1958; 1972). Low back pain is likely when lifting is carried out by groups who are unaccustomed to physical effort (for example American immigrants to Israel [Magora and Taustein, 1969]); there is associated weakness of the trunk musculature (Alston et al., 1966), although it is difficult to be certain whether this is cause or effect. Nevertheless, in the context of heavy industry, it is often desirable not only to develop cardio-respiratory power, but also to provide specific exercises for the abdominal and spinal muscles.

Finally, in many industries, much time and more production is lost through minor absenteeism. One cause is uncertified illness. An improvement of a man's total working capacity could thus play a role in checking absenteeism by bringing his physique to the point where he felt capable of coping with both a day's work and a minor ailment. In practice, absenteeism among certain types of workers can be correlated with fitness scores (Lindén, 1969; Buzina, 1972).

9
Nutrition and fitness

In this chapter, we shall look briefly at the topics of health foods and cholesterol. However, our main concern will be over-nutrition. We have already noted (Chapter 5) that in the affluent western nations the majority of older adults have an excessive body weight. We shall now examine how far this burden is due to over-eating, and how far it represents lack of exercise. Effects upon the cost of body movement will also be discussed briefly.

Health foods and the diet of the athlete
Athletes and their trainers have searched for a 'super diet' with an enthusiasm matched only by the quest of the alchemists for the philosopher's stone. A recent survey of contestants in the World Masters' Championships (Kavanagh and Shephard, 1976b) showed that 66 of 135 competitors were taking vitamins and other dietary supplements. One 47-year-old man who was attempting a cross-Canada run included in his rations wheat germ, Granola, Special K (a fortified cereal), rice-polishings, liver extract, celery leaf powder, yeast, ascorbic acid tablets, and Vitamin E (Shephard, Kavanagh, et al., 1976). Other unfortunate contestants have been persuaded to swallow such peculiar 'ergogenic aids' as queen bee extract, seaweed cakes, and various specific vitamin supplements (Bourne, 1948; Yakovlev, 1958; Cureton, 1959). Such is the power of faith that performance has sometimes improved! However, any gains have a purely psychological basis; there is no substantial evidence that physiological performance is improved thereby (Buskirk, 1967; Bailey et al., 1970; Sharman et al., 1971; W.P. Morgan, 1972; Ellis and Nasser, 1973; Shephard, Campbell, et al., 1974; Shephard, Kavanagh et al., 1976). If a person is in good health, there is no advantage in departing from a normal mixed diet. This should provide an adequate intake of calories, a reasonable balance of protein, fat, and carbohydrate, and no more than the natural content of vitamins and minerals.

The total calorie requirement of the athlete is typically 3750–4350 kcal (15,675–18,190 kJ) per day (Ferro-Luzzi et al., 1975), and he often eats twice as much protein as a more sedentary subject (2.5–3.0 g/kg of body weight). There is no great harm in this; indeed, there have been suggestions that during intensive training body protein formation is helped by a minimum protein intake of 2 g/kg (about 14% of a 4000 kcal, 16,700 kJ diet), and that if this minimum is not provided the haemoglobin level and blood protein concentration fall (Yamaji, 1951). Others maintain that on a marginal diet the total energy intake is more important than the proportion of protein (Callaway, 1975). Although some authors have suggested there is no protein usage in endurance activity (Hedman, 1957; P.O. Åstrand, 1967b), our observations indicate a combustion of at least 50 g over a marathon race (Kavanagh and Shephard, 1975b,c). To this figure must be added increases in muscle bulk, sometimes as much as 20 kg over the course of a season. It is thus hardly surprising that very intense activity can burn away muscle from regions of the body that are not contributing actively to a sport (Wright, Nicoletti, and Shephard, 1976), particularly if the athlete is still growing and his protein intake is limited.

There is some evidence that the mechanical efficiency of exercise is greater if carbohydrate is used as a fuel rather than fat; however, the difference is small (less than 5%) and difficult to document (Gemmill, 1942). The relative proportions of carbohydrate and fat consumed vary with the intensity and duration of exercise (Bock et al., 1928; Christensen and Hansen, 1939; Hultman, 1971; Pruett, 1970), the state of training of the individual (Holloszy, 1973), and blood levels of fatty acids (Bremer, 1967; Paul, 1970). In vigorous activity, at least 75% of the fuel is carbohydrate (Pruett, 1970; Hultman, 1971), but with more moderate work 50–60% of the energy may be derived from fat. If effort is prolonged, the usage of fat increases progressively, mainly because the muscle stores of carbohydrate (glycogen) are becoming depleted (Hultman, 1967, 1971; Bergstrom et al., 1973; Gollnick et al., 1974). On the other hand, if the work is severe enough to involve the oxygen debt mechanism, an increased proportion of energy is necessarily derived from carbohydrate.

The muscle glycogen stores are not exhausted with less than 60–90 min of vigorous exercise (Hultman, 1967; 1971); depletion occurs first in smaller muscles (Bergstrom et al., 1973) and slow fibres (Gollnick et al., 1974). The relative proportions of fat and carbohydrate in the diet thus have little influence on performance in brief events, but become critical when work is sustained for several hours. Scandinavian authors (Saltin and Hermansen, 1967; Åstrand, 1967b) have suggested a suitable dietary regimen for boosting the glycogen content of the muscles prior to an endurance event. This comprises (1) an exhausting run one week before competition, (2) a diet rich in fat and protein for the next three days, and (3) a carbohydrate-rich diet throughout the remaining period of preparation (R.H. Johnson and Rennie, 1973).

Irrespective of the duration of the event, it is unwise to eat a large meal less than three or four hours prior to heavy exercise (Van Itallie et al., 1960). A combination of the excitement of the contest and vigorous work may induce vomiting, while performance is also impaired by diversion of blood flow from the active muscles to the intestines. Both fatty foods and concentrated solutions of glucose delay emptying of the stomach (Fordtran and Saltin, 1967; Costill, 1972; Shephard, Kavanagh, et al., 1976); the best form of food to take before sustained work is thus a dilute solution of sugar. During exercise up to 800 ml of a 2.5% solution of glucose can be ingested per hour (Costill, 1972); at most this will yield 80 kcal (334 kJ) of energy. If prolonged work is performed in a hot climate, the most pressing need is to make good water losses in the sweat (Kavanagh, Shephard, and Pandit, 1974; Shephard, Kavanagh, et al., 1976). The plasma concentration of mineral ions (sodium and potassium) does not fall during competition, and on grounds of simplicity there is much to commend the use of pure water as a replacement fluid. Following activity, salt losses in the sweat must be replenished either by deliberate salting of food or by the use of fruits and beverages with high mineral contents.

Low cholesterol diets
We have seen that fatty plaques are formed in the walls of the blood vessels in the early stages of atherosclerotic arterial disease, and that a high cholesterol level in the blood stream is associated with a high risk of a coronary attack. It is thus tempting to assume that health would be improved by resorting to a low cholesterol diet, replacing such items as butter, cream, and eggs by vegetable oils (Stamler, 1971; Blackburn, 1974). Certainly, one can show a striking correlation between the percentage of the national calorie consumption that is derived from saturated fats and the incidence of new episodes of coronary heart disease (Keys, 1970). In Japan, a twofold increase of fat consumption from 1950 to 1968 has been associated with a fourfold increase of cholesterol intake (Wen and Gershoff, 1973). If a population is affluent and is consuming large amounts of saturated fat and cholesterol, a substantial reduction in these two components of diet will reduce the serum cholesterol level of most individuals. A reduction in the intake of animal fat seems particularly wise for patients with pathological elevation of serum cholesterol (the various forms of hyperlipoproteinaemia [Kuo, 1972]). However, dietary modifications often have remarkably little effect on the blood cholesterol level of a more average person (Van Itallie and Hashim, 1965), and differences of habitual diet explain less than 3% of variations in individual serum cholesterol levels (Medalie, 1970). This is not altogether surprising, since more

cholesterol is synthesized in the liver and the intestines than is derived directly from the diet (Ho et al., 1970). If a subject eats no cholesterol, the blood level drops for two or three weeks until it stands at about half the normal resting value. Thereafter, it gradually returns towards its initial reading, presumably because synthesis within the body is increased (Goode, Firstbrook, and Shephard, 1966).

Since much of the blood cholesterol is derived from carbohydrate, there is good reason to suppose that synthesis can be increased by an excessive intake of either fat or carbohydrate; conversely, the logical basis of control is to strike a better balance between the total calorie intake and habitual activity patterns. Observations on both animals and human subjects tend to confirm this view. The nomads of Somalia, Kenya, and Tanzania eat mainly milk, meat, and blood, yet they remain thin, with a low serum cholesterol level; suggested explanations include freedom from 'stress' and a high level of physical activity, although unfortunately both are poorly documented (Mann et al., 1955, 1964). Traditional Eskimos also show a low serum cholesterol level despite a very high fat diet (Draper, 1976; Sayed et al., 1976), many of the group have high activity levels (Godin and Shephard, 1973a), but it has been argued further that much of the fat they consume is unsaturated.

There is some evidence that a low cholesterol diet reduces the chance of a coronary attack in the 'high-risk' type of patient (Joliffe et al., 1959). Several extensive inter-university tests of this hypothesis are currently underway. Smaller studies of a mental institution in Finland (Turpeinen et al., 1968), a veterans' hospital in Los Angeles (Dayton et al., 1969), and men attending a cancer detection clinic in New York (Rinzler, 1968) have all shown advantages of marginal statistical significance to subjects consuming a low fat diet. On the basis of current knowledge, it is therefore desirable to restrict the intake of both animal fat and refined sugars in patients where a coronary episode appears imminent. There seems less justification for modifying the diet of entire populations. Moderation is particularly important with respect to the replacement of animal fat by vegetable oils, since there is little information on the long-term safety of such a change; indeed, at least one animal study has suggested that an excessive use of rape-seed oil could itself produce degenerative changes in the heart muscle.

Activity and the control of obesity
Many people who are overweight claim with pathos that 'they never eat a thing.' Are such claims true, or do the obese eat more than those who are slim? There have been suggestions of an enzyme defect in chronic obesity (Galton, 1966), but it is unlikely that the fat person has discovered a new basis for the synthesis of matter! As in other mortals, the body weight of an obese subject represents the cumulative balance between intake of food and water and expenditures in

physical work. A person who gains 10 kg of fat between the ages of 30 and 40 must therefore have overeaten relative to his average daily activity for the same period. Several factors explain the pathetic denials of the typical obesity clinic:

1. Account must be taken not only of the size of meals but of the nature of intervening snacks. Those who 'never eat a thing' often fortify their spartan life by frequent doses of sweets (candy), chocolate, biscuits (cookies), baked goods, syrupy tea or coffee, soft drinks, and alcohol. This is not to imply that frequent meals are intrinsically a bad idea: indeed, by curbing peaks and troughs of blood sugar, they can help to reduce overeating (Leveille and Romsos, 1974). One study showed more obese children in a school that provided three meals a day than in a rival establishment where seven meals a day were available (British Medical Journal, 1972b). However, care must be taken to include all sources of nutrients when calculating the daily dietary intake.

2. The extent of overeating need be only slight. Ten kilograms of tissue fat has an energy equivalent of 7100 kcal* (29,700 kJ), less than three days' supply of food. If 10 kg of fat has accumulated over 10 years, then the extent of over-eating on an average day may have been no more than 0.1%, within the standard error of even an expert chef!

3. The obese person may eat no more than his slimmer friends. His problem could arise rather from a low level of habitual activity; the elevator is taken instead of a flight of stairs, and the tram (streetcar) is ridden to avoid walking three blocks. Laziness of this order, repeated daily for 10 years, is equivalent to 10 kg of fat.

4. Available calories may be used a little more efficiently by the obese person. With a serious attitude to meals, the fat gourmand may absorb food more completely than the nervous individual who snatches a sandwich as he continues working. A taste for sweet foods may lead to the use of carbohydrate rather than fat as a metabolic fuel, with a greater energy yield per calorie eaten. Gross hormonal disturbances are unlikely, but a small reduction of thyroid secretion could lead to less 'uncoupling' of the linkage between carbohydrate usage and the formation of high-energy phosphate bonds in the tissues. Finally, a solid layer of subcutaneous fat conserves body heat, and less energy must be dissipated to keep an obese person warm when he is at rest.

Once a person becomes obese, activity is usually further restricted (Bruch, 1940). Leaving aside the question of possible changes in the discharge of activity centres in the hypothalamus (Mayer, 1972; Lepkovsky, 1973; Panksepp, 1974), there are several more immediate practical reasons for this. The energy cost of

---

* The energy equivalent of dietary fat is 9 kcal (37.6 kJ) per gram; however, tissue fat also includes a fair amount of water.

movement is increased (see the following section). Usually the level of endurance fitness is also low, and exertion leaves the fat member of any group hot and breathless. Lastly, if sports are suggested, an obese person may be self-conscious regarding the ungainly figure he cuts as he struggles into shorts that are bursting at the seams. Several authors have documented the laziness of the obese. In one study from Philadelphia (Chirico and Stunkard, 1960) a pedometer was used to estimate the total distance walked per day. Obese men covered an average of 5.9 km (3.7 miles), compared with 9.6 km (6.0 miles) in non-obese controls of similar occupation and social background; in women, the corresponding figures were 3.2 km (2.0 miles) and 7.8 km (4.9 miles) per day. Another approach has been to obtain a cinematograph film of group activity. Stefanik et al. (1959) compared 14 obese and 14 normal boys attending a vacation camp in the U.S. The obese boys had a lower food intake, but also participated much less in active pursuits. Bullen et al. (1964) watched adolescent girls at a similar camp. They found that the well-padded specimens spent 70% of swimming time, 80% of volleyball time, and 55% of tennis time merely standing or sitting. The girls of normal weight were inactive for a much lower percentage of the time allocated to the various sports (swimming, 25%; volleyball, 50%; tennis, 20%). Durnin (1967b) reached parallel conclusions from dietary and diary surveys in Scotland; none of his adult subjects were performing much heavy work, but the proportion of the day spent in moderate activity (3.5–5.4 kcal min^{-1}, 14.6–22.6 kJ min^{-1}) was much lower in plump women than in those of average build. In children (Durnin, 1966), there was no difference of activity between 'thin' and 'normal' individuals, but the 'plump' girls of his sample devoted less time than their thinner counterparts to both 'very heavy' exercise at school and 'moderate' exercise in their leisure hours. In Japan, the proportion of obese children is increasing (Ishiko et al., 1968), particularly in urban areas; the fat students claim to enjoy swimming and games such as dodge-ball and baseball, but express a firm dislike of running and gymnastics. All of these studies point to the conclusion that a person with long-standing obesity can eat less than his friends and yet remain fat because he deliberately avoids endurance-type activities.

The treatment of obesity is based on the simple principle of striking a new balance between food intake and energy expenditure. In many patients the change of living pattern need not be extreme. A 5% increase in activity, or a corresponding adjustment of diet can correct body weight by 10 kg (22 pounds) over the course of three months. Weight loss of this order should not require drugs or specific medical help; it can be achieved by simple discretion. Larger changes are more difficult to realize and maintain, and the advice of a specialist is then desirable.

While greater activity, restricted diet, or a combination of the two measures may be prescribed, many physicians prefer to emphasize dietary controls and appetite-suppressing drugs. This may be partly because they are taught more about medication than exercise, and partly because the obese patient seems a 'poor risk' from the viewpoint of suggesting sustained endurance effort. However, greater emphasis should be given to an active regimen for several reasons:

1. The success rates of conventional weight control programs are abysmally low. A careful study from England reported only 16 successes in 75 patients, and 8 of the 16 later relapsed (Innes et al., 1974). In the U.S., Sohar and Sneh (1973) re-examined 38 obese patients 14 years after weight reduction by dieting; 33 of the group had regained all of the lost fat, and the remaining 5 patients were quite obese at the time of re-examination.

The effectiveness of any weight-control program depends upon the co-operation of the patient. Exercise is more enjoyable to most people than a course of water and dry rolls. Indeed, vigorous activity has a mood-elevating effect, which counteracts the depression of dietary restriction even more effectively than drugs such as 'dexedrine.' In any event, use of the amphetamines is now banned in many countries, including Canada, because drug-dependence is rapidly acquired.

2. When body weight is reduced, protein is lost as well as fat. This tendency is minimized when the fat is lost through vigorous exercise (Keys et al., 1950; Babirack et al., 1974) – indeed in children fat may be replaced by muscle without change of body weight (Parizkova, 1964).

3. As much as three-quarters of the potential benefit of dietary restriction may be lost because it is typically accompanied by a reduction in daily activity (Behnke and Wilmore, 1974).

4. Vigorous exercise has the immediate effect of inhibiting both appetite and food intake (Edholm et al., 1955; Thomas and Miller, 1958; Mayer, 1960). Thus, if a person who is attempting to lose weight feels hungry, it is often helpful to go for a brisk run. The mechanism of relief is probably triggered because exercise increases the blood sugar level.

The hazards of obesity
The unfavourable influence of obesity upon cardiovascular mortality has already been discussed (Chapter 8). A rich and excessive diet increases the blood cholesterol level, and in some way not yet fully understood, this increases the risk of a coronary incident. In early childhood, over-feeding apparently increases the number of fat cells in the body, adding to problems of weight control in later life (Angel, 1974; Bjorntorp et al., 1973). An excess of body fat in the adult has other adverse effects on life expectancy (Table 28). Surgery becomes more diffi-

TABLE 28

Mortality of grossly obese* men and women, classified by disease,
and expressed as percentages of standard values for subjects of the same sex,
aged 15–69 years (based on data of Society of Actuaries, 1959)

Condition	Men			Women		
	D	E	F	D	E	F
Diabetes	179	385	629	270	242	250
Vascular diseases of brain	136	183	215	143	142	210
Heart and circulation	131	155	185	175	178	217
Pneumonia and influenza	128	103	242	148	110	–
Digestive diseases	147	197	298	140	200	225
Kidney diseases	146	230	298	93	122	–
Accidents and homicides	109	126	120	85	98	–
Suicides	71	104	142	47	–	–
All conditions	123	145	168	130	138	178

* The excess weight varies somewhat with stature. Three categories are recognized (D, E,
and F). For men, the averages are +24 kg (D), +33 kg (E), and +42 kg (F). For women,
the corresponding figures are +28 kg (D), +37 kg (E) and +46 kg (F).

cult when the organs requiring operative treatment are deeply embedded in fat.
The abdominal wall is more difficult to suture and takes longer to heal. Bed rest
is thus prolonged, and this together with the natural lethargy of the obese person
leads to post-operative complications – chest infections, thromboses of the leg
veins, and so on.

The cost of physical activity is usually increased in the obese. Many authors
(Passmore and Durnin, 1955; McKee and Bolinger, 1960; Malhotra et al., 1962;
J.R. Brown, 1966; Godin and Shephard, 1973b; Hanson, 1973) have discussed
the relationship between energy expenditure (E) and body weight (W). Some
have assumed a direct relationship, of the type

(15) $E = b(W)$,

where b is a constant. Brown (1966) suggested use of an equation of the form

(16) $E = a + b(W)^n$,

where a and b are constants and n is a power function variously set at 0.75 to
1.00. Taking $n = 1$, he calculated average values of the constant b for various segments of a mixed industrial population working an eight-hour shift. In sedentary
employees such as clerks, it amounted to 5 ml of oxygen per kg of body weight.

When the work was heavy or very heavy, the constant increased to about 12 ml min^{-1} kg^{-1}; on the other hand, in certain occupations that involved only sitting or standing (for example, hand-press operators) b was not statistically significant. Godin and Shephard (1973b) pointed out that the total energy expenditure had two main components. One was related to basal energy expenditure; this was proportional to the surface area of the body, and thus was a power function of body weight ($W^{0.75}$). The second component related the basic cost of the task to the added cost of supporting and moving the body against gravitational forces. In most sedentary workers, the basal component was dominant, but much of any additional activity was performed against gravity (getting up, climbing stairs, and so on). However, in press operators, a substantial amount of work was performed against the resistance of the press, the required effort being relatively independent of gravity; in equation (16), this would increase a rather than b, thus masking the effect of weight on basal energy expenditure. In most forms of heavy work, the body was moved against gravity, and this reinforced the effect of body weight on basal energy expenditures. Accordingly, it was suggested that energy expenditures be calculated as the sum of a two-component equation

$$(17) \quad E = a(W)^{0.75} + b(W)^1.$$

The first term corresponds to basal energy expenditure. The second term corresponds to the added cost of performing the chosen activity; the exponent n thus varies from near zero in activities such as cycling to close to 1.0 in activities where the body weight must be raised and lowered (Godin and Shephard, 1973b; Hanson, 1973).

The effects described so far could arise irrespective of the basis of body weight (muscle or fat). We must now consider whether there are penalties specific to obesity. Heat dissipation is necessarily hampered by a thick layer of subcutaneous fat; the fat person must therefore direct a larger proportion of his total cardiac output to the skin during work, with an inevitable reduction of maximum oxygen intake (Haymes et al., 1974). Some authors have found no difference of mechanical efficiency between normal and obese subjects during such activities as walking on a treadmill (Turrell et al., 1964) and operating a pulley system while lying supine (McKee and Bolinger, 1960). Others have reported a low efficiency of cycling in the grossly obese (Dempsey et al., 1966; Davies et al., 1975). Dempsey et al. attributed this in part to the increased friction imposed by the pendulous skinfolds, and in part to an increase of postural work. The energy cost of supporting the body and moving the legs is not normally considered in calculating the efficiency of cycling, but from the work of Dempsey et al. it would seem that at least in the untrained this can be an important unmeasured variable. In the experiments of Godin and Shephard (1973b), the weight exponent n became progressively smaller as subjects became familiar with the bicycle ergometer test. A further factor influencing efficiency is the general level of muscular and cardio-respiratory training. In an obese person, the body musculature is often relatively inadequate to move the large body mass, and this predisposes to a clumsy and inefficient pattern of movement. The unfavourable ratio of fat to muscle is commonly associated with a low level of cardio-respiratory fitness (Dempsey et al., 1966), and this again leads to a clumsy and inefficient pattern of movement during exhausting exercise. It also means that during an emergency more work must be performed by a poorly prepared heart, and this added stress on the cardiovascular system is one further reason why heavy subjects have an above average liability to coronary attacks.

In fairness to the overweight, their one advantage should be noted – death by drowning is less likely. Not only does the buoyancy of fat decrease the need for active swimming, but its insulating properties preserve life long after the thinner victims of a shipwreck have died of cold exposure. 'Cross-channel' and other long-distance swimmers can be quite fat (Pugh et al., 1960), although obesity is not a common characteristic of swimmers competing over shorter distances (P.O. Åstrand, Engstrom, et al., 1963; Shephard, Godin, and Campbell, 1973).

10
Endurance fitness and the body musculature

Reference has already been made to muscular training and isometric exercise at various points in this book. It has been suggested that in general the development of muscle bulk and strength do little for endurance fitness, and that in certain circumstances both the immediate response of the body to such exercises and the resultant 'top-heavy' muscular development can be a disadvantage to health. The present chapter will amplify this viewpoint, while noting also specific situations where muscular training may be beneficial.

Muscular contraction and blood flow
While the general effect of exercise is to cause a constriction of arteries supplying the body muscles (Shepherd, 1963), a variety of local mechanisms sufficiently outweigh central effects to cause a dilatation of the vessels to the active tissues (Duling and Pittman, 1975; Haddy and Scott, 1975). Nevertheless, an increase of muscular blood flow is not always realized, because mechanical effects of the contraction (nipping of the artery where it penetrates the fascial sheath of the muscle and direct compression of smaller vessels within the belly of the muscle) may impede the circulation. The problem was first described by Gaskell (1877). Difficulty can arise during either rhythmic (isotonic) or sustained (isometric) contraction, with a relative deficiency or a complete obstruction of blood flow for such time as the contraction is maintained. With rhythmic exercise, a fair measure of compensation is achieved through a high rate of flow between contractions (Barcroft and Dornhorst, 1949; Barcroft, 1963; Shepherd, 1963), although if a sufficiently intense effort is sustained for more than a third of a movement cycle some deficit of flow may be anticipated. This is shown (1) by failure of local blood flow to increase linearly with work load (Clausen, 1973), (2) by an accumulation of lactic acid in the blood (Kay and Shephard, 1969), and (3) by a large increase of blood flow at the end of effort (Barcroft and

Dornhorst, 1949). With sustained isometric exercise, the only possible basis of meeting the oxygen needs of the muscles is to increase the mean arterial pressure and thus the effective pressure driving blood through the contracting tissues.

If the muscular effort is relatively weak, the rise of blood pressure may be sufficient to maintain the blood flow to the muscle. The critical force of contraction where the circulation is first impeded can be determined by observing the ability to sustain contractions of differing intensity; if the blood supply is adequate, fatigue does not occur for many minutes (Royce, 1959; Röhmert, 1960, 1968; Shephard, 1974e). The findings are essentially similar for small muscles (such as those concerned in the hand grip) and large muscles (such as those concerned in extension of the knee joint). Contraction at less than 10% of maximum force can be sustained almost indefinitely. Some limitation is first seen at 15% of maximum force, and at 20% of maximum the endurance time is shortened to 4-6 minutes. At 50% of maximum, the contraction can be held for only 1-2 minutes. With a further increase to 70% of maximum force, the contraction is apparently sufficiently powerful to stop all arterial flow to the muscle, since the time to fatigue is no longer shortened by mechanical compression of the artery external to the muscle.

Lind and his colleagues have made extensive measurements of limb flow, blood pressure, and cardiac output during isometric exercise (Lind and McNicol, 1967). Their observations confirm and extend the empirical deductions made by Royce (1959) and Röhmert (1960, 1968) on the basis of times to fatigue. Some rise of mean arterial tension occurs even with weak isometric contractions, but if the intensity of effort is less than 15% of maximum voluntary force, a new and higher equilibrium is soon reached; this is sufficient to maintain the supply of blood to the muscles. No equilibrium is possible during more vigorous efforts; the blood pressure continues to rise until the point of fatigue is reached. The terminal blood pressure (systolic 220-240 mm Hg, 29-31 kPa; diastolic 120-140 mm Hg, 16-18 kPa) is relatively constant in a given individual, but with more vigorous contractions the rate of rise of pressure is faster and the time to fatigue is shorter. The stimulus to the rise of blood pressure is apparently some by-product of activity that accumulates within the muscles. The response is unaltered if the outflow of blood from the active muscles is blocked by a cuff, but it is abolished when the sensory nerves are destroyed (as in the disease syringomyelia). The precise chemical nature of the stimulus has yet to be determined. Lind and McNicol (1967) argued that the time relationships of the rise in blood pressure were well matched by the efflux of potassium ions from the active muscle; this seems a plausible explanation, since the potassium ion is also a prime candidate for the mediation of local vascular dilatation within contracting muscle (Haddy and Scott, 1975). Other possible stimuli, such as oxygen lack, carbon dioxide excess, and lactate accumulation, all seem 'out of phase' with the changes in blood pressure (Duling and Pittman, 1975). However, the phase relationships have to date been studied for venous blood samples, and this does not necessarily indicate conditions at receptor sites within the muscles.

The heart rate and blood pressure often return to their resting value within one minute of ceasing an isometric contraction, but blood flow is increased for the first 10–15 minutes of the recovery period, and even an hour later the time to fatigue of the muscle concerned is still substantially shorter than normal. Exhaustion is due to an accumulation of anaerobic metabolites rather than to total usage of glycogen reserves; nevertheless, a series of 10–12 fatiguing contractions greatly deplete muscle stores of carbohydrate (Shephard, 1974e).

The rise of blood pressure during an isometric contraction does not lead to an excessive blood flow through inactive tissues, since these are protected by reflex adjustments in the calibre of their arterial vessels. However, there are two exceptions: the weakly contracting muscle and the brain. If a muscle is contracting weakly, then its blood supply can be improved by the more vigorous isometric contraction of a second muscle elsewhere in the body; the response to the contraction of several muscles is not additive, but rather coincides with that produced by the most vigorous contraction when this occurs alone. The blood supply to the brain is regulated more by arterial pressure than by changes in the calibre of its vascular supply. Thus any points of weakness in the brain vessels must bear the immediate brunt of the rise of pressure induced by static exercise. However, if the contraction is sustained, the pressure soon rises inside the skull, so that the risk of cerebral vessel rupture returns to its normal level.

Rhythmic exercise may give rise to some oxygen lack in the most active muscles, particularly if the effort is intense, rest periods are short, and perfusion pressures are reduced by holding the active part above the heart. As the exercise is continued, the muscle concerned becomes painful or weak, and if the total bulk of active tissue is sufficient, an accumulation of lactate can be demonstrated in the blood stream, with an accompanying disproportionate increase of ventilation (Issekutz et al., 1962; Shephard, 1975d). Following exercise, the blood flow is greatly increased for several minutes. However, the cumulative oxygen debt is usually insufficient to cause a substantial rise of mean arterial blood pressure. The systolic pressure rises because of the increase in cardiac output, but the diastolic pressure either remains constant or declines (Figure 34).

The potentially harmful effects of isometric exercise arise in part from the stress that the rise of arterial pressure places upon the walls of the blood vessels, and in part from the resultant large increase in the work of the heart. Since the rise in blood pressure is a progressive phenomenon, fatalities are most common when work with a substantial isometric element (such as carrying a heavy suitcase or shovelling snow) has been performed for a substantial time. In the context of training, prolonged isometric contractions are not necessary. As with other forms of training, duration is less important to the development of strength than is the intensity of effort. Hettinger (1961) suggested that strength could be developed by holding a contraction at 70% of maximum voluntary force for only six seconds per day. While this conclusion is not yet universally accepted (Rasch, 1964; 1971), it does suggest the possibility of carrying out isometric training for strength (if not endurance) without causing a disastrous rise of blood pressure.

Isometric exercise and endurance fitness

The development of muscular strength has very little influence upon cardio-respiratory performance. Nagle and Irwin (1960) trained 40 students for eight weeks, using a high and low resistance weight-lifting program. At the end of this period, the students' performance on a bicycle ergometer test was unchanged relative to a control group who had engaged simply in light recreational activity.

In some circumstances, isometric training may even have a negative impact on cardio-respiratory health. A subject may feel he has done his duty by fitness once he has completed a brief muscle-building routine, dissipating time and interest that should have been directed to cardio-respiratory endurance work. Furthermore, if muscle weight is increased without parallel development of the cardio-respiratory system, the aerobic power per unit of body weight is inevitably diminished.

The absence of any cardio-respiratory benefits from isometric training is hardly surprising in view of the low oxygen cost of such activity. Josenhans (1967) made a detailed study of knee extension. His subjects were able to extend both knees with a force of 40 kg (30% of maximum voluntary contraction) for a total of 150 seconds. The over-all oxygen cost of this exertion was about 2.3 litres, less than 1 l. min^{-1}, and only about a third of aerobic power. The same subjects could have developed a similar oxygen consumption by climbing the standard double 9-inch (22.9-cm) step only 11 or 12 times per minute. Although the final heart rates were quite rapid in reaction to compression of the muscle vessels, the same amount of isotonic work could have been performed at a steady heart rate of 100–105 beats per minute; such exercise is plainly insufficient to produce cardio-respiratory training even in sedentary subjects.

The need for muscle

The average sedentary worker rarely taxes his arm and shoulder muscles. Development of bulk in this region looks impressive, but it merely presents the body with an added burden, to be carried by what is often a rather poor and inadequate cardio-respiratory system.

Is the same true for the endurance athlete? A coach will commonly point to the swaying figure of a tired distance runner, and comment that if the muscles in the upper part of the body were better developed, the effort wasted by the swaying motion could be put to more effective use. However, the conclusion seems unjustified. Even if the shoulder muscles are weak, the fraction of their total power used in controlling posture is small and unlikely to compromise their blood supply. Body sway reflects general circulatory inadequacy, and can be remedied only by improving the function of the cardio-respiratory system.

A more important argument in favour of some muscle development is that a heavy course of endurance training can lead to a substantial loss of strength in muscles not heavily involved in the prime activity (Shephard, Campbell, et al., 1974; Wright, Nicoletti, and Shephard, 1976). Some long distance runners apparently have almost no muscle in the upper half of their bodies. This may help them to win specific competitions, but seems undesirable from the viewpoint of general health. Strong muscles can also enhance the speed of the thrower and the sprinter, and give an ability to sustain fast throwing over a long period (Clarke, 1974).

In certain forms of endurance exercise such as hand-cranking and cycling, the end-point tends to be local weakness and fatigue of the muscles (page 114). A fair proportion of the total muscle mass is involved in both forms of exercise, but electromyography shows that an undue proportion of the work load is carried by one specific muscle group, the biceps and the quadriceps respectively. These muscles are exercised at such a fraction of their maximum voluntary force that the local circulation is limited during their contraction phase; the deficit of blood flow cannot be made good during the remainder of the movement cycle, and lactic acid accumulates. Strengthening of the biceps and quadriceps may thus be helpful to the performance of these types of exercise, permitting the subject to reach a work load where the cardio-respiratory system is fully taxed before local circulatory problems arise. If the muscles are stronger, it may also be possible to sustain submaximum exercise for a much longer period; this could be one reason why training often leads to only a small improvement of maximum oxygen intake but a large improvement of endurance time.

Several practical applications of these findings may be noted. With an arm-specific sport such as swimming, the maximum oxygen intake developed in the water is usually lower than that measured on the treadmill (P-O. Åstrand, Engstrom, et al., 1963). However, the top-level athlete with optimal development of his arm muscles comes very close to the treadmill figure while he is swimming (J.F. Faulkner, 1966; Holmer, 1972). One useful measure of training in such sports is thus the proportion of the treadmill aerobic power that can be developed under competitive conditions.

Cardiac patients who use their arms at work may find that such activity is provoking anginal pain or is causing severe ST segmental depression of the electrocardiogram. A return to previous employment may then be helped by exercises to strengthen the working muscles.

Finally, the development of specific muscles can minimize the risk of injury. In some situations such as in contact sports, physical bulk can protect a joint (Ryan, 1960), but more commonly the muscle is required to play an active role. Development of the knee and ankle muscles, for example, decrease the chances of injuring these joints (K.K. Klein, 1959). Again, if sedentary subjects are required to lift a heavy load, weakness of the spinal muscles can predispose to prolapse of an inter-vertebral disc, while weakness of the abdominal muscles increases the risk of hernia formation (J.R. Brown, 1958, 1972; Alston et al., 1966; Magora and Taustein, 1969).

11
The use of drugs and
related procedures

It is now well documented that smoking in general, and cigarette consumption in particular has an adverse long-term effect upon health (National Health and Welfare, Canada, 1964; U.S. Public Health Service, 1964, 1967; Terry, 1967, 1970; Royal College of Physicians, 1971). The risk of developing respiratory ailments (chronic bronchitis, emphysema, and asthma), cardiovascular diseases (coronary and other forms of atheroma, thrombo-angiitis obliterans, and hypertension) and cancer (carcinoma of the mouth, larynx, bronchi, and bladder) are all increased in direct proportion to the daily consumption of cigarettes. The harmful effects of urban air pollutants and many industrial dusts such as asbestos, cotton dust, and uranium are greatly enhanced in the smoker (Gilson, 1973; Merchant et al., 1973; Meurman et al., 1974). In women, the possibility of premature birth and other perinatal complications is increased by smoking (Meyer et al., 1974), and the growth of their children is impaired for at least 11 years (Butler and Goldstein, 1973). Thus, in the sense that smoking interferes with normal growth and increases the chance of disease, it has an adverse influence upon the fitness of the individual. Unfortunately, many people have little interest in avoiding illness 20 or 30 years hence; when considering whether to smoke or not, they are concerned with more immediate rewards (Shephard et al., 1973c), particularly the immediate effects of their habit upon health and fitness.

The experience of trainers has varied (Karpovich and Hale, 1951). Some have found non-smokers to be more proficient athletes than smokers, especially in endurance events; others have found no adverse effect in sportsmen who smoked frequently and openly or occasionally and surreptitiously. Direct experiment is difficult; persistent smokers cannot be trusted to abandon their habit, and even if it were justifiable to ask non-smokers to smoke, it would be difficult to persuade them to inhale. Karpovich and Hale concluded that the endurance time was a little shorter immediately following the smoking of one or two cigarettes, but that in many individuals the loss of performance was small and statistically insignificant. Glassford and Howell (1969) had their subjects perform a standard treadmill task (uphill running); again, the endurance of the smokers (13 minutes) was a little shorter than that of the non-smokers (16 minutes).

The physiological responses to cigarette smoke are such that some immediate deterioration of cardio-respiratory fitness would be anticipated. Factors to be considered include the formation of a compound between carbon monoxide and haemoglobin (carboxyhaemoglobin), an increase of heart rate, a constriction of peripheral blood vessels, and bronchial spasm.

Formation of carboxyhaemoglobin
The blood level of carboxyhaemoglobin is substantially increased in the smoker. Police officers, customs officers, parking garage attendants, and others exposed to automobile exhaust (Ramsey, 1967; Godin et al., 1972; Wright et al., 1975) often claim they are being poisoned by vehicular fumes, but personal air pollution by the cigarette is responsible for at least three-fourths of the carboxyhaemoglobin found in the blood of those who smoke cigarettes (Lawther, 1967; Rode et al., 1972). In closed cars and poorly ventilated public buildings the accumulation of cigarette smoke can even increase carboxyhaemoglobin levels in non-smokers (Sebben et al., 1976; Pimm and Shephard, 1976). Assuming that there is no further exposure to cigarette smoke or other high concentrations of carbon monoxide, about a half of the retained carbon monoxide is eliminated from the blood stream within three to four hours (Goldsmith et al., 1963; Rode et al., 1972; Godin and Shephard, 1972). The concentration of carboxyhaemoglobin is thus a useful guide to recent smoking history; in a heavy smoker, figures of 5-10% are common (Table 29). If an infra-red carbon monoxide analyser is available, the blood carboxyhaemoglobin level can be estimated very simply by the brief rebreathing of oxygen. Application of this technique to a group of 180 patients who claimed to have given up smoking showed that almost 10% of the sample were untruthful. When confronted with the objective evidence of their misdeeds, the majority of the group admitted that they had not wished to disappoint the clinic staff by reporting an inability to conquer their cigarette addiction.

Carbon monoxide has approximately 200 times the affinity of oxygen for haemoglobin. Unless there is a compensatory increase in the haemoglobin reading, the effective oxygen-carrying capacity of the blood (λ) is thus reduced by 5-10% in the cigarette smoker. The curve relating the oxygen content of the air to the oxygen content of the blood (the oxygen dissociation curve) is also displaced to

TABLE 29

Blood levels of carboxyhaemoglobin (smoking prohibited for 1½ hours before testing)

	Group A (n = 18)	Group B (n = 10)	Group C (n =10)	Group D (n = 34)	Group E Boys (n = 33)	Group E Girls (n = 35)
First visit	4.34 ± 2.29%	1.31 ± 0.65%	2.69 ± 1.82%	5.05 ± 2.34%	1.12% ± 0.48	1.09% ± 0.29
Second visit	1.80 ± 1.70%	0.83 ± 0.31%	4.77 ± 1.64%	5.41 ± 2.46%	–	–

Group A. Smoking at first visit, not smoking one year later.
Group B. Gave up smoking 1–3 days before first visit, not smoking one year later.
Group C. Gave up smoking 1–3 days before first visit, reverted to smoking one year later.
Group D. Smoking at both visits.
Group E. School children aged 10–12 (omitting two who confessed to smoking).
Data obtained by author and his associates at Riverdale Smoking Withdrawal Centre and University of Toronto.

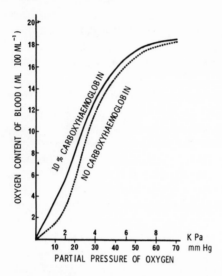

Figure 39 The influence of carbon monoxide exposure on the solubility of oxygen in the blood (after Åstrup et al., 1966).

the left following exposure to carbon monoxide (Figure 39). Given a fixed extraction of oxygen from the blood (Astrup et al., 1966), the effect of this displacement is to decrease the tissue oxygen pressure, thus increasing the chance that symptoms of oxygen lack may develop in the active tissues and in the heart muscle. Finally, the red pigment of the muscles (myoglobin) is also poisoned by carbon monoxide; the rate of saturation and desaturation is slower than for haemoglobin (Godin and Shephard, 1972), but ultimately some 10% of the inhaled carbon monoxide is found in the muscle pigment. The oxygen-storing capacity of the muscle fibres is thus reduced, and there is a corresponding decrease in the ability of the subject to make sudden and powerful movements.

From the basic conductance equations (page 68), it follows that a change in λ due to the formation of carboxyhaemoglobin produces an almost proportionate decrease in the maximum oxygen intake (Apthorp et al., 1958; Ekblom and Huof, 1972; Pirnay, Dujardin, et al., 1972a; Vogel and Gleser, 1972). Conversely, a few hours of abstinence from cigarettes leads to a 5-10% gain in endurance fitness.

Circulation

Changes in the responses of the heart and blood vessels following smoking are generally attributed to absorption of nicotine. A traditional 1-g cigarette contained some 20 mg of nicotine; of this total, 2-3 mg was volatilized and about 1 mg was absorbed in the lungs (Comroe, 1964). Several countries now require cigarette manufacturers to specify the average nicotine yield of their cigarettes, and in consequence new brands have been introduced with the nicotine yield cut to about 1 mg. The smoking public fondly imagine they are using safer cigarettes. However, since they are usually addicted to the nicotine, they either take more puffs per cigarette or smoke a larger total number of low nicotine cigarettes (Russell et al., 1975), the latter possibility being of some interest to the manufacturers! Further, a low nicotine cigarette does not yield a low concentration of carbon monoxide, and since it is likely this gas that causes atherosclerosis (Wald et al., 1973), the last state of the 'safe' smoker may be worse than the first.

Comroe (1964) has argued that the absorbed fraction of nicotine acts mainly upon the chemosensitive tissues of the carotid body, but the more usually accepted explanation of immediate circulatory changes is that nicotine releases the hormone noradrenaline (Burn, 1960), both locally (in the heart muscle and the walls of the blood vessels) and more generally (by stimulating the rate of secretion from the adrenal medulla).

In the resting subject, the smoking of a single cigarette produces quite marked changes. The heart rate is increased by 15–20 beats per minute and there is an associated rise of cardiac output and systemic blood pressure (Thomas et al., 1956; Regan et al., 1961; Irving and Yamamoto, 1963). Blood flow to the skin is diminished, particularly if the rate of smoking is rapid (Shepherd, 1951), while the flow to the muscles is increased (Rottenstein et al., 1960). Finally, the increased level of circulating noradrenaline makes the heart muscle more irritable, so that the heavy smoker is liable to abnormalities of cardiac rhythm. All of these disturbances are reversed progressively over some six hours of abstinence (Rode et al., 1972).

The net effect of the immediate circulatory changes is to increase the work of the heart. The rise in mean blood pressure initially yields a matching increase of coronary flow; however, the latter is not sustained, perhaps because smoking stimulates the secretion of vasopressin, a posterior pituitary hormone that constricts the coronary vessels (Regan et al., 1961). Thus, if the blood flow to the heart muscle is already compromised by coronary atherosclerosis, smoking can enhance the tendency to oxygen lack; possible manifestations include a deterioration of contractility in the heart muscle (negative inotropic effect), electrocardiographic changes (depression of the ST segment), and cardiac (anginal) pain (Aronow et al., 1974). Under resting conditions, acute changes are not seen in the average patient, but they are readily revealed by having the subject exercise.

Exercise itself stimulates the secretion of noradrenaline, and perhaps for this reason some of the acute effects of smoking are less obvious in an active subject. The heart rate averages about 5 beats per minute faster in the smoker than in the non-smoker at a given intensity of moderate work (Chevalier et al., 1963; Blackburn et al., 1960); however, the difference is by no means consistent, and in maximal effort the heart rate is the same in smokers and non-smokers. As under resting conditions, the effects upon the performance of submaximum work disappear with about six hours of abstinence from cigarettes (Rode et al., 1972). There is some evidence that the oxygen debt is larger in smokers than in non-smokers (Chevalier et al., 1963). However, it is difficult to interpret this finding as a pharmacological response to nicotine, since the acute effect of smoking is to increase rather than to decrease muscle blood flow. Furthermore, if a smoker is persuaded to exercise immediately following inhalation from one or two cigarettes, his oxygen debt is no different from that observed in a comparable experiment after abstinence from tobacco (Henry and Fitzhenry, 1950). Thus, it has yet to be proved that the difference in debt is due to smoking as such; if confirmed, it may reflect a long-term adverse effect on the blood supply to the leg muscles.

We may therefore conclude that although the smoking of one or two cigarettes can produce striking physiological changes during rest and submaximum exercise, these changes have no acute influence upon the circulatory component of endurance fitness apart from a possible increase in the size of the oxygen debt. Smoking affects the circulatory component mainly through long-term effects on the calibre of the blood vessels supplying the heart and skeletal muscle (Herbert, 1975).

Respiratory function

Tobacco smoke depresses the function of the cilia lining the trachea, increases mucus secretion by the goblet cells, and causes a variable amount of bronchial spasm. The cilia show a transient phase of stimulation, and their rate of movement is then depressed for 30 or 40 minutes (Dalhamn, 1966; Camner et al., 1973; Thomson and Pavia, 1973; Wanner et al., 1973); the removal of mucus and particulate matter from the airway is thus slowed. This has no direct influence upon endurance fitness, but if the particles include viruses, bacteria, cancer-producing tars, or harmful industrial dusts such as asbestos, health can be adversely affected; colds, for example, cause symptoms for 36 days in smokers, but only 17 days in non-smokers (British Medical Journal, 1974). The increased secretion of mucus by goblet cells lining the airway (Reid, 1960; Ebert and Terracio, 1975) is widely recognized as the 'smoker's cough' of the early chronic bronchitic; again, this has no acute influence upon endurance fitness, although in the long term the poor gas mixing and obstructed airways of chronic chest disease lead to a marked loss of cardio-respiratory performance (Mertens et al., 1976; Shephard, 1976f).

Bronchial spasm does not seem a specific effect of nicotine; a similar increase of airway resistance is produced by both normal (2%) and low (0.5%) nicotine content cigarettes (Comroe, 1964); the spasm is readily reversed by subcutaneous injections of atropine (Sterling, 1967) and enhanced by propranolol (Zuskin et al., 1974). It may be either a reflex response to the dense cloud of particles in cigarette smoke (Dautrebande and DuBois, 1958; McDermott, 1962), or an effect of irritant aldehydes found in the vapour phase of the smoke (Guillerm et al., 1972). The intensity of response probably varies with the sensitivity of the individual's bronchi (Gayrard et al., 1974), but in a normal (non-allergic) subject it is usual to find an immediate doubling of airway resistance, with a gradual return to normal over the next 30 or 40 minutes. A change in airflow resistance of this order has little practical significance for the resting subject; breathing does not seem difficult until the airway resistance is four or five times normal. On the other hand, during maximum exercise the work of breathing accounts for at least 10% of the total oxygen consumed (Shephard, 1966e); if the airway resistance is doubled, there is an almost proportionate increase in the oxygen cost of respiration (Rode and Shephard, 1971b) and a corresponding decrease in the oxygen available for external work. In the young smoker the added cost is resolved by a couple of days of abstinence from cigarettes, but with a longer history of smoking chronic bronchitis persists, and it may then take several years of abstinence for the oxygen cost of breathing to drop to the level of a non-smoker.

Tobacco particles are so fine (average size about 0.25 μ) that they penetrate to the smaller branches of the bronchial tree. Modern tests of small-airway function such as the frequency dependence of lung compliance, the critical closing volume, and modification of airflow by helium/oxygen mixtures (Dosman et al., 1975; Martin, Lindsay, et al., 1975) suggest that the prime site of spasm is in the small muscular bronchioles. Since these contribute relatively little to the total airway resistance, the disturbance of lung function is rather greater than the doubling of resistance might suggest. Gas distribution is impaired by the narrowing of the small airways (Wilson et al., 1960; Ross et al., 1967), and this increases the dead space/tidal volume ratio, making a given ventilation less effective in terms of gas exchange. Chronic exposure to cigarette smoke over many years can lead to gross abnormalities of gas distribution, but in an acute sense the influence of small-airway spasm upon endurance fitness is less important, since ventilation contributes relatively little to the over-all conductance of oxygen (Chapter 3).

Weight control
Many women claim that they smoke mainly to curb their appetite. There is some physiological basis for this claim, since hunger is associated with a falling blood sugar, and nicotine injection produces a temporary increase of blood sugar. It is less certain that the nicotine mechanism retains its effectiveness when it is used

TABLE 30

Maximum oxygen intake, skinfold thickness, body weight, and smoking

Group	Maximum oxygen intake l.min^{-1} STPD			ml kg^{-1} min^{-1}			Skinfold thickness (total, 8 folds, mm)			Body weight (kg)		
	First visit	Second visit	Difference	First visit	Second visit	Difference	First visit	Second visit	Difference	First visit	Second visit	Difference
A (n = 18)	2.76 ±0.54	2.79 ±0.64	+0.03 ±0.39	34.5 ±5.2	32.2 ±7.9	-2.3 ±5.4	107.8 ±38.9	146.5 ±54.6	+38.7 ±33.0	81.2 ±12.5	85.5 ±14.1	+4.3 ±4.0
B (n = 10)	3.02 ±0.47	2.85 ±0.42	-0.17 ±0.40	40.9 ±7.7	35.4 ±5.6	-5.5 ±6.2	93.1 ±29.2	148.1 ±41.5	+55.0 ±28.7	75.6 ±8.1	81.7 ±6.8	+6.1 ±2.0
C (n = 10)	2.66 ±0.57	2.62 ±0.57	-0.04 ±0.36	35.6 ±7.7	34.4 ±6.7	-1.2 ±3.9	87.4 ±26.1	98.5 ±25.8	+11.2 ±11.5	75.3 ±9.9	76.4 ±10.1	+1.1 ±2.7
D (n = 34)	2.61 ±0.44	2.65 ±0.46	+0.04 ±0.33	36.5 ±6.7	36.4 ±6.9	-0.1 ±4.6	94.1 ±40.8	112.9 ±46.3	+18.8 ±27.0	72.4 ±9.8	73.7 ±9.8	+1.3 ±2.5

Group A. Smoking at first visit, not smoking one year later.
Group B. Gave up smoking 1-3 days before first visit, not smoking one year later.
Group C. Gave up smoking 1-3 days before first visit, reverted to smoking one year later.
Group D. Smoking at both visits.
Data obtained by author and his associates at Riverdale Smoking Withdrawal Centre, Toronto.

40 or 50 times per day. However, in one cross-sectional study (Khosla and Lowe, 1972), 40-year-old non-smokers were on average 5.4 kg heavier than smokers of the same age. Again, there is often a substantial rise of body weight (Table 30) and parallel increments in skinfold readings within a few months of giving up smoking. It is tempting to invoke as an explanation the need to reset hypothalamic blood sugar regulating mechanisms that are no longer repeatedly bombarded with nicotine. However, other factors are also involved. As the taste-buds of the tongue recover from chronic nicotine poisoning, even ordinary items of food gain a long-forgotten piquancy, while the psychological cravings previously satisfied by cigarettes are commonly transferred to other indulgences such as chocolates.

From the viewpoint of endurance fitness, the early increase of body weight soon counterbalances any gain of maximum oxygen intake due to reduction of blood carboxyhaemoglobin level, so that the aerobic power per unit of body weight remains constant or may even diminish (Rode et al., 1972). However, if the patient is not discouraged by this development, a new balance is soon established between activity and food intake, and once the cigarette habit has been firmly abandoned any gain in weight can also be corrected. The need seems to be a concerted approach to life-style modification. Smoking, diet, exercise, and the psychological approach to the demands of work and leisure are all related items, and for a successful reduction of coronary risk all must be treated in a coordinated manner. It is also worth emphasizing that although fat reduces life expectancy (Table 38), a moderate increase of body weight is far less lethal than the continued consumption of cigarettes.

ALCOHOL

It has been recognized for many years that persistent heavy drinking can have an adverse effect upon the health of the liver, the central nervous system, and the heart muscle. The typical victim, such as the alcoholic clergyman in a poor parish, spends a major part of his income on alcohol, and the main basis of tissue malfunction is nutritional. The energy requirements of the body are met by alcohol instead of food, and there is a serious shortage of vitamins, particularly vitamin B_1.

Such patients obviously have a poor cardio-respiratory performance. In the heavy drinker who still maintains a reasonably balanced diet, obesity is a common problem. The tippler eats equally with his friends, but fails to take account of the energy content of his liquid refreshment. Further, a drowsy state is induced by his heavy lunchtime session at the bar, and while his friends enjoy a brisk noon-hour walk, the drinker is often reduced to a low level of activity.

Moderate amounts of alcohol produce a dilatation of the blood vessels in the skin, but the blood flow to muscle is either unchanged (Gillespie, 1967) or reduced (Graf and Ström, 1960). The heart rate and cardiac output may thus be greater than normal at rest and during moderate exercise, both immediately after the ingestion of alcohol (Hebbelinck, 1959; Blomqvist et al., 1970) and during any subsequent 'hangover' (Karvinen et al., 1962). However, the anticipated response is by no means consistently reported (Garlind et al., 1960; Wendt et al., 1966; Gould, 1970), and one may suspect that in a subject who is initially nervous the local circulatory effects of alcohol are outweighed by its depressant action on the higher centres of the brain. During heavy exercise the skin vessels are dilated without alcohol, so that in these circumstances small amounts of the drug are unlikely to influence either the magnitude or the distribution of cardiac output. During maximum effort, Blomqvist et al. (1970) found no alcohol-induced change of maximum heart rate, stroke volume, or arterio-venous oxygen difference. While animal experiments suggest that large doses of alcohol can impair the contractility of the heart muscle (Gould, 1970), the response to doses encountered in industry and in competitive performance falls more in the realm of the psychologist than the physiologist.

Alcohol depresses brain function. It is thus sometimes taken by athletes to counteract the excessive arousal produced by international competition. As such, it has been regarded as a form of 'doping,' and two Swedish pistol shooters were disqualified on this count in the Mexico City Olympics. While confidence is increased, skill, judgment, and reaction time are impaired, and loss of neuromuscular control may give a less efficient pattern of movement (M.H. Williams, 1974). The relative importance of these various changes depends on the nature of the performance subsequently expected of the subject, and since both the taste and the likely effects of alcohol are universally known, it is almost impossible to carry out controlled experiments. Some authors have hypothesized that by releasing inhibitions alcohol might improve the force of brief muscular movements and extend the time to fatigue in endurance work; however, laboratory experiments do not support these views (Asmussen and Bøje, 1948; Williams, 1974). In field tests, Hebbelinck (1963) noted a 10% deterioration in times for an 80-metre dash 30 minutes after drinking a small quantity of alcohol, but it is difficult to be certain that the subjects did not 'wish' this effect upon themselves.

The combination of vasodilatation and mild sedation after ingestion of alcohol leads to a decrease of resting systemic blood pressure. This may reduce the chance of a vascular accident in a tense, anxious patient, and thus it could be argued that the taking of a small dose of alcohol has improved health. However, it is dangerous to treat anxiety by a dependence-inducing drug, particularly when the patient has unlimited access to the proposed remedy. Anxiety and tension can probably be relieved with greater benefit to the individual by the taking of a few minutes of vigorous exercise.

Provided that the specific hazard of obesity is avoided, we may conclude that moderate amounts of alcohol have little influence upon endurance fitness. Men will continue to regard alcohol as a mocker or the gift of the gods; their decision between these opposing verdicts must be based on the statistics for alcoholism (2-6% incidence among North American adults) and traffic accidents (alcohol implicated in more than 50% of incidents) rather than upon any supposed effects of alcohol upon cardio-respiratory performance.

'ERGOGENIC AIDS'

We have already discussed the search for a diet that would improve endurance and thus the performance of the athlete in distance events (Chapter 9). The rules of most sports meetings are such that drugs may be supplied only to prevent or alleviate disease. Nevertheless, incidents have arisen in a number of international competitions where contestants were persuaded to take various potent drugs in the belief that their performance would be improved thereby.

d-Amphetamine

One of the more commonly used illicit pills has been 'dexedrine,' properly described as *d*-amphetamine (Golding, 1972; Dirix, 1973; Shephard, 1976c). This compound is one of a series of synthetic products with some structural similarity to adrenaline:

$$CH(OH)-CH_2-\overset{H}{N}-CH_3 \qquad CH_2CH(NH_2)CH_3$$

ADRENALINE   AMPHETAMINE

Until prescription was controlled, the drug was widely used by physicians to suppress appetite. Small quantities of amphetamines are still found in some self-administered remedies for the common cold where they are mixed with antihistamines to counteract the depressant effect of the latter class of drug. One Canadian bronze medallist in the Mexico City Pan-American games (1975) was disqualified on the grounds that she had treated a cold with a mixture containing the related drug phenylephrine two days before her race.

Administration of d-amphetamine alone increases the arousal of the subject, and excessive doses lead to sleeplessness and a confused mental state. The resting systemic blood pressure is raised, through a diminution in the circulation to the skin and an increase in the tone of the venous reservoirs. These are effects that some have thought might improve physical performance. However, in sustained near-maximal exercise, the blood flow to the skin is required for heat dissipation, and any restriction of such flow exposes the athlete to a dangerous heat stress (Hardinge and Peterson, 1964; Shephard, 1976c). Further, even if such medication were permitted in a contest, there is no good reason to suppose that an improvement of performance would result. A wide variety of amines were tested during World War II, when the experts of aviation medicine were seeking a wonder drug for pilots exposed to added gravitational stress. The plan was to augment the tone of the leg veins, but after exhaustive trials it was concluded that none of the drugs examined were of benefit (Stewart, 1941). Both exercise (Von Euler and Hellner, 1952; Von Euler, 1974) and gravitational stress stimulate the natural secretion of adrenaline and noradrenaline, and it would be surprising if the introduction of additional amines into the body were to benefit performance.

Athletes are very open to suggestion, and in some experiments claiming improvement of performance by drugs such as d-amphetamine, controls were plainly inadequate. Equally dramatic changes are sometimes produced by a bland lactose tablet! When appropriate controls have been arranged, d-amphetamine has had no effect on maximum oxygen intake or maximum heart rate (Margaria, Aghemo, and Novelli, 1964; Pirnay, Petit, et al., 1968b; Wyndham, Rogers, et al., 1971) and there has been little change in endurance performance (Karpovich, 1959; Golding and Barnard, 1963; Bättig, 1965). Such improvement as has been noted could result from the small gains in strength and vigilance that accompany greater arousal (Hurst et al., 1968) and from an elevation of mood that overcomes poor motivation and fatigue (Bättig, 1965); this last factor could account for reports that after amphetamine treatment there is a greater production of lactate in exhausting effort (Pirnay et al., 1968b; Hueting and Poulus, 1970).

Other stimulants of the central nervous system
Caffeine, one of the active compounds present in the tea and coffee, has a direct stimulating action on the central nervous system, increasing irritability, shortening reaction time, and relieving sensations of physical and mental fatigue. Muscle strength is also increased. Small doses have no effect on the circulation, but larger doses produce a general constriction of blood vessels and a rise of blood pressure. At the same time, the coronary blood flow is improved and the stroke volume of the heart is increased. It would seem that this class of compound inhibits the de-

struction of 3-5 cyclic adenosine monophosphate (AMP), a ubiquitous enzyme activator.

The older published data suggested that relatively large doses of the caffeine class of stimulants could increase physical performance (Weiss and Laties, 1962). Graf (1930), for example, reported that cola (a mixture of caffeine and the related compound theobromine) increased the work output on a bicycle ergometer by 20-30%, and Asmussen and Bøje (1948) concluded that caffeine was helpful in overcoming the inhibitory effects of fatigue in prolonged maximal effort. Some more recent experiments have failed to support these observations. Thus Margaria et al. (1964) found no changes of either maximum oxygen intake or endurance time when subjects were given 250 mg caffeine. Again, Ganslen et al. (1963) found no change in either aerobic power or the response to submaximal work when his subjects were given a small dose (200 mg) of caffeine. However, when the same dose was combined with another central nervous stimulant (400 mg metrazol), there was an increase of stroke volume during submaximum work and a small gain of aerobic power.

Attempts to regulate the use of caffeine and related stimulants is difficult, since they are present in so many beverages. A strong cup of coffee may well contain the average therapeutic dose of caffeine. Tea contains caffeine and the related compound theophylline. Cola, cocoa, and chocolate all contain theobromine. The simplest approach seems to be to allow athletes to drink as much as they wish of these compounds in beverage form, while prohibiting the administration of pharmacological preparations.

From the standpoint of the average citizen, interest has been aroused by reports that the risks of myocardial infarction are increased by drinking coffee. In one report, risks rose 60% with the drinking of one to five cups per day, and 120% with the drinking of more than six cups per day (Jick et al., 1973). An excessive consumption of coffee can give many of the symptoms of an anxiety state (British Medical Journal, 1975), including irritability, tremor, palpitations, an irregular pulse, disturbed sleep, and gastro-intestinal disturbances. However, it is difficult to be certain whether the heavy consumption of coffee is not itself a sign of an underlying disturbance of personality (Bishop and Reichert, 1970), and a single cup of coffee (158 mg of caffeine) produces only minimal changes in the performance of the heart in the post-coronary patient (Gould et al., 1973).

CAFFEINE   THEOPHYLLINE   THEOBROMINE

Cocaine is best known as a local anaesthetic. However, it also has a general stimulating effect on the central nervous system. The blood pressure, pulse, and respiration rate are increased, as are the blood sugar and body temperature; the last effect arises in part from constriction of blood vessels supplying the skin, and in part from a direct action on the temperature-regulating centres of the brain.

Cocaine is greatly valued by the natives of the Amazon valley and parts of Peru and Bolivia. It is obtained by chewing the leaves of the coca tree (*Erythroxylon coca*), and it has been reputed to permit great feats of endurance with little food or rest (Karpovich, 1959). However, as with so many supposed ergogenic aids, it is hard to duplicate these effects during moderate periods of exercise in the laboratory. Hanna (1970) studied both chewing and non-chewing Quechua Indians of Peru; his only findings were a higher heart rate in submaximal work and an insignificantly longer time to exhaustion when the subjects were chewing coca leaves. Older reports had suggested that small doses of cocaine increased both the capacity to sustain muscular work on an ergograph and endurance on the bicycle ergometer; however, the methodology of these experiments makes their interpretation suspect (M.H. Williams, 1974).

From the practical viewpoint, the dangers of addiction are such that cocaine is no longer used even as a local anaesthetic. It certainly has no role in attempts to improve human performance.

Drugs modifying the heart rate. Some authors have attached an almost mystical significance to the slow resting heart rate of the athlete. In the experimental animal, stimulation of the vagus nerve slows the heart, while stimulation of the sympathetic fibres causes cardiac acceleration. It has thus been postulated that the athlete has a high vagal tone (a frequent traffic of impulses passing down his vagus nerve), while the person who is unfit suffers from an excess of sympathetic tone (Raab, 1964; Raab and Krzywanek, 1966). Some have made a further daring leap of faith, and assumed that if the resting heart rate were slowed by a drug such as propranolol, which blocks the response of the heart muscle to sympathetic nerve impulses, an improvement of physical performance would result. Unfortunately for the men of faith, the eventual response of the heart to exercise is almost normal in dogs where both vagal and sympathetic nerves have been surgically excised (Donald and Shepherd, 1964). The whole fantasy of 'vagal tone' and the athlete thus seems unsound. Further, propranolol does more than slow the heart – it blocks the slow response of the remainder of the body to noradrenaline. Measurements of working capacity made after the administration of propranolol may thus show somewhat poorer performance than in the control state (Cumming and Carr, 1967); certainly, cardiac output is reduced, although the maximum oxygen intake measured during brief exhausting effort may be unchanged (P.O. Åstrand, Ekblom, and Goldberg, 1971).

Propranolol is commonly given to the post-coronary patient to reduce the frequency of abnormal heart rhythms. The failure of the heart rate to increase appreciably during exercise makes it difficult to use normal submaximum and maximum stress test protocols. One possibility is to arrange with the patient's physician for withdrawal of the drug prior to testing. However, this must be done gradually, as the sudden cessation of treatment can itself occasionally provoke ventricular fibrillation.

Digitalis

Digitalis and its purified derivatives digitoxin and digoxin are widely used for the clinical treatment of congestive heart failure. The active principle of the drug has several effects upon the heart muscle. The frequency of impulses generated at the cardiac pacemaker is decreased, and a partial blockage of conduction from the atrium to the ventricle further slows the heart rate. The force of individual contractions is increased, and the ventricles tend to empty more completely. In a patient with heart failure, administration of digitalis leads to an increase of both stroke volume and cardiac output, but in the normal subject resting cardiac output is diminished by 20–35% following digitalization.

There have been reports that the swimming time of rats with weighted tails is increased by administration of digitalis (Falkenhahn et al., 1967). However, therapeutic doses have no effect on either static muscular endurance or the performance of maximum work in normal, healthy subjects (Nordstrom-Ohrberg, 1964; Bruce et al., 1968). In addition, the drug is dangerous and potentially toxic, and there seems no justification in administering it to other than cardiac patients.

Buffers

The size of the oxygen debt is normally limited by the accumulation of lactic acid in the muscles and the bloodstream; a decrease of intra-muscular pH inhibits the enzymes involved in glycogen breakdown, with accompanying sensations of pain, fatigue, weakness, and breathlessness. It is therefore conceivable that, if the capacity of the tissues to buffer acid were increased, a larger oxygen debt could be accumulated, with a resulting gain of performance in exercise of brief duration.

A decrease of buffering capacity can certainly arise when a patient with poliomyelitis is overventilated in a Drinker respirator, or when a healthy young subject moves from sea level to high altitude. However, in both these cases, the ventilatory pace is forced over a long period. In the absence of ventilatory pacing, the acidity of the body fluids is closely regulated. If an 'alkali' such as sodium bicarbonate is given, the body quickly adjusts the excretion of carbon dioxide from the lungs and the reabsorption of bicarbonate ions in the distal tubes of the kidneys, so that any gain of buffering capacity is only transitory. An increase of tissue buffer capacity can further have an adverse effect upon oxygen transport, altering the sensitivity of the respiratory centres to carbon dioxide accumulation, and causing a leftward shift of the oxygen dissociation curve, thus hampering release of oxygen from the blood to the tissues. Nevertheless, early reports suggested that during the phase of acute alkalosis, substantial increases of oxygen debt (up to 20%) and endurance times could be demonstrated (Dill et al., 1932, Denning et al., 1931, 1937). In more recent experiments, the subjects have been well trained, and smaller doses of alkali have been administered much closer to the commencement of field (W. Johnson and Black, 1953) and laboratory (Margaria, Aghemo, and Sassi, 1971) tests. Under such circumstances, performance and blood lactate levels have remained unchanged.

Many interesting questions remain unanswered. Is it possible to boost the buffering capacity of the tissues naturally by repeated intensive exercise of the 'interval training' type? And if a natural increase is produced through a suitable training program, does this preclude additional benefit from deliberate ingestion of alkalis? Finally, can a more long-lasting change in buffering capacity be produced by administration of a less readily excreted organic buffer such as 'THAM' (tris-hydroxymethyl-aminomethane [Nahas, 1962])? If so, does this help performance, or are the gains in pH outweighed by the decrease in blood volume caused by the diuretic action of this compound?

'Anabolic' compounds
Most of the drugs so far discussed have a relatively brief period of action. However, certain anabolic compounds have been given to athletes for longer periods. The materials in question include the anabolic steroids and aspartates.

The best known of the anabolic steroids is testosterone, a male sex hormone secreted by the testes. Testosterone has two main effects: it causes the development of masculinity and it promotes the synthesis of protein within the body. Several synthetic derivatives of testosterone (methandrostenolone, 'Dianabol'; norethandrolone; oxandrolone) are now available. In these compounds, the masculinizing effects have been reduced and the protein-synthesizing (anabolic) effects have been enhanced (Fox et al., 1962). Compounds of this type are reputedly taken by a high proportion of strength athletes (Golding, 1972; Williams, 1974; Shephard, 1976c). It is likely that such drugs play a useful role in restoring the fitness of an older person whose muscles have wasted from prolonged bed rest, but it would be more surprising if the anabolic steroids were of benefit to young men whose testes are initially secreting a normal amount of testosterone.

Animal experiments (Murphy and Eagan, 1971; Brown and Pilch, 1972; Wydra, 1972) have generally shown no benefit from the administration of anabolic compounds. However, it has been argued that the type of exercise possible with small mammals (treadmill running or forced swimming) is not conducive to muscle building, and indeed often leads to a negative caloric balance. Some studies with human subjects (for example, Fowler et al., 1965; Fahey and Brown, 1972) have again shown no response. Other recent workers who have combined steroids with progressive resistance exercises and a high protein diet have succeeded in increasing both body weight (Casner et al., 1971; L.C. Johnson et al., 1972) and strength (Bowers and Reardon, 1972; Ariel, 1973). Part of the increase in weight is probably due to water retention (Casner et al., 1971), but there also appears to be an increase of muscle mass. This is without benefit in terms of the oxygen transporting system (Bowers and Reardon, 1972; Johnson et al., 1972), and competitive swimmers show no gains of speed or endurance (O'Shea and Winkler, 1970).

Since any gains of muscle mass persist for some time after the drugs have been discontinued, international regulation by athletic organizations is difficult. One proposal has called for weekly weight records on all strength competitors, with 'spot' checks of the urine where surprising gains are being registered.

The steroids are dangerous compounds. In young athletes, they can cause precocious puberty and premature closure of the epiphyses of the long bones. In the adult, they lead to testicular atrophy, depressed sperm counts, and occasional liver damage. Many athletes are well aware of these risks but yet fear that they will not succeed in international competition unless they also join the drug-taking craze.

TESTOSTERONE   METHANDROSTENOLONE   NORETHANDROLONE

Aspartic acid is a naturally occurring amino acid, and is thus on the border line between a drug and a food. It forms one of the links between protein and carbohydrate metabolism. If the diet contains adequate amounts of protein and carbohydrate, it is not immediately clear why the administration of an excess of this 'bridge' substance should be helpful. Golding (1972) has suggested it may help clearance of ammonia from the blood after effort. There have been reports that salts of aspartic acid extend the swimming times of rats (Rosen et al., 1962; Cutinelli et al., 1970) and relieve fatigue in man (Shaw et al., 1962), extending endurance times by up to 50% (Ahlborg et al., 1968), but others have been unable to confirm these observations (Consolazio et al., 1964; Fallis et al., 1963).

COOH
|
CH$_2$
| ASPARTIC ACID
CH(NH$_2$)
|
COOH

OXYGEN

It is well recognized that oxygen has a beneficial effect upon the performance of endurance exercise if it is administered during the working period. The heart rate and respiratory minute volume are decreased at any given submaximal work load. Maximum heart rate is unchanged, but the oxygen debt is diminished (Cunningham, 1966) and the duration of exhausting exercise can be extended by the use of oxygen mixtures (Asmussen and Nielsen, 1946; Miller, 1952; Bannister and Cunningham, 1954; Cunningham, 1966; Hagerman et al., 1968). These benefits are further extended if the oxygen is supplied at somewhat greater than atmospheric pressure (Taunton et al., 1970; Wyndham, Strydom, et al., 1970), although if the pressure is too high the negative effects of oxygen poisoning can lead to a deterioration of performance (Kaijser, 1970). The carriage of oxygen is not considered seriously for athletic events, but it has been used with substantial benefit by patients whose exercise tolerance is limited by chronic respiratory disease (Cotes, 1965).

Early work suggested that the administration of oxygen prior to exercise augmented performance. Thus Hill and Flack (1910) gave air or oxygen for a total of five minutes before a bout of stair-climbing. In the oxygen experiments there were gains in both endurance and the speed of pulse recovery, with a lessening of shortness of breath. The 1932 Japanese Olympic swimming team breathed oxygen before their races, apparently with great success, and stimulated by their victories Karpovich (1934) carried out further experiments, giving oxygen one, two or three minutes before a period of combined running and breath-holding. Considerable benefit was observed in the one-minute experiments and slight benefit in the two-minute tests, but there was no advantage when the oxygen was given three minutes before exercise.

More recently, Miller (1952) has argued that the apparent effects of oxygen have a psychological basis, since they can be reproduced by telling the athletes that they have inhaled oxygen. On theoretical grounds, it has been suggested that arterial blood is almost completely saturated with oxygen, and that any oxygen in the chest is eliminated within one or two breaths, so that the advantage to an athlete is inevitably dissipated before the start of a contest. The oxygen stored in lung gas is certainly lost very quickly. However, if the oxygen mixture has been inhaled for a substantial period of time, smaller quantities of oxygen are also stored in the blood and tissues. This additional gas, 80–100 ml in excess of normal body stores, is not eliminated for several minutes, and it can boost the total tissue oxygen expenditure by as much as 1% during the first minute of vigorous exercise, surely more than enough to influence the outcome of a closely matched contest.

Several investigators have shown that the administration of oxygen after exercise has no influence on the rate of recovery of heart rate, blood pressure, or blood lactate (Miller, 1952; Elbel et al., 1961; Bjorgum and Sharkey, 1966; Hagerman et al., 1968). The oxygen intake soon drops to 50% or less of the maximum oxygen intake during recovery, and it would be surprising if the facilitation of oxygen transport were helpful at this stage.

HYPNOSIS

Some authors have found that hypnotic suggestion of heavy exercise can induce increases of heart rate, ventilation, and oxygen consumption of the order anticipated for actual performance of the task (W.P. Morgan, 1972). Equally, suggestions of a heavy loading during effort can increase the heart rate and the perceived effort, delaying attainment of a steady state.

However, the effects on subsequent physical performance are much less clearly established. The current consensus seems that hypnosis usually has little influence on a well-trained and well-adjusted normal subject. On the other hand, the exercise tolerance of many less fit members of the community is limited by half-conscious fears, often dating back to childhood. Parents may have uttered solemn warnings about the dangers of straining the heart, or (in girls) of becoming too masculine and damaging the reproductive organs. If such fears can be resolved by hypnosis or other forms of psychotherapy, then the individual concerned will undoubtedly show a gain in both immediate effort tolerance and also in the capacity to accept a strenuous training regimen. Equally, hypnosis may be helpful in correcting the pre-competitive anxieties of an over-aroused athlete.

The fear of exercise is particularly strongly entrenched in patients who have sustained a myocardial infarction, and in the first year following the critical incident many patients respond as well to hypnotherapy as to a program of physical rehabilitation (Kavanagh, Shephard, et al., 1970).

12
A financial postscript

In this final chapter, we shall attempt to assess the cost of lack of endurance fitness to a 'western'-type nation. There are many imponderables in such an analysis, and the conclusions that can be drawn at the present time are somewhat tentative. Nevertheless, we live in an age when all national expenditures are increasingly judged in terms of their 'cost-effectiveness' (Dorfman, 1965), and the potential impact upon an economy of research and other support for a physical fitness campaign is an important question that merits careful consideration.

Much of the information to be presented refers to the United States. The reason for this bias is that the economic costs of chronic ill-health have been the subject of detailed scrutiny in that country (Klarman, 1964; DeBakey, 1965; Special Committee on Aging, 1966; Rice, 1967). Application of such findings to the economies of other nations (Shephard, 1974h) is complicated by some aging of the data themselves and by substantial differences in the age distribution of populations, the incidence and patterns of disease, the types and costs of medical care, and the levels of employment and productivity. Nevertheless, the total cost per capita in other western nations is unlikely to differ from the U.S. estimates by more than a factor of two or three.

CALCULATING THE COSTS OF ILL-HEALTH

Three main items must be evaluated: the morbidity and mortality rates for the disease in question, the direct costs of health care, and the indirect impact of mortality and morbidity upon the economy.

Rates of occurrence
It is by no means easy to establish the rate of occurrence of a disease process. A proportion of those affected may not realize that they are unwell or are wrongly informed regarding the nature of their illness, while a further substantial propor-

tion know they are unwell but fail to report their disability. If the usual type of household survey were carried out in a population of 1000 people, it has been estimated that 150 would have some type of heart disease, but only 60 of the 150 would report their illness (White and Ibrahim, 1963). The approach used in many U.S. studies has been to administer a standard one-visit medical examination to a representative sample of the population. The occurrence rate thus found is substantially higher than that obtained from household surveys, but unless precautions are taken to include elderly and institutionalized patients and exhaustive tests are applied, the prevalence of a given disease is still underestimated. Mortality figures can also be misleading. Thus, the frequency of coronary deaths can be somewhat overestimated from death certificates; if a middle-aged patient dies suddenly, and a post-mortem examination reveals no other disease process, it is common to attribute death to a coronary attack. Almost everyone over the age of 40 has some atheromatous disease of the coronary vessels, and should a pathologist wish to 'explain' the manner of death, he can usually find a suitable plaque to blame.

In 1967 it was estimated that 87 million of the U.S. population were affected by one or more forms of chronic illness, and of this total, 22.6 million had reported some limitation of activity (Rice, 1967). In the specific context of fitness, the group of greatest interest is patients with cardiovascular disease. A survey covering the period 1960 to 1962 reported that cardiovascular disease was definitely present in 13.2% of U.S. adults, and it was suspected in a further 11.7%; a high blood pressure (hypertension) or coronary atherosclerosis accounted for more than 90% of the cases with proven disease and over half of those where disease was suspected (DeBakey, 1965). Over the same period, a total of 968,000 U.S. citizens died of cardiovascular disease (DeBakey, 1965). Of these deaths, 599,000 were attributed to 'arteriosclerotic and other diseases of the heart,' 197,000 to strokes, and 75,000 to hypertension. A major part of both chronic ill-health and premature deaths is thus attributable to forms of cardiovascular disease where an increase of physical activity could conceivably be beneficial.

The annual incidence of 'heart attacks' in the United States has been set at about 700,000; 500,000 coronary patients die each year, 100,000 before a physician can be summoned (Haskell, 1968). Unfortunately, many coronary episodes occur at the most productive period of life, and each year 150,000 people in the U.S. die of coronary disease before they have reached the age of retirement (Rice, 1967).

Direct costs
The direct costs of ill-health include expenditures for personal services and supplies – hospital care, services of physicians and nurses, and provision of drugs – together with expenditures on non-personal items such as research, training, pub-

lic health services, capital construction, and insurance schemes. The U.S. figures for 1962 set the direct costs of cardiovascular disease at $3.07 billion, $2.58 billion for personal services and $0.49 billion for non-personal items. Hospital care accounted for a large proportion of the direct costs. Attempts to apportion hospital costs between the different forms of cardiovascular disease are not especially fruitful, because such expenses vary markedly with the intensity of care provided and the number of days of hospitalization required; a typical infarct patient may spend at least three weeks in hospital, at a cost of $100 or more per day. Nevertheless, direct costs are small relative to the indirect costs.

Indirect costs
The indirect costs of disease include losses of production due to ill-health, premature death, and grief. Several assumptions are necessary in putting a dollar figure to such losses. The services of a housewife must first be priced; in some surveys, the worth of a wife has been assumed equal to the average earnings of a full-time domestic servant, but this is certainly a conservative measure. The loss of output from an employed person must also be evaluated. This is usually set at the average income of the labour force; economists argue that for our present purpose the average personal income is a more realistic figure than a per capita proportion of the gross national product, since the latter includes also the workings of capital. Finally, the rate of employment of the labour force must be known; in the U.S. studies of the early 1960s, 96% was assumed, although under current conditions 93–94% might be more accurate.

In the case of premature death, account must also be taken of anticipated real gains in productivity (typically 1–2% per annum), and the bank rate or discount rate (5–7% in the early 1960s, currently higher; this figure expresses the relationship between the productivity of an investment and the reluctance of society to sacrifice current for future consumption). Most previous calculations have made no allowance for the potential consumption of goods and services by a person dying prematurely. However, it would seem an inescapable fact that if an equal number of productive years are lost, a person who is permanently crippled makes a greater charge upon the economy than a person who dies at an early age. Some economists go even further and argue that a fatal coronary attack at the age of 65 spares the economy a possible 20 or 30 years of pension payments plus final geriatric care!

It is particularly difficult to calculate the economic cost of pain, suffering, and orphanhood. Klarman (1964) estimated that the ravages of cardiovascular disease would cause 3% of children to become paternal orphans before the age of 18. This certainly would have some adverse effect upon their subsequent development and productivity. A large proportion of the adult population also labour with a burden of recent or continuing sorrow and anxiety. The influence of such personal problems upon productivity is certainly greater than zero, but in the absence of reliable information 'intangible losses' are often omitted from calculations. Klarman (1964) set the total cost of intangible losses for the U.S. as high as $5.2 billion per year.

The expected cumulative loss of earnings by all U.S. citizens dying of cardiovascular disease was estimated from standard life insurance tables at about $17.6 billion per year. This was a conservative figure, since the tables used in the calculations included patients dying of all forms of cardiovascular disease. The error was partially offset by the risk that a patient spared a coronary attack might have incurred some other illness that would have kept him from a full working life. Nevertheless, the true cost to the U.S. economy of premature 'cardiovascular' deaths, measured in 1962 dollars, was probably as high as $19.4 billion. Losses of output due to prolonged illness accounted for a further $3.0 billion, bringing the total indirect costs to $27.6 billion per year (Klarman, 1964).

Total costs
The total impact of cardiovascular disease upon the U.S. economy may be recapitulated as follows (in billions of dollars):

Direct costs	
Personal services	$ 2.6
Non-personal services	0.5
Indirect costs	
Premature death	19.4
Loss of output from illness	3.0
Loss of output from intangibles	5.2
TOTAL	$30.7

In current (1976) dollars, the $30.7 billion of 1962 could be approximately doubled to $60 billion. Dividing this among a population of 200 million, there would be an annual charge of $300 per capita, or about $600 per wage-earner. Over a working life of 50 years, cardiovascular disease would thus rob each employee of some $30,000.

Figures for a smaller western nation (Canada) were computed by Armstrong (1965). At the time of his study, the prevalence of cardiovascular disease was about 2.5 million cases in a total population of a little over 20 million. The proportion was slightly lower than in the U.S., probably because the Canadian population was somewhat younger. The cost of personal services for cardiac patients was set at $120 million, a lower per capita figure than in the U.S. Basic hospital and medical costs were then (and remain) lower in Canada, and less expensive forms of treatment were used. Armstrong set the loss of output due to cardiovascular disease at $80 million, a substantially lower per capita figure than for the U.S., even taking into account differences in earning power between the two nations. He gave no estimate of costs attributable to the use of non-personal services, losses of productivity from premature deaths, and intangible losses; if these had been set at 60% of the U.S. figures (to allow for differences in the average earning power and age of the two populations), the total annual cost to the Canadian economy would have been $1.7 billion in 1965, and perhaps $3 billion at 1976 prices (about $150 per capita, or $300 per wage-earner).

THE INFLUENCE OF ACTIVITY

We would not avoid the above losses entirely if the activity of all 'sedentary' workers were increased. Nevertheless, a major part of the present heavy toll of cardiovascular disease is attributable to conditions such as atherosclerosis, hypertension, and 'strokes,' where we suspect that exercise may play a useful preventive role. Evidence regarding the beneficial effects of physical activity is discussed in Chapter 8. The mortality from coronary disease is about 50% lower in occupations calling for heavy physical work. It is less certain that the same differential benefit extends to hypertension and 'strokes'; however, some effect is likely through the control of obesity and other risk factors. Even if the over-all effect of increased activity were only a 25% reduction of cardiovascular costs, the annual savings to the economy would amount to some $15 billion dollars in the U.S. and $0.75 billion dollars in Canada.

IMPLICATIONS FOR POLICY

Much more research is needed before any precision can be attached to the above estimates. However, the probable costs of cardiovascular disease are so large that expenditures on both research and the promotion of fitness should be reviewed critically.

U.S. expenditures on cardiovascular research were estimated at $112 million in 1962 and $122 million in 1963; some 86% of this total was provided from government funds. About 40% of the available support was directed to specific research on arteriosclerotic heart disease, strokes, and hypertension (DeBakey, 1965), but a large fraction of the cardiovascular contribution was applied to problems of secondary and tertiary care rather than the prevention of disease. In Canada, government analysts have recently reviewed the distribution of expenditures by the Department of National Health and Welfare (Table 1, Lalonde,

1974). During the fiscal year 1969/70, allocations for the improvement of all areas of life-style were a mere $12 million, compared with $1256 million for health care. By the fiscal year 1973/4, there had been some redistribution of funds, but questions of life-style still only received $45 million, compared with $2320 million for health care. In most nations, the proportion of the national resources devoted to the promotion of positive health still seems small in relation to the probable importance of the subject.

What is an appropriate amount of money to spend on the promotion of 'fitness' and the provision of facilities for sport and recreation? If a serious national campaign were undertaken to mould public opinion in favour of increased personal activity, this could in itself cost much of the potential saving to the economy in terms of health care costs. The average citizen is currently so saturated by advertising that campaigns such as that mounted by the Canadian crown corporation Participaction are hard pressed even to change public awareness of the fitness problem. An effective program of mass persuasion could have an annual cost of at least $100 million in Canada and $1 billion in the United States. On the other hand, the response of public behaviour to persistent conditioning is consistent, and as the owners of some commercial gymnasia have found, attitudes to fitness can be changed in a substantial segment of the community if an adequate sum is given to a suitable advertising agency. One large chain of commercial gymnasia has about 130,000 members in Southern Ontario. It is reputed to spend about $1.5 million per year on advertising. About $50 seems enough to recruit one further person who will sign a three-year membership contract. It is, of course, less certain that enthusiasm for exercise will persist throughout the three-year period, and if a gymnasium is small and overcrowded, the cynic may suspect that the operators will not be heart-broken if a proportion of the new recruits soon become 'drop-outs.'

Many forms of activity are relatively expensive when viewed on a national scale. Thus the annual cost to the consumer of a Canadian business men's gymnastic course ranges from about $100 per head in the spartan surroundings of the YMCA to $500 in the luxury of some commercial 'spas.' Given a choice, the average business man might well prefer exercise to heart disease, but in a statistical sense heart disease is cheaper than attendance at a commercial spa. The cost per head of all forms of gymnastics could no doubt be reduced if facilities were used by a higher percentage of the population. Nevertheless, the typical 'fitness class' is currently regarded as 'too expensive' by the typical 'working-class' family. In Hamilton, it has proved necessary to offer not only a free program but also free parking to steel company employees exercising after a heart attack.

Many good sports are costly to the community, if not to the individual, because they require a large acreage of land (Table 31). If all of the population of a

TABLE 31

Relative capital costs of providing facilities for simultaneous exercise
in a population of 2.4 million people (figures based on approximate data
for the metropolitan Toronto region, 1976)

Sport	Costs		
	Construction ($ billion)	Land ($ billion)	Total ($ billion)
Football/soccer	1.0	10.0	11.0
Tennis (doubles, 3 shifts)	1.4	1.3	2.7
Conservation park (swimming)	–	–	0.32
Urban swimming (360/pool)			
Outdoor	1.2	6.0	7.2
Indoor	3.7	6.0	9.7
Urban Skating (1000/rink)			
Outdoor	0.8	3.0	3.8
Indoor	1.5	3.0	4.5

metropolitan region such as Toronto (2.4 million people) were to play soccer on Saturday mornings, there would be a need for 110,000 fields covering an area of 300 square miles. The Lea marsh development in central London (McIntosh, 1963) provides a small-scale example of what would be required. The cost of levelling and turfing the necessary number of soccer fields would be a mere $1 billion, but within the confines of a large city such as Toronto a suitable tract of land could cost as much as $10 billion even without access roads. A system of tennis courts covering some 22 square miles could serve the same population in three one-hour shifts. The cost of constructing some 200,000 courts would be about $1.4 billion; in this instance, the land used would likely be potential housing plots, with a higher cost, perhaps $1.3 billion. Conservation-type parks are cheaper, since they are situated farther from urban centres and the nature of the terrain may be unsuitable for residential or industrial development. A park of 400 acres provides reasonable amenities for 10,000 people. The combined cost of land and preparation is perhaps $1.3 million per park, so that a total expenditure of $0.32 billion (plus any necessary access roads) would permit the simultaneous recreation of 2.4 million people. The operating costs of a conservation area are relatively low (perhaps 30 cents per visitor), and this can often be covered by admission and parking fees. Most conservation areas include facilities for swimming, and about three-quarters of those visiting a park enter the water on a fine day; the number that swim is more problematical! In an urban area, an outdoor pool accommodating a maximum of 300–400 people per afternoon costs about $180,000 for construction and a further $900,000 for land and parking. The total cost for our hypothetical population of 2.4 million is thus $7.2 billion. An indoor pool of the same size has a construction cost of about $560,000. The total cost of facilities to permit the entire city to swim would then be $9.7 billion, with the advantage that the pool could be used throughout the year. Skating arenas have a price tag similar to that for swimming pools. The construction costs (exclusive of land) are about $320,000 for an outdoor artificial rink and $640,000 for an indoor arena. However, as many as 1000 people may use a skating rink during public skating periods, and it seems possible to schedule minor league hockey at all times from the small hours of the morning until late at night. Thus, although an indoor arena operates for only about seven months a year, it may represent a better investment to a community than a swimming pool. It is heavily used when open, and provides exercise at a time when many forms of outdoor activity are less enjoyable.

Costs for the various forms of recreation are summarized in Table 31. All are high. Indeed, with the exception of conservation parks and tennis courts, projected expenditures exceed the total estimated costs of heart disease. The tennis courts fare relatively well in this comparison, partly because town-planners permit a court or a pair of courts to be built without parking facilities, and partly because we have assumed that local community organizations will manage the courts well enough to ensure play in three shifts on a typical afternoon. The latter assumption may be unrealistic in the warmer periods of the summer. The swimming pool or skating arena draws a larger total number of people, and it is thus constructed on a site of at least five acres, with parking for perhaps 100 cars.

All of the figures that have been cited are somewhat artificial, since it is most unlikely that every man, woman, and child would insist simultaneously on his right to participate in a given form of exercise. However, the calculations serve to emphasize that the outdoor sports enjoyed by the more active members of the middle-class depend in a substantial measure upon the disinterest of the populace at large. It would be wrong to restrict public spending on recreation to the anticipated yield from increases in productivity and health. Nevertheless, a substantial increase of municipal taxation and/or a more rigid control of land speculation would be needed to provide adequate facilities for the majority of sports.

Some cities may argue that they have neither the money to satisfy the land speculators nor the intestinal fortitude needed to regulate such speculation. However, defeatism is unnecessary, even in communities where the 'developer' is king, since elaborate facilities are by no means essential to an increase of activity on a community-wide basis. Educational programs should emphasize forms of exercise that have a high cost-effectiveness ratio. This takes us back to the beginning of our book, where we referred to the value of active domestic hobbies and pastimes. In many schools the emphasis has been upon the exotic and the star performer in team sports. Although such interests have their place, more attention should be paid to forms of exercise that can be taken in the home and with the family – domestic handiwork, gardening, manual lawn-mowing, walking, jogging, running, cycling, and cross-country skiing. Some of these activities may provide one answer to both the gasoline crisis and the polluted air of our cities – if traffic-free zones are established, the existing road network could become a vast open air 'gymnasium.' A number of European cities have now established very attractive central shopping precincts to which vehicles have limited access, and this idea shows signs of taking root even in North America. Here we have a unique opportunity to convince metropolitan man of the virtues of physical activity – through the creation of cities where the only permissible modes of transport between widely spaced subway stations are walking, jogging, cycling, and invalid chairs. Let us see that we do not lose this opportunity through the design of micro-electric cars that will carry us nearer to both our immediate destinations and our ultimate graves.

Glossary of symbols
and abbreviations

Complicated symbols and abbreviations have been deliberately avoided in this book. However, the use of a systematic 'shorthand' is becoming increasingly popular in literature devoted to fitness. A brief list of the more common symbols and abbreviations is thus given here. Where several abbreviations have the same or similar meanings, the preferred symbols are underlined. The reasons governing this choice are discussed elsewhere (Shephard, 1967d; Ellis, 1971).

UNITS OF 'WORK': $\underline{\text{kN-m min}^{-1}}$, kg-m min^{-1}, kp-m min^{-1}, ft-lb min^{-1}, watts (W), $\underline{\text{kJ min}^{-1}}$, kcal min^{-1}

Activity is usually expressed as a rate of working (that is, a power). Mechanical, electrical, or heat units may be employed. The common mechanical units of kg-m min^{-1} are now being replaced by $\underline{\text{kN-m min}^{-1}}$ (kilonewton-metres per minute, a slightly more precise term, one being equivalent to 101.9 kg-m min^{-1} in a normal gravitational field). Other units are the kilopond-metre per minute (too often confused with pounds) and the foot-pound per minute. Electrical units (watts, W) are sometimes used, particularly when work is performed on an electrically braked bicycle ergometer. Thermal units (kilojoules per minute, $\underline{\text{kJ min}^{-1}}$, and kilocalories per minute, kcal min^{-1}) may be chosen when the work performed is deduced from measurements of dietary intake or oxygen consumption. The various units of power are readily interconvertible:

4.19 kN-m min^{-1} = 427 kg-m min^{-1} = 427 kp-m min^{-1} = 3088 ft-lb min^{-1} = 69.8 W = 1.0 kcal min^{-1} = 4.19 kJ min^{-1}.

AEROBIC POWER: $\dot{V}_{O_2(max)}$, maximum oxygen intake, aerobic capacity; predicted $\dot{V}_{O_2(max)}$

Many authors have described the $\dot{V}_{O_2(max)}$ as the aerobic capacity. However, this is dimensionally incorrect. Oxygen intake is an expression of power rather than capacity. The value obtained depends on the period of effort involved. The $\dot{V}_{O_2(max)}$ is traditionally measured for exercise of about five minutes' duration. It may be expressed in absolute units (litres per minute STPD, or millimoles per minute) or it may be related to body weight or fat-free weight (ml kg^{-1} min^{-1}; mmol kg^{-1} min^{-1}); 1 ml STPD = 22.4 mmol oxygen. The predicted $\dot{V}_{O_2(max)}$ is an estimate of the individual's true $\dot{V}_{O_2(max)}$ derived from measurements of pulse or heart rate and oxygen consumption or work rate during submaximum effort.

Note that the pulse rate refers to a cardiac frequency determined by palpation of the wrist or neck, while the heart rate refers to a measurement made at the heart (stethoscope over the apex beat, or electrocardiogram). On occasion, a centrally recorded heart beat may fail to generate a detectable peripheral pulse beat.

'WORKING CAPACITY': PWR_{170}, PWR_{150}, PWC_{170}, W_{170}; $\dot{V}_{O_2,170}$; LPI; oxygen pulse; MR; Met

If it is not possible to conduct a maximum exercise test, the predicted $\dot{V}_{O_2(max)}$ is commonly used as a measure of 'working capacity.' However, some authors prefer to state the oxygen consumption ($\dot{V}_{O_2,170}$) or the rate of working at a fixed heart rate (170 min^{-1} in young subjects and 150 min^{-1} in older subjects). The latter is variously described as the predicted work rate ($\overline{PWR_{170} \text{ or } PWR_{150}}$), physical working capacity (PWC_{170} or PWC_{150}), or work rate ($\overline{W_{170} \text{ or } W_{150}}$).

The *Leistungspulsindex* (LPI) is the increase of pulse rate that occurs when the work load is increased by 60 kg-m min^{-1} or 0.588 kN-m min^{-1}. The oxygen pulse is the increase in oxygen consumption (ml min^{-1} STPD) for a unit increase of pulse rate. Both indices are popular in some parts of Germany. They reflect the slope of the heart rate/work load relationship.

The terms MR (metabolic rate) and Met (ratio of observed to basal metabolic rate) are sometimes used, particularly in experiments where subjects exercise in a hot environment. One advantage claimed for the Met is that the energy cost of a given activity is relatively independent of body weight. This has some attraction when formulating a simple clinical exercise prescription.

ANAEROBIC POWER: ATP, ADP, CP, phosphagen, lactic acid, excess lactate, R, RQ, ΔR

In the absence of oxygen, the body derives energy from the phosphate bonds of adenosine triphosphate (ATP) and creatine phosphate (CP). The breakdown of one gram-molecule of either compound is associated with the transfer of 10-12 kcal (42-50 kJ) of energy to muscle proteins. ATP is converted to adenosine diphosphate (ADP), while CP is converted to creatine (C). Both reactions are reversible, and the high-energy phosphate bonds are thus resynthesized when oxygen becomes available. Phosphagen is an alternative name for the total store of ATP and CP (or in some books CP alone).

The total amount of energy stored in phosphate bonds is relatively small. A larger amount of anaerobic power is obtained through the incomplete breakdown of glycogen to lactic acid. The concentration of lactic acid in the blood and tissue fluids is now increasingly expressed as gram-molar or equivalent concentrations (m mol $l.^{-1}$, mEq $l.^{-1}$) although some authors still use the traditional mg per 100 ml of fluid; 1 m mol = 1 mEq = 90 mg lactic acid. A few authors have reported results as 'excess lactate.' Lactic acid concentrations are influenced by the coexisting concentrations of pyruvate; the excess lactate is thus the quantity of lactate above that predicted from the pyruvate concentration.

Anaerobic work is associated with an increase in the ratio of carbon dioxide to oxygen in expired gas (the respiratory exchange ratio, R), but the ratio of metabolic carbon dioxide production to oxygen consumption (the true respiratory quotient, RQ) remains unchanged. Under steady-state conditions, R = RQ. The increase of the respiratory exchange ratio (ΔR) above an arbitrary resting level is sometimes used in the prediction of maximum oxygen intake (Issekutz et al., 1962; Shephard, 1975d).

VENTILATORY CAPACITY: VC, FRC, RV, TLC, TLV, V_T

The vital capacity (VC) is the maximum volume that can be expired after a full inspiration. The functional residual capacity (FRC) is the volume of gas remaining in the lungs at the end of a normal expiration, while the residual volume (RV) is the volume remaining in the lungs at the end of a forceful expiration. The total lung capacity (TLC, TLV) is equal to the sum of VC + RV. The tidal volume (V_T) is the gas volume displaced in each respiratory cycle.

VENTILATORY POWER: MVV_{100}, MBC_{100}, AGW; $FEV_{1.0}$; MVV_{40}; PEF; $\dot{V}_{E,max}$

The maximum voluntary ventilation (MVV_{100}) is the maximum volume that a subject can respire at the rate specified by the subscript; the period of hyperventilation is fixed, usually at 15 seconds, but occasionally at 12, 20, or 30 seconds. The MVV is also known as the maximum breathing capacity (MBC) and the *Atemgrenzwert* (AGW). The MVV_{100} is normally substantially greater than the respiratory minute volume during maximum exercise ($\dot{V}_{E,max}$).

An alternative and less exhausting index of ventilatory power commonly adopted in clinical practice is the forced expiratory volume (FEV); this is measured from full inspiration, and is the maximum volume that a subject can expire over the interval specified by the subscript. The maximum voluntary ventilation at 40 breaths per minute (MVV_{40}) is sometimes predicted by multiplying the $FEV_{0.75}$ by an arbitrary constant (40). Another simple clinical test of ventilatory power is to measure the peak expiratory flow rate (PEF), the maximum ventilatory flow that can be sustained for 10 milliseconds.

STANDARDIZATION OF GAS VOLUMES: ATPS, BTPS, STPD

Gas volumes are normally measured experimentally at ambient temperature and pressure, saturated with water vapour (ATPS). Measurements of ventilatory capacity and ventilatory power are converted to equivalent volumes at body temperature and pressure, saturated with water vapour (BTPS). On the other hand, measurements of gas transfer are expressed as the equivalent volume of dry gas under standard conditions of temperature and pressure (1 STPD or mmol).

GAS TRANSFER: $\dot{V}_E$; $\dot{V}_A$; $\underline{\dot{D}_L}$, T_L; $\dot{Q}_c$; λQ; $\dot{D}_t$; C_{I,O_2}; F_{I,O_2}; P_{i,O_2}; $\dot{G}_{O_2}$

Although the symbols used to represent gas transfer look complicated, there is an underlying and relatively simple system of logic. The dot above a symbol indicates a time derivative; thus V is a static volume but $\dot{V}$ represents the same volume displaced in unit time. The subscript characterizes the site of measurement; thus $\dot{V}_E$ is the volume of gas expired per minute and $\dot{V}_A$ is the alveolar ventilation per minute. Capital subscripts refer to the gas phase and lower case subscripts indicate the blood phase; thus $\dot{Q}$ is the total cardiac output per minute and $\dot{Q}_c$ is the slightly smaller volume of blood flowing through the pulmonary capillaries. The solubility coefficient λ is introduced to reflect the ability of unit volume of blood to carry differing quantities of different gases.

The 'pulmonary diffusing capacity' ($\dot{D}_L$ or D_L) may be defined as the over-all rate of transfer of gas between the alveoli and pulmonary capillary blood per unit gradient of partial pressure. It is also described as the transfer factor (T_L), and is sometimes broken down into components corresponding to membrane diffusion ($\dot{D}_M$) and the rate of reaction rate θ between the transferred gas and the blood content of the pulmonary capillaries ($\underline{Q_c}$ or V_c). Thus:

$$\frac{1}{\dot{D}_L} = \frac{1}{\dot{D}_M} + \frac{1}{\theta Q_c}.$$

A tissue-diffusing capacity $(\dot{D}_t)$ may also be calculated. This describes gas exchange between the tissue capillaries and the active tissues in similar units.

The driving pressure governing the rate of gas transfer may be represented in terms of concentration (C, with units of ml $l.^{-1}$), fractional concentration (F), or partial pressure gradient (P, measured in kPa, Torr, or mm Hg; 1 kPa = 7.5 Torr = 7.5 mm Hg). The subscripts applied to these abbreviations refer to the site of measurement and the gas concerned. Thus C_{I,O_2} is the concentration of oxygen in the inspired gas, F_{A,CO_2} is the fractional concentration of CO_2 in alveolar gas, and $P_{a.N_2}$ is the partial pressure of nitrogen in arterial blood. A bar above a symbol is used to designate the mean value; thus $C_{\bar{v},O_2}$ is the concentration of oxygen in mixed venous blood.

$\dot{G}$ is the symbol proposed for the over-all conductance or gas transfer coefficient characterizing exchange between the atmosphere and the active tissues. Thus, for oxygen:

$$\dot{V}_{O_2} = \dot{G}_{O_2}(C_{I,O_2} - C_{t,O_2}).$$

CIRCULATORY CAPACITY AND POWER: Qs, SV; $\underline{f_h}$, HR; BV; THb; AVD; $\dot{Q}$, $\dot{Q}_{max}$, CO, q

As with the respiratory system, the circulation has characteristic capacities and their corresponding time derivatives. The stroke volume (Q_s, SV) is the quantity of blood expelled by the heart per beat. The product of Qs and the heart rate per minute (f_h, F, HR) is thus the cardiac output or cardiac minute volume $(\dot{Q}, CO, q)$.

The total blood volume (BV) is the value obtained by equilibration of a known volume of a non-diffusible marker substance throughout the vascular system. The total haemoglobin (THb) is the weight of circulating haemoglobin, currently expressed in grams (156 g $l.^{-1}$ = 2.44 mmol $l.^{-1}$). The heart volume (HV) is a figure derived from measurements of the cardiac shadow in chest radiographs. The arterio-venous difference (AVD) is essentially a concentration gradient, and is better expressed in symbols compatible with the ventilatory equations $(C_{a,O_2} - C_{\bar{v},O_2})$.

STANDARDIZATION OF SYMBOLS

In the past many different symbols have been used to represent the same quantity. There are now several definitive documents on the standardization of symbols and abbreviations (Pappenheimer, 1950; Cotes, 1965; Shephard, 1967d; Ellis, 1971). The enthusiast is advised to consult these sources before inventing further terminology!

References

Adams, F. 1844. Paulus Aegineta, the Seven Books of. London: Sydenham Soc.
(cited by Ryan, 1974).

Adams, F.H., Bengtsson, E., Berven, H., and Wegelius, C. 1961. The physical
working capacity of normal school children. II. Swedish City and Country.
Pediatrics 28, 243-57.

Adams, W.C., Fox, R.H., Fry, A.J., and MacDonald, I.C. 1975. Thermo-
regulation during marathon running in cool, moderate and hot environments.
J. appl. Physiól. 38, 1030-7.

Adamson, G.T., and Cotes, J.E. 1967. Static and explosive muscle force:
relationship to other variables. J. Physiol. 189, 76-77p.

Adolph, E.F. 1964. Perspectives of adaptation. Some general properties.
In Handbook of Physiology, Section 4: Adaptation to the Environment.
Ed. D.B. Dill. Washington, D.C.: Amer. Physiol. Soc.

Adrian, E.D. 1925. Interpretation of the electromyogram. Lancet (ii),
1229-33, 1283-6.

Ahlborg, B., Ekelund, L.G., and Nilsson, C.G. 1968. Effect of potassium-
magnesium aspartate on the capacity for prolonged exercise in man. Acta
physiol. Scand. 74, 238-45.

Ahlquist, R., Taylor, J., Rawson, G., and Sydow, V. 1954. Comparative
effects of epinephrine and levarterenol in intact anaesthetized dog.
J. Pharm. exp. Therap. 110, 352-60.

Allen, J.G. 1966. Aerobic capacity and physiological fitness of Australian men.
Ergonomics 9, 485-94.

Alpert, J.S., Bass, H., Szues, M.M., Banas, J.S., Dalen, J.E., and Dexter, L.
1974. Effects of physical training on hemodynamics and pulmonary function
at rest and during exercise in patients with chronic obstructive pulmonary
disease. Chest 66, 647-51.

Alpert, N.R., and Root, W.S. 1954. Relationship between excess respiratory metabolism and utilization of intravenously infused sodium racemic lactate and sodium ℓ (–) lactate. Amer. J. Physiol. *177*, 455–62.

Alston, W., Carlson, K.E., Feldman, D.J., Grimm, Z., and Gerontinos, L. 1966. A quantitative study of muscle factors in the chronic low back syndrome. J. Amer. Geriatr. Soc. *14*, 1041–7.

Altman, P.L., and Dittmer, D.S. 1971. Respiration and Circulation. Bethesda, Md.: Federation of Amer. Soc. Exp. Biol.

Altshuler, B. 1961. The role of the mixing of intrapulmonary gas flow in the deposition of aerosol. In: Inhaled Particles and Vapours. Ed. C.N. Davies. Oxford: Pergamon Press.

American Association for Health, Physical Education and Recreation 1958. Youth Fitness Test Manual. Washington, D.C.: National Educational Assoc.

– 1965. Youth Fitness Test Manual, rev. ed. Washington, D.C.: National Education Assoc.

American Heart Association 1967. Report of committee on electrocardiography (chairman C.E. Kossmann). Recommendations for standardization of leads and of specifications for instruments in electrocardiography and vectorcardiography. Circulation *35*, 583–602.

American Medical Association 1966. Committee on Exercise and Physical Fitness. Chicago: Amer. Med. Assoc.

Andersen, H.T., and Barkve, H. 1970. Iron deficiency and muscular work performance. Scand. J. clin. Lab. Invest. *25*, Suppl. *114*, 1–62.

Andersen, K.L. 1964. Physical fitness – studies of healthy men and women in Norway. In: International Research in Sport and Physical Education. Ed. E. Jokl and E. Simon. Springfield, Ill.: C.C. Thomas.

– 1967a. Ethnic group differences in fitness for sustained and strenuous muscular exercise. In: Proc. Int. Symp. on Physical Activity and Cardiovascular Health. Canad. Med. Assoc. J. *96*, 832–5.

– 1967b. Work capacity of selected populations. In: The Biology of Human Adaptability. Ed. P.T. Baker and J.S. Weiner. Oxford: Clarendon Press.

Andersen, K.L., Elsner, R.E., Saltin, B., and Hermansen, L. 1962. Physical fitness in terms of maximal oxygen intake of nomadic Lapps. Fort Wainwright, Alaska. U.S.A.F. Arctic Med. Lab., Tech. Rept. AAL TDR–61–53.

Andersen, K.L., and Hart, J.S. 1963. Aerobic working capacity of Eskimos. J. appl. Physiol. *18*, 764–8.

Andersen, K.L., and Magel, J.R. 1970. Physiological adaptation to a high level of habitual physical activity during adolescence. Int. Z. angew. Physiol. *28*, 209–27.

Andersen, K.L., Shephard, R.J., Denolin, H., Varnauskas, E., and Masironi, R. 1971. Fundamentals of exercise testing. Geneva: W.H.O.

Anderson, S.D., Silverman, M., and Walker, S.R. 1972. Metabolic and ventilatory changes in asthmatic patients during and after exercise. Thorax 27, 718–25.

Anderson, T.W. 1973. The vulnerable myocardium. Lancet (2), 1084–5.

Anderson, T.W., and Le Riche, W.H. 1970. Ischaemic heart disease and sudden death, 1901–1961. Brit. J. prev. soc. Med. 24, 1–9.

Anderson, T.W., and Shephard, R.J. 1968a. A theoretical study of some errors in the measurement of pulmonary diffusing capacity. Respiration 26, 102–15.

– 1968b. Physical training and exercise diffusing capacity. Int. Z. angew. Physiol. 25, 198–209.

– 1968c. The effects of hyperventilation and exercise upon the pulmonary diffusing capacity. Respiration 25, 465–84.

Andrew, G.M., Becklake, M.R., and Guleria, J.S. 1972. Heart and lung function in swimmers and non-athletes during growth. J. appl. Physiol. 32, 245–51.

Anend, B.K. 1961. Nervous regulation of food intake. Physiol. Rev. 41, 677–708.

Angel, A. 1974. Patho-physiology of obesity. Canad. Med. Assoc. J. 110, 540–8.

Antel, J., and Cumming, G.R. 1969. Effect of emotional stimulation on exercise heart rate. Res. Quart. 40 (2), 5–10.

Apthorp, G.H., Bates, D.V., Marshall, R., and Mendel, D. 1958. Effect of acute carbon monoxide poisoning on work capacity. Brit. Med. J. (ii), 476–8.

Arch. d. Gabinete Medico del Comite Nacional de Deportes 1947. LaPaz, Bolivia.

Ariel, G. 1973. The effect of anabolic steroid upon muscular contractile force. J. Sports Med. Phys. Fitness 13, 187–90.

Armstrong, J.B. 1965. In: Notes on Public Health and Preventive Medicine. Department of Public Health, University of Toronto, Toronto.

Arnott, W.M., Cumming, G., and Horsfield, K. 1968. Alveolar ventilation. Ann. Int. Med. 69, 1–12.

Aronow, W.S., Cassidy, J., Vangrow, J.S., March, H., Kern, J.C., Goldsmith, J.R., Khemka, M., Pagano, J., and Vawter, M. 1974. Effect of cigarette smoking and breathing carbon monoxide on cardiovascular hemodynamics in anginal patients. Circulation 50, 340–7.

Arstila, M. 1972. Pulse-conducted trangular exercise – e.c.g. test. Acta med. Scand. Suppl. 529.

Asclepiades. 1955. Asclepiades, His Life and Writing (translated by R.M. Green). New Haven, Conn.: Licht (cited by Ryan, 1974).

Ashley, F.W., and Kannel, W.B. 1974. Relation of weight change to changes in atherogenic traits: the Framingham study. J. Chr. Dis. 27, 103–14.

Asmussen, E. 1973. Ventilation at transition from rest to exercise. Acta physiol. Scand. *89*, 68–78.

Asmussen, E., and Bøje, O. 1948. The effects of alcohol and some drugs on the capacity for work. Acta physiol. Scand. *15*, 109–18.

Asmussen, E., and Christensen, E.H. 1939. Einfluss der Blutverteilung auf den Kreislauf bei körperlicher Arbeit. Skand. Arch. Physiol. *82*, 185–92.

– 1967. Kompendium: Legemsövelsernes Specielle Teori. Københavns Universitets Fond til Tilvejebringelse af Läremidler, Copenhagen.

Asmussen, E., and Heebøll-Nielsen, K. 1961. Isometric muscle strength of adult men and women. Comm. Test. and Obs. Inst., Hellerup, Denmark *11*, 3–44.

– 1962. Isometric muscle strength in relation to age in men and women. Ergonomics *5*, 167–9.

Asmussen, E., and Mathiasen, P. 1962. Some physiologic functions in physical education students reinvestigated after twenty-five years. J. Amer. Geriatr. Soc. *10*, 379–87.

Asmussen, E., and Molbech, S.V. 1959. Methods and standards for evaluation of the physiological working capacity of patients. Comm. Test. and Obs. Inst., Hellerup, Denmark, *4*.

Asmussen, E., and Nielsen, M. 1946. Studies on the regulation of respiration in heavy work. Acta physiol. Scand. *12*, 171–87.

– 1955a. Physiological dead space and alveolar gas pressures at rest and during muscular exercise. Acta physiol. Scand. *38*, 1–21.

– 1955b. Cardiac output during muscular work and its regulation. Physiol. Rev. *35*, 778–800.

Åstrand, I. 1960. Aerobic work capacity in men and women with special reference to age. Acta physiol. Scand. *49*, Suppl. *169*, 1–92.

– 1967. Degree of strain during building work as related to individual aerobic work capacity. Ergonomics *10*, 293–303, 1967.

– 1971a. Estimating the energy expenditure of housekeeping activities. Amer. J. clin. Nutr. *24*, 1471–5.

– 1971b. Circulatory responses to arm exercise in different work positions. Scand. J. clin. Lab. Invest. *27*, 293–97.

Åstrand, I., Åstrand, P-O, Christensen, E.H., and Hedman, R. 1960. Intermittent muscular work. Acta physiol. Scand. *48*, 448–53.

Åstrand, I., Åstrand, P-O., Hallback, I., and Kilbom, A. 1973. Reduction in maximal oxygen intake with age. J. appl. Physiol. *35*, 649–54.

Åstrand, I., Gahary, A., and Wahren, J. 1968. Circulatory responses to arm exercise with different arm positions. J. appl. Physiol. *25*, 528–32.

Åstrand, P.O. 1952. Experimental Studies of Physical Working Capacity in Relation to Age and Sex. Copenhagen: Munksgaard.

- 1967a. Commentary. In: Proc. Int. Symp. on Physical Activity and Cardio-vascular Health. Canad. Med. Assoc. J. *96*, 730.
- 1967b. Diet and athletic performance. Fed. Proc. *27*, 1772-1777.
- 1967c. Concluding remarks. In: Proc. Int. Symp. on Physical Activity and Cardiovascular Health. Ed. R.J. Shephard. Canad. Med. Assoc. J. *96*, 907-11.
- 1973. Physiological bases for sport at different ages. In: Sport in the Modern World - Chances and Problems. Ed. O. Grupe, D. Kurz, and J.M. Teipel. Berlin: Springer Verlag.

Åstrand, P.O. Cuddy, T.E., Saltin, B., and Stenberg, J. 1964. Cardiac output during sub-maximal and maximal work. J. appl. Physiol. *19*, 268-74.

Åstrand, P.O., Ekblom, B., and Goldberg, A.N. 1971. Effects of blocking the autonomic nervous system during exercise. Acta physiol. Scand. *82*, 18A.

Åstrand, P.O. Ekblom, B., Messin, R., Saltin, B. and Stenberg, J. 1965. Intra-arterial blood pressure during exercise with different muscle groups. J. appl. Physiol. *20*, 253-6.

Åstrand, P-O., Engström, L., Eriksson, B., Karlberg, P., Nylander, I., Saltin, B., and Thoren, C. 1963. Girl swimmers. With special reference to respiratory and circulatory adaptation and gynaecological and psychiatric aspects. Acta Paediatr. Suppl. *147*, 1-75.

Åstrand, P.O., and Rodahl, K. 1970. A Textbook of Work Physiology. New York: McGraw-Hill.

Åstrand, P.O., and Ryhming, I. 1954. A nomogram for calculation of aerobic capacity (physical fitness) from pulse rate during sub-maximal work. J. appl. Physiol. *7*, 218-21.

Åstrand, P.O., and Saltin, B. 1961a. Oxygen uptake during the first minutes of heavy muscular exercise. J. appl. Physiol. *16*, 971-6.

- 1961b. Maximal oxygen uptake and heart rate in various types of muscular activity. J. appl. Physiol. *16*, 977-81.

Åstrup, P., Hellung-Larsen, P., Kjeldsen, K., and Mellemgaard, K. 1966. The effect of tobacco smoking on the dissociation curve of oxyhaemoglobin. Scand. J. clin. Lab. Invest. *18*, 450-7.

Auchincloss, J.H., and Gilbert, R. 1973. Estimation of maximum oxygen uptake with a brief progressive stress test. J. appl. Physiol. *34*, 525-6.

Aurelianus, C. 1950. On Chronic Diseases. Transl. I.E. Drabkin. Chicago: University of Chicago Press (cited by Ryan, 1974).

Babirack, S.P., Dowell, R.T., and Oscai, L.B. 1974. Total fasting and total fasting plus exercise: effects on body composition of the rat. J. Nutr. *104*, 452-7.

Badeer, H.S. 1968. Metabolic basis of cardiac hypertrophy. Progress Cardiovasc. Dis. *11*, 53-63.

Bailey, D.A., Carron, A.V., Teece, R.G., and Wehner, H.J. 1970. Vitamin C supplementation related to physiological response to exercise in smoking and non-smoking subjects. Amer. J. clin. Nutr. 23, 905–12.

Bailey, D.A., Ross, W.D., Weese, C., and Mirwald, R.L. 1974. A dimensional analysis of aerobic power in boys. Proc. VIth Int. Symp. on Work Physiology, Sec, Czechoslovakia.

Bailey, D.A., Shephard, R.J., and Mirwald, R.L. 1976. Validation of a self-administered home-test of cardio-respiratory fitness. Canad. J. appl. Sports Sci. 1, 67–78.

Bailey, D.A., Shephard, R.J., Mirwald, R.L., and McBride, G.A. 1974. Current levels of Canadian cardio-respiratory fitness. Canad. Med. Assoc. J. 111, 25–30.

Bake, B., Bjure, J., and Widimsky, J. 1968. The effect of sitting and graded exercises on the distribution of pulmonary blood flow in healthy subjects studied with the 133 xenon technique. Scand. J. clin. Lab. Invest. 22, 99–106.

Baker, J.A., Humphrey, S.J.E., and Wolff, H.S. 1967. Socially acceptable monitoring instruments (SAMI). J. Physiol. 188, 4p.

Baker, L.G., Ultman, J.S., and Rhoades, R.A. 1974. Simultaneous gas flow and diffusion in a symmetric airway system: a mathematical model. Resp. Physiol. 21, 119–38.

Balke, B. 1954. Optimale korperliche Leistungsfahigkeit, ihre Messung und Veränderung infolge Arbeitsermüdung. Int. Z. angew. Physiol. 15, 311–23.

Banister, E.W. 1971. Energetics of muscular contraction. In: Frontiers of Fitness. Ed. R.J. Shephard. Springfield, Ill.: C.C. Thomas.

Banister, E.W., and Jackson, R.C. 1967. The effect of speed and load changes on oxygen intake for equivalent power outputs during bicycle ergometry. Int. Z. angew. Physiol. 24, 284–90.

Banister, E.W., and Taunton, J.E. 1971. A rehabilitation programme after myocardial infarction. Brit. Columbia Med. J., Oct.

Bannister, R.G., Cotes, J.E., Jones, R.S., and Meade, F. 1960. Pulmonary diffusing capacity on exercise in athletic and non-athletic subjects. J. Physiol. 152, 66–67p.

Bannister, R.G., and Cunningham, D.J.C. 1954. The effects on the respiration and performance during exercise of adding oxygen to the inspired air. J. Physiol. 125, 118–37.

Barach, J.H. 1914. The energy index, cardiovascular energy as indicated by the arterial pressure per minute. J. Amer. Med. Assoc. 62, 525.

Barcroft, H. 1963. Circulation in skeletal muscle. In: Handbook of Physiology, Section 2: Circulation, Vol. 2. Ed. W.F. Hamilton. Washington, D.C.: Amer. Physiol. Soc.

Barcroft, H., and Dornhorst, A.C. 1949. Blood flow through the human calf during rhythmic exercise. J. Physiol. 109, 402–411.

Barcroft, J. 1914. The respiratory function of the blood. Cambridge, U.K.: University Press.

Barker, S.B., and Summerson, W.H. 1941. The colorimetric determination of lactic acid in biological material. Amer. J. Biol. *138*, 535–54.

Barnard, R.J., Gardner, G.W., Diaco, N.V., et al. 1973. Cardiovascular responses to sudden strenuous exercise – heart rate, blood pressure and ECG. J. appl. Physiol. *34*, 833–7.

Barnard, R.J., MacAlpin, R.N., Kattus, A.A., and Buckberg, G.D. 1973. Ischemic response to sudden strenuous exercise in healthy men. Circulation *48*, 936–42.

Barney, R.K. 1972. An historical reinterpretation of the forces underlying the first State legislation for physical education in the public schools of the United States, with special attention to the role played by the early California Turnvereine. Proc. 2nd Canad. Symp. on the History of Sport and Physical Education, Windsor, Ont.

Bar-Or, O., and Shephard, R.J. 1971. Cardiac output determination in exercising children – methodology and feasibility. Acta Paed. Scand. Suppl. *217*, 49–52.

Bar-Or, O., and Zwiren, L.D. 1973. Physiological effects of increased frequency of physical education classes and of endurance conditioning on 9 to 10 year old girls and boys. In: Paediatric Work Physiology. Proc. 4th Int. Symp. Ed. O. Bar-Or. Natanya, Israel: Wingate Inst.

Barringer, T.B. 1917. Studies of the heart's functional capacity. Arch. Int. Med. *20*, 830–9.

Bartels, R., Billings, C.E., Fox, E.L., Mathews, D.K., O'Brien, R., Tauz, D., and Webb, W. 1968. Abstracts, AAHPER Convention, p. 13 (cited by Pollock, 1973).

Bartlett, R.G., Brubach, H.F., and Specht, H. 1958. Some factors determining the maximum breathing capacity. J. appl. Physiol. *12*, 247–54.

Bass, H., Whitcomb, J.F., and Forman, R. 1970. Exercise training: therapy for patients with chronic obstructive pulmonary diseases. Dis. Chest *57*, 116–21.

Bassey, E.J., and Fentem, P.H. 1974. Extent of deterioration in physical condition during post-operative bed rest and its reversal by rehabilitation. Brit. Med. J. (iv), 194–6.

Bates, D.V. 1962. Respiratory disorders associated with impairment of gas diffusion. Ann. Rev. Med. *13*, 301–18.

Bates, D.V., Boucot, G., and Dormer, A.E. 1955. The pulmonary diffusing capacity in normal subjects. J. Physiol. *129*, 237–52.

Bättig, K. 1965. Modellversuche an der Ratte über die Art der Amphetamin-wirkung bei verscheiden strukturierten Leistungen. Schweiz. Z. f. Sportmedizin *13*, 99–116.

Beard, E.F., and Owen, C.A. 1973. Cardiac arrhythmias during exercise testing in healthy men. Aerospace Med. *44*, 286–9.

Beaver, W.L., and Wasserman, K. 1970. Tidal volume and respiratory rate changes at start and end of exercise. J. appl. Physiol. *29*, 872–6.

Bedford, T. 1948. Basic principles of ventilation and heating. London: H.K. Lewis.

Beeckmans, J., and Shephard, R.J. 1967. A theoretical basis for the partitioning of maximal cardio-respiratory performance. Canad. J. Physiol. Pharm. *45*, 185–90.

– 1971. Computer calculations of exercise dead space: the role of laminar flow and development of a clinical prediction formula. Respiration *28*, 232–52.

Behnke, A.R., and Wilmore, J.H. 1974. Evaluation and Regulation of Body Build and Composition. Englewood Cliffs, N.J.: Prentice-Hall.

Belding, H.S., Hertig, B.A., Kraning, K.K., Roets, P.P., and Nagata, H. 1966. Use of a water bath for study of human heat tolerance. In: Human Adaptability and Its Methodology, pp. 115–21. Ed. H. Yoshimura and J.S. Weiner. Tokyo: Japanese Soc. for the Promotion of Sciences.

Belloc, N.B., and Breslow, L. 1972. Relationship of physical health status and health practices. Prev. Med. *1*, 409–21.

Bergmann, J. 1884. Über die Grösse des Herzens bei Menschen und Tieren. Inaug. Diss., Univ. München. Munich: Wolf and Sohn.

Bergstrom, J. 1967. Local changes of ATP and phosphorylcreatine in human muscle tissue in connection with exercise. Circ. Res. (Suppl. to Vols. *20* and *21*) I, 91–6.

Bergstrom, J., Hultman, E., and Saltin, B. 1973. Muscle glycogen consumption during cross-country skiing (the Vasa ski race). Int. Z. angew. Physiol. *31*, 71–5.

Berridge, M.E. 1974. The structure and future of CAHPER. CAHPER J. *40* (5), 53–9.

Berson, A.S., and Pipberger, H.V. 1966. The low frequency response of electro-cardiographs, a frequent source of recording errors. Amer. Heart J. *71*, 779–89.

Bettmann, O.L. 1956. A Pictorial History of Medicine. Springfield, Ill.: C.C. Thomas.

Bevegard, B.S., and Shepherd, J.T. 1967. Regulation of the circulation during exercise in man. Physiol. Rev. *47*, 178–213.

Bevegard, S., Freyschuss, V., and Strandell, T. 1966. Circulatory adaptation to arm and leg exercise in supine and sitting position. J. appl. Physiol. *21*, 37–46.

Bevegard, S., Holmgren, A., and Johnsson, B. 1960. The effect of body position on the circulation at rest and during exercise, with special reference to the influence of stroke volume. Acta physiol. Scand. *49*, 279–98.

Bink, B. 1962. The physical working capacity in relation to working time and age. Ergonomics *5*, 25–8.

Bishop, L.F., and Reichert, P. 1970. The inter-relationship between anxiety and arrhythmia. Psychosomatics *11*, 331–4.

Bishop, W.H. 1970. Greek athletics in ancient Rome. Proc. 1st Canad. Symp. on the History of Sport and Physical Recreation, Edmonton, Alta.

Bjorgum, R.K., and Sharkey, B.J. 1966. Inhalation of oxygen as an aid to recovery after exertion. Res. Quart. *37*, 462–7.

Bjorntorp, P., de Jounge, K., Krotkiewski, M., Sullivan, L., Sjöström, L., and Steinberg, J. 1973. Physical training in human obesity: 3. Effects of long term physical training on body composition. Metabolism *22*, 1467–75.

Blackburn, H. 1974. Progress in the epidemiology and prevention of coronary heart diseases. In: Progress in Cardiology. Ed. P.N. Yu and J.F. Goodwin. Philadelphia: Lea & Febiger.

Blackburn, H., Brozek, J., and Taylor, H.L. 1960. Common circulatory measurements in smokers and non-smokers. Circulation *22*, 1112–24.

Blackburn, H., Taylor, H.L., Okamoto, N., Rautaharju, P., Mitchell, P.L., and Kerkhof, A. 1967. Standardization of the exercise electrocardiogram. A systematic comparison of chest lead configurations employed for monitoring during exercise. In: Physical Activity and the Heart. Ed. M.J. Karvonen and A.J. Barry. Springfield, Ill.: C.C. Thomas.

Blackburn, H., Taylor, H.L., Hamrell, B., Buskirk, E., Nicholas, W.C., and Thorsen, R.D. 1973. Premature ventricular complexes induced by stress testing. Amer. J. Cardiol. *31*, 441–9.

Blomqvist, G. 1974. Exercise physiology related to diagnosis of coronary artery disease. In: Coronary Heart Disease: Prevention, Detection, Rehabilitation with Emphasis on Exercise Testing. Ed. S. Fox. Denver, Col.: Int. Med. Corp.

Blomqvist, G., Saltin, B., Dean, W.F., and Mitchell, J.H. 1970. Acute effect of ethanol ingestion on the response to submaximal and maximal exercise in man. Circulation *42*, 463–70.

Blumchen, G., Roskamm, H., and Reindell, H. 1966. Herzvolumen und körperliche Leistungsfähigkeit. Kreislaufforschung *55*, 1012–16.

Boas, E.P., and Goldschmidt, E.F. 1932. The Heart Rate. Springfield, Ill.: C.C. Thomas.

Bobbert, A.C. 1960. Physiological comparison of three types of ergometer. J. appl. Physiol. *15*, 1007–14.

Bock, A.V. 1928. Dynamic changes occurring in man at work. J. Physiol. *66*, 136–61.

Bock, A.V., Vancaulaert, C., Dill, D.B., Fölling, A., and Hurxthal, L. 1928. Studies in muscular activity, part 4: 'Steady State' and the respiratory quotient during work. J. Physiol. *66*, 162–74.

Bohr, C. 1909. Über die spezifische Tätigkeit der Lungen bei der respiratorischen Gasaufnahme. Skand. Arch. Physiol. *22*, 221–80.

Boning, D., Schweigart, V., Tibes, V., Hammer, B., and Meier, V. 1974. Oxygen transport of the exercise muscle – importance of the 'in vivo'- oxygen dissociation curve. I.U.P.S. Satellite Symp. on Exercise Physiology, Patiala, India.

Bonjer, F.H. 1966. Measurement of working capacity by assessment of the aerobic capacity in a single session. Fed. Proc. 25, 1363–5.

– 1968. Relationships between physical working capacity and allowable caloric expenditure. In: Int. Coll. on Muscular Exercise and Training. Ed. H. Rohmert. Darmstadt: Gentner Verlag.

Bonstingl, R.W., Morehouse, C.A., and Niebel, B.W. 1975. Torques developed by different types of shoe on various playing surfaces. Med. Sci. Sports 7, 127–31.

Bookwalter, K.W. 1950. Grip strength norms for males. Res. Quart. 21, 249–73.

Booth, F.W., and Gould, E.W. 1975. Effects of training and disuse on connective tissue. Exercise Sport Sci. Rev. 3, 83–112.

Booth, F.W., and Kelso, J.R. 1973. Cytochrome oxidase of skeletal muscle-adaptive response to chronic disease. Can. J. Physiol. 51, 679–81.

Borg, G. 1971. The perception of physical performance. In: Frontiers of Fitness. Ed. R.J. Shephard. Springfield, Ill.: C.C. Thomas.

Boslooper, T. 1971. The image of woman in classical antiquity. Proc. 2nd World Symp. on the History of Sport, Banff, Alta.

Bottin, R., Deroanne, R., Petit, J.M., Pirnay, F., and Juchmes, J. 1966. Comparaison de la consommation maximum d'O_2 mésurée à celle prédite en fonction de la fréquence cardiaque, au moyen du nomogramme d'Astrand. Rev. educ. Phys. 6, 224–9.

Bottin, R., Petit, J.M., Deroanne, R., Juchmes, J., and Pirnay, F. 1968. Mésures comparées de la consommation maximum d'O_2 par paliers de 2 ou de 3 minutes. Int. Z. angew. Physiol. 26, 355–62.

Bottin, R., Pirnay, F., Deroanne, R., Juchmes, J., and Petit, J.M. 1971. Les consommations maximum d'O_2 avec charges. Arch. Int. Physiol. Biochim. 79, 711–16.

Bouchard, C., Godbout, P., Landry, F., Mondor, J.C., Houde, P., and Levesque, C. 1973. Une étude sur le taux de generalité et de specificité de la puissance aerobique maximale lors d'efforts en vita maxima. First Canadian Pluri-Disciplinary Congress on Sport and Physical Activity, Montreal.

Bouchard, C., Hollmann, W., Venrath, H., Herkenrath, G., and Schlüssel, H. 1966. Minimalbelastungen zur Pravention kardiovaskularer Erkrankungen. Sportarzt und Sportmedizin 7, 348–57.

Bourne, G.H. 1948. Vitamins and muscular exercise. Brit. J. Nutr. 2, 261–3.

Bowers, K.D., and Martin, R.B. 1975. Cleat-surface friction on new and old Astroturf. Med. Sci. Sports 7, 132–5.

Bowers, R., and Reardon, J.F. 1972. Effects of methadrostenolone (Dianabol) on strength development and aerobic capacity. Med. Sci. Sports 4, 54.

Boylan, J.W. 1971. Founders of Experimental Physiology. Munich: Lehmanns Verlag.

Brashear, R.E., and Ross, J.C. 1968. Splenic contributions to pulmonary diffusing capacity in dogs and man. J. appl. Physiol. 25, 48–51.

Bremer, J. 1967. In: Cellular Compartmentalization and Control of Fatty Acid Metabolism, pp. 65–8. Ed. J. Bremer and F.C. Gran. New York: Academic Press.

British Medical Journal 1972a. Haemoglobinometry in new units. Brit. Med. J. (iii), 129–30.

– (Ed.) 1972b. To nibble or gorge? Brit. Med. J. (iii), 716–17.

– (Ed.) 1973a. Significance of ectopic beats. Brit. Med. J. (ii), 191–2.

– (Ed.) 1973b. Editorial – Pilot error. Brit. Med. J. (ii), 258–9.

– (Ed.) 1973c. Obesity and coronary heart disease. Brit. Med. J. (i), 566–7.

– (Ed.) 1974. Smoking and colds. Brit. Med. J. (iii), 594.

– (Ed.) 1975. Anxiety symptoms and coffee drinking. Brit. Med. J. (i), 296–7.

Brooke, J.D., and Firth, M. 1972. Changes in cardiac responses of sportsmen from hours of prolonged severe exercise. Brit. J. Sports Med. 6, 121–4.

Brooks, G.A., Hittelman, K.J., Faulkner, J.A., and Beyer, R.E. 1971. Temperature, skeletal muscle mitochondrial functions and oxygen debt. Amer. J. Physiol. 220, 1053–9.

Brouha, L. 1943. The step test: a simple method of measuring physical fitness for muscular work in young men. Res. Quart. 14, 31–6.

Brown, B., and Pilch, A. 1972. The effects of exercise and Dianabol upon selected performances and physiological parameters in the male rat. Med. Sci. Sports 4, 159–65.

Brown, J.R. 1958. Factors involved in the causation of weight-lifting accidents. Ergonomics 2, 117–18.

– 1966. The metabolic cost of industrial activity in relation to weight. Med. Serv. J. Canada 22, 262–72.

– 1972. Manual Lifting and Related Fields. An Annotated Bibliography. Ontario: Labour Safety Council.

Brown, J.R., and Crowden, G.P. 1963. Energy expenditure ranges and muscular work grades. Brit. J. industr. Med. 20, 277–83.

Brown, J.R., and Shephard, R.J. 1967. Some measurements of fitness in older female employees of a Toronto department store. Canad. Med. Assoc. J. 97, 1208–13.

Brown, R.C. 1967. Commentary. In: Proc. Int. Symp. on Physical Activity and Cardiovascular Health. Canad. Med. Assoc. J. *96*, 727.

Brozek, J. (consulting ed.). 1963. Body composition, pts. I and II. Ann. N.Y. Acad. Sci. *110*, 1-1018.

- 1965. Human Body Composition. Oxford: Pergamon Press.

Bruce, R., Lind, A.R., Franklin, D., Muir, A.L. Macdonald, H.R., McNicol, G.W., and Donald, K.W. 1968. The effects of digoxin on fatiguing static and dynamic exercise in man. Clin. Sci. *34*, 29-42.

Bruch, H. 1940. Obesity in childhood: Energy expenditure of obese children. Amer. J. dis. Childh. *60*, 1082-1109.

Brunner, B.C. 1969. Personality and motivating factors influencing adult participation in vigorous physical activity. Res. Quart. *40*, 464-9.

Bryan, A.C., Bentivoglio, L.G., Beerel, F., MacLeish, H., Zidulka, A., and Bates, D.V. 1964. Factors affecting regional distribution of ventilation and perfusion in the lung. J. appl. Physiol. *19*, 395-402.

Bullen, B.A., Reed, R.B., and Mayer, J. 1964. Physical activity of obese and non-obese adolescent girls. Appraised by motion picture samples. Amer. J. clin. Nutr. *14*, 211-23.

Burger, G.C.E. 1964. Permissible load and optimal adaptation. Ergonomics *7*, 397-417.

Burger, H.C., Loopman, L.J., and Van Loon, P. 1967. Work and effort. J. appl. Physiol. *22*, 913-22.

Burke, W.E., Tuttle, W.W., Thompson, C.W., Janney, C.D., and Weber, R.J. 1953. The relationship of grip strength and grip strength endurance to age. J. appl. Physiol. *5*, 628-30.

Burn, J.H. 1960. The action of nicotine on the peripheral circulation. Ann. N.Y. Acad. Sci. *90*, 81-4.

Burt, J.J., and Jackson, R. 1965. The effects of physical exercise on the coronary collateral circulation of dogs. J. Sports Med. Phys. Fitness *5*, 203-6.

Burton, A.C. 1965. Physiology and Biophysics of the Circulation. Chicago: Year Book Medical Publishers.

Buskirk, E.R., and Taylor, H.L. 1957. Maximal oxygen intake and its relation to body composition, with special reference to chronic physical activity and obesity. J. appl. Physiol. *11*, 72-8.

Buskirk, E.R. 1967. Commentary. In: Proc. Int. Symp. on Physical Activity and Cardiovascular Health, Toronto. Canad. Med. Assoc. J. *96*, 719.

- 1968. Problems related to conduct of athletes in hot environments. In: Physiological Aspects of Sports and Physical Fitness. Chicago: Athletic Inst.

Buskirk, E.R., Kollias, J., Piconreatigue, E., Akers, R., Prokop, E., and Baker, P. 1967. In: Int. Symp. on the Effects of Attitude on Physical Performance. Ed. R.F. Goddard. Chicago: Athletic Inst.

Butler, N.R., and Goldstein, H. 1973. Smoking in pregnancy and subsequent child development. Brit. Med. J. (iv), 573-5.

Buzina, R. 1972. Nutrition status, working capacity and absenteeism in industrial workers. 1st Int. Symp. on 'Alimentation et Travail.' Paris: Masson et Cie.

Byrne-Quinn, E., Weil, J.V., Sodal, I.E., Filley, G.F., and Grover, R.F. 1971. Ventilatory control in the athlete. J. appl. Physiol. 30, 91-8.

Callaway, D.H. 1975. Nitrogen balance of men with marginal intakes of protein and energy. J. Nutr. 105, 914-23.

Camner, P., Philipson, K., and Arvidsson, T. 1973. Withdrawal of cigarette smoking: a study on tracheobronchial clearance. A.M.A. Arch. Env. Health 26, 90-2.

Campbell, W.R., and Pohndorf, R.H. 1961. Physical fitness of British and United States children. In: Health and Fitness in the Modern World. Ed. L.A. Larson. Washington, D.C.: Athletic Inst.

Canadian Association for Health, Physical Education and Recreation 1966. Fitness Performance Test Manual. Toronto: Canad. Assoc. for Health, Physical Education and Recreation.

Carey, P., Stensland, M., and Hartley, L.H. 1974. Comparison of oxygen uptake during maximal work on the treadmill and the rowing ergometer. Med. Sci. Sports 6, 101-3.

Carlsten, A. 1972. Influence of leg varicosities on the physical work performance. In: Environmental Effects on Work Performance. Ed. G.R. Cumming, A.W. Taylor, and D. Snidal. Ottawa: Canad. Assoc. of Sports Sciences.

Carrow, R.E., Brown, R.E., and Van Huss, W.D. 1967. Fiber sizes and capillary to fiber ratios in skeletal muscle of exercised rats. Anat. Record 159, 33-40.

Carswell, S. 1975. Changes in aerobic power in patients undergoing elective surgery. J. Physiol. 251, 42-3p.

Carter, C.O. 1961. The inheritance of congenital stenosis. Brit. med. Bull. 17, 251-4.

Casner, S.W., Early, R.G., and Carlson, R.R. 1971. Anabolic steroid effects on body composition in normal young men. J. Sports Med. Phys. Fitness 11, 98-103.

Celander, O. 1954. The range of control exercised by the sympathico-adrenal system. Acta physiol. Scand. 32, Suppl. 116.

Cermak, J. 1973. Changes of the heart volume and of the basic somatometric indices in 12-15 years old boys with an intense exercise regime. A long term study. Brit. J. Sports Med. 7, 241-4.

Chance, B. 1957. Cellular oxygen requirements. Fed. Proc. 16, 671-80.

Chance, B., and Pring, M. 1968. Logic in the design of the respiratory chain. In: Biochimie des Sauerstoffs, pp. 120-30. Ed. B. Hess and H. Standinger. Berlin: Springer Verlag.

Cheraskin, E., and Ringsdorf, W.M. 1971. Predictive medicine, X. Physical activity. J. Amer. Geriatr. Soc. *19*, 969–73.

Chevalier, R.B., Bowers, J.A., Bondurant, S., and Ross, J.C. 1963. Circulatory and ventilatory effects of exercise in smokers and non-smokers. J. appl. Physiol. *18*, 357–60.

Chiang, B.N., Perlman, L.V., Ostrander, L.D., and Epstein, F.H. 1969. Relationship of premature systoles to coronary heart disease and sudden death in the Tecumseh epidemiologic study. Ann. Int. Med. *70*, 1159–66.

Chirico, A.M., and Stunkard, A.J. 1960. Physical activity and human obesity. New Engl. J. Med. *263*, 935–40.

Choquette, G., and Ferguson, R.J. 1973. Blood pressure reduction in 'borderline' hypertensives following physical training. Canad. Med. Assoc. J. *108*, 699–703.

Christensen, E.H. 1932. Beiträge zur Physiologie schwerer körperlicher Arbeit. VI Mitteilung: Der Stoffwechsel und die respiratorischen Funktionen bei Schwerer körperlicher Arbeit. Arbeitsphysiologie *5*, 463–78.

Christensen, E.H., and Hansen, O. 1939. Methodik der respiratorischen quotient – Bestimmungen in Ruhe und bei Arbeit. Skand. Arch. Physiol. *81*, 137–51.

Christensen, E.H., and Hoberg, P. 1950. Physiology of skiing. Int. Z. angew. Physiol. *14*, 292–303.

Christie, D. 1968. Physical training in chronic obstructive lung disease. Brit. Med. J. (ii), 150–1.

Clarke, H.H. 1966. Muscular Strength and Endurance in Man. Englewood Cliffs, N.J.: Prentice-Hall.

– 1974. Strength development and motor-sports improvement. Physical Fitness Research Digest *4* (4), Oct.

– 1975. Athletes: their academic achievement and personal-social status. Phys. Fitness Research Digest *5* (3), 1–23.

Clausen, J.P. 1973. Muscle blood flow during exercise and its significance for maximal performance. In: Limiting Factors of Physical Performance. Ed. J. Keul. Stuttgart: Georg Thieme.

Clausen, J.P., Klausen, K., Rasmussen, B., and Trap-Jensen, J. 1971. Effects of selective arm and leg training on cardiac output and regional blood flow. Acta physiol. Scand. *82*, 35–6A.

– 1973. Central and peripheral circulatory changes after training of the arms and legs. Amer. J. Physiol. *225* (3) 675–682.

Clausen, J.P., Trap-Jensen, J., and Lassen, N.A. 1970. The effects of training on the heart rate during arm and leg exercise. Scand. J. clin. Lab. Invest. *26*, 295–301.

Cluver, E.H., de Jongh, T.W., and Jokl, E. 1942. Manpower (South Africa) *1*, 39 (cited by Sloan, 1966).

Coburn, R.F., and Mayers, L.B. 1971. Myoglobin O_2 tension determined from measurements of carboxymyoglobin in skeletal muscle. Amer. J. Physiol. *220*, 66–74.

Colley, J.R.T. 1974. Obesity in school children. Brit. J. Prev. Soc. Med. *28*, 221–5.

Comfort, A. 1964. Ageing: The Biology of Senescence. New York: Holt, Rinehart & Winston.

Comroe, J.H. 1964. The physiological effects of smoking. Physiology for Physicians *2*, 1–6.

Consolazio, C.F., Matoush, L.O., Nelson, R.A., Torres, J.B., and Isaac, G.J. 1963. Environmental temperature and energy expenditures. J. appl. Physiol. *18*, 65–8.

Consolazio, C.F., Nelson, R.A., Matoush, L.O., and Isaac, G.J. 1964. Effects of aspartic acid salts (Mg + K) on physical performance of men. J. appl. Physiol. *19*, 257–61.

Cooper, K.H. 1968. Aerobics. New York: Evans.

– 1970. Guidelines in the management of the exercising patient. J. Amer. Med. Assoc. *211*, 1663–7.

Cormack, R.S., and Heath, J.R. 1974. New techniques for calibrating the Lloyd-Haldane apparatus. J. Physiol. *238*, 627–38.

Cosentino, F. 1970. A history of physical education in Canada. Proc. 1st Canad. Symp. on the History of Sport and Physical Education, Edmonton, Alta.

Costill, D. 1972. Fluid replacement during and following exercise. In: Fitness and Exercise. Ed. J.F. Alexander, R.C. Serfass, and C.M. Tipton. Chicago: Athletic Inst.

Costill, D.L. 1967. The relationship between selected physiological variables and distance running performance. J. Sports Med. Fitness *7*, 61–6.

Cotes, J.E. 1965. Lung Function: Assessment and Application in Medicine. Oxford: Blackwell.

– 1966. Occupational Safety and Health Series, Rept. *6*. Geneva: I.L.O.

– 1974. Genetic factors affecting the lung. Genetic component of lung function. Bull. physio-pathol. Resp. *10*, 109–17.

Cotes, J.E., Berry, G., Burkinshaw, L., Davies, C.T.M., Hall, A.M., Jones, P.R.M., and Knibbs, A.V. 1973. Cardiac frequency during submaximal exercise in young adults; relation to lean body mass, total body potassium and amount of leg muscle. Quart. J. exp. Physiol. *58*, 239–50.

Cotes, J.E., and Woolmer, R.F. 1962. A comparison between twenty seven laboratories of the results of analysis of an expired gas sample. J. Physiol. *163*, 36–7p.

Cotes, J.E., Dobbs, J.M., Elwood, P.C., Hall, A.M., McDonald, A., and Saunders, M.J. 1969. The response to submaximal exercise in adult females; relationship to haemoglobin concentration. J. Physiol. *203* (1), 79p.

Cotton, F.S., and Dill, D.B. 1935. On the relationship between the heart rate during exercise and that of the immediate post-exercise period. Amer. J. Physiol. *111*, 554–8.

Cournand, A., and Richards, D.W. 1941. Pulmonary insufficiency. I. Discussion of a physiological classification and presentation of clinical tests. Amer. Rev. Tuberc. *44*, 26–41.

Coustry-Degré, C., Collard, L., Grevisse, M., and Denolin, H. 1975. Facteurs psycho-sociaux favorisant le declanchement de l'infarctus du myocarde. Manuscript in preparation.

Cox, A. 1970. Sport in Canada 1868–1900. Proc. 1st Canad. Symp. on the History of Sport and Physical Education, Edmonton, Alta.

Crampton, C.W. 1905. A test of condition. Medical News *87*, 529–35.

Crone, P.B., and Tee, G.H. 1974. Staphylococci in swimming pool water. J. Hyg. (Camb.) *73*, 213–20.

Cruz-Coke, R., Donoso, H., and Barrera, R. 1973. Genetic ecology of hypertension. Clin. Sci. Mol. Med. *45*, 55–65s.

Cullumbine, H. 1949/50. Relationship between body build and capacity for exercise. J. appl. Physiol. *2*, 155–68.

Cumming, G., Crank, J., Horsfield, K., and Parker, I. 1966. Gaseous diffusion in the airways of the human lung. Resp. Physiol. *I*, 58–74.

Cumming, G., Horsfield, K., and Preston, S.B. 1971. Diffusion equilibrium in the lungs examined by nodal analysis. Resp. Physiol. *12*, 329–45.

Cumming, G.R. 1967. Current levels of fitness. In: Proc. Int. Symp. on Physical Activity and Cardiovascular Health. Canad. Med. Assoc. J. *96*, 868–77.

– 1970. Fitness Testing of Athletes. Canad. Fam. Phys. (Aug.), 48–52.

– 1971. Correlation of physical performance with laboratory measures of fitness. In: Frontiers of Fitness. Ed. R.J. Shephard. Springfield, Ill.: C.C. Thomas.

– 1972. The frequency and possible significance of ischemic S-T changes in the exercise electrocardiogram. In: Training. Scientific Basis and Application. Ed. A.W. Taylor. Springfield, Ill.: C.C. Thomas.

– 1973. Exercise testing. Newsletter, Amer. Coll. Sports Med. Madison, Wis., Oct.

– 1974. Attempts at maximal exercise testing in 3-6 year old children. Proc. Canad. Assoc. Sports Sciences, Edmonton, Alta, Sept.

– 1975. Put graded exercise testing in your medical office. Canad. Fam. Phys. (March), 102–13.

– 1976. Supine exercise hemodynamics in children after total repair of Fallot's Tetralogy. In: Proc. VIIth Int. Symp. of Pediatric Work Physiology. Ed. R.J. Shephard. Quebec City: Pelican Press.

Cumming, G.R., and Alexander, W.D. 1968. The calibration of bicycle ergometers. Canad. J. Physiol. Pharm. *46*, 917–19.

Cumming, G.R., and Borysyk, L.M. 1972. Criteria for maximum oxygen uptake in men over 40 in a population survey. Med. Sci. Sports *4*, 18–22.

Cumming, G.R., Borysyk, L., and Dufresne, C. 1972. The maximal exercise e.c.g. in asymptomatic men. Canad. Med. Assoc. J. *106*, 649–53.

Cumming, G.R., and Carr, W. 1967. Hemodynamic response to exercise after beta-adrenergic and parasympathetic blockade. Canad. J. Physiol. Pharm. *45*, 813–19.

Cumming, G.R., and Friesen, W. 1967. Bicycle ergometer measurement of maximal oxygen uptake in children. Canad. J. Physiol. Pharm. *45*, 937–46.

Cumming, G.R., Goodwin, A., Baggley, G., and Antel, J. 1967. Repeated measurements of aerobic capacity during a week of intensive training at a youth's track camp. Canad. J. Physiol. Pharm. *45*, 805–11.

Cumming, G.R., Goulding, D., and Baggley, G. 1969. Failure of school physical education to improve cardiorespiratory fitness. Canad. Med. Assoc. J. *101*, 69–73.

Cumming, G.R., and Keynes, R. 1967. A fitness performance test for school children and its correlation with physical working capacity and maximal oxygen uptake. Canad. Med. Assoc. J. *96*, 1262–9.

Cunningham, D.A. 1966. Effects of breathing high concentrations of oxygen on treadmill performance. Res. Quart. *37*, 491–4.

Cunningham, D.A., and Eynon, R.B. 1973. The working capacity of young competitive swimmers, 10–16 years of age. Med. Sci. Sports *5*, 227–31.

Cunningham, D.A., Goode, P.B., and Critz, J.B. 1975. Cardiorespiratory response to exercise on a rowing and a bicycle ergometer. Med. Sci. Sports *7*, 37–43.

Cunningham, D.A., and Paterson, D. 1976. A comparison of methods of calculating cardiac output by the CO_2 rebreathing technique. In press.

Cuomo, A.J., Tisi, G.M., and Moser, K.M. 1973. Relationship of $D_{L,CO}$ and K^{M-I} to lung volume and partition of pulmonary perfusion. J. appl. Physiol. *35*, 129–35.

Cureton, T.K. 1936. Analysis of vital capacity as a test of condition.for high school boys. Res. Quart. *7*, 80–92.

– 1945. Physical Fitness Appraisal and Guidance. St Louis: Mosby.

– 1959. Diet related to athletics and physical fitness. J. Phys. Educ. *57*.

Cutinelli, L., Sorrentino, L., Tramonti, C., Salvatore, F., and Cedrangolo, F. 1970. Protection by ornithine-aspartate of the effects of physical exercise. Arzheim-Forsch. *8*, 1064–7.

Dahlstrom, H. 1964. Reliability and validity of some fitness tests. In: International Research in Sport and Physical Education. Ed. E. Jokl and E. Simon. Springfield, Ill.: C.C. Thomas.

Dalhamn, T. 1966. Effect of cigarette smoke on ciliary activity. Amer. Rev. Resp. Dis. *93*, 108–14.

Damez, M.K., Dawson, P.M., Mathis, D., and Murray, M. 1926. Cardiovascular reactions in athletic and non-athletic girls. J. Amer. Med. Assoc. *86*, 1420–2.

Damoiseau, J., Deroanne, R., and Petit, J.M. 1963. Consommation maximale d'oxygène aux differents ergomètres. J. Physiol. (Paris) *55*, 235–6.

Danforth, W.H. 1965. Activation of glycolytic pathway in muscle. In: Control of Energy Metabolism. Ed. B. Chance, R.W. Estabrook, and J.R. Williamson. New York: Academic Press.

D'Angelo, E., and Torelli, G. 1971. Neural stimuli increasing respiration during different types of exercise. J. appl. Physiol. *30*, 116–21.

Darling, R.C. 1946. The significance of physical fitness. Arch. Phys. Med. *28*, 140–5.

Dautrebande, L., and DuBois, A.B. 1958. Acute effect of breathing inert dust particles and of carbachol aerosol on the mechanical characteristics of the lungs in man. Changes in response after inhaling sympathomimetic aerosols. J. clin. Invest. *37*, 1746–55.

Davies, C.T.M. 1967. Submaximal tests for estimating maximum oxygen intake. Commentary. In: Proc. Int. Symp. on Physical Activity and Cardiovascular Health. Canad. Med. Assoc. J. *96*, 743–4.

– 1968. Limitations to the prediction of maximum oxygen intake from cardiac frequency measurements. J. appl. Physiol. *24*, 700–6.

– 1972a. Maximum aerobic power in relation to body composition in healthy sedentary adults. Human Biol. *44*, 127–39.

– 1972b. The oxygen-transporting system in relation to age. Clin. Sci. *42*, 1–13.

– 1972c. The effects of schistosomiasis, anaemia and malnutrition on the responses to exercise in African children. J. Physiol. *230*, 27p.

– 1973. The contribution of leg (muscle plus bone) volume to maximum aerobic power output: the effects of anaemia, malnutrition and physical activity. J. Physiol. *231*, 108p.

Davies, C.T.M., Barnes, C., and Sargeant, A.J. 1971. Body temperature in exercise. Effect of acclimatization to heat and habituation to work. Int. Z. angew. Physiol. *30*, 10–19.

Davies, C.T.M., Chukweumeka, A.C., and Van Haaren, J.P.M. 1973. Iron deficiency anaemia: its effect on maximum aerobic power and responses to exercise in African males aged 17–40 years. Clin. Sci. *44*, 555–62.

Davies, C.T.M., Cotes, J.E., and John, C. 1967. Relationship of oxygen uptake, ventilation and cardiac frequency to body weight during different forms of standardized exercise. J. Physiol. *190*, 29p.

Davies, C.T.M., Godfrey, S., Light, M., Sargeant, A.J., and Zeidifard, E. 1975. Cardiopulmonary responses to exercise in obese girls and young women. J. appl. Physiol. *38*, 373–6.

Davies, C.T.M., and Knibbs, A.V. 1971. The training stimulus. The effects of intensity, duration and frequency of effort on maximum aerobic power output. Int. Z. angew. Physiol. *29*, 299–305.

Davies, C.T.M. and Sargeant, A.J. 1974a. Physiological responses to standardized arm work. Ergonomics *17*, 41–9.

– 1974b. Physiological responses to exercise following fracture of the leg and subsequent rehabilitation. J. Physiol. *242*, 134–5p.

– 1974c. Physiological responses to one- and two-leg exercise breathing air and 45% oxygen. J. appl. Physiol. *36*, 142–8.

– 1975. Circadian variation in physiological responses to exercise on a stationary bicycle ergometer. Brit. J. industr. Med. *32*, 110–14.

Davies, C.T.M., Tuxworth, W., and Young, J.M. 1970. Physiological effects of repeated exercise. Clin. Sci. *39*, 247–58.

Davies, C.T.M., and Van Haaren, J.P.M. 1973. Effect of treatment on physiological responses to exercise in East African industrial workers with iron deficiency anaemia. Brit. J. industr. Med. *30*, 335–40.

Davis, E.C., Logan, G.A., and McKinney, W.C. 1961. Biophysical Values of Muscular Activity, p. 51. Dubuque, Iowa: W.C. Brown.

Davis, R.H., Jacobs, A., and Rivlin, R. 1967. Dietary iron and haematological status in normal subjects. Brit. Med. J. *3*, 711–12.

Dayton, S., Hashimoto, S.D., Dixon, W.J., and Tomiyasu, W. 1969. A controlled clinical trial of a diet high in unsaturated fat in preventing complications of atherosclerosis. Circulation *40*, Suppl. II, 1–63.

DeBakey, M.E. 1965. Chairman: The President's Commission on Heart Disease, Cancer and Stroke. Report to the President. Vol. 2. Washington, D.C.: U.S. Government Printing Office.

de Coster, A. 1971. Present concepts of the relationship between lactate and oxygen debt. In: Frontiers of Fitness. Ed. R.J. Shephard. Springfield, Ill.: C.C. Thomas.

de Coster, A., Denolin, H., and Englert, M. 1958. Etude de la ventilation alvéolaire et de l'espace mort physiologique au repos et à l'effort chez les sujets normaux et pathologiques. Acta med. Scand. *162*, 47–60.

Defares, J.G. 1956. A study of the carbon dioxide time course during rebreathing. Ph.D. Thesis, University of Utrecht, Utrecht, Holland.

Dehn, M., and Bruce, R.A. 1972. Longitudinal variations in maximal oxygen intake with age and activity. J. appl. Physiol. *33*, 805–7.

Delhez, L., Botton-Thonon, A., and Petit, J.M. 1967–68. Influence de l'entrainment sur la force maximum des muscles respiratoires. Soc. Med. Belg. Ed. Phys. *20*, 52–63.

de Marées, H., and Barbey, K. 1973. Änderung der peripheren Durchblutung durch Ausdauertraining. Z. f. Kardiol. *62*, 653–63.

Demedts, M., and Anthonisen, N.R. 1973. Effects of increased external airway resistance during steady-state exercise. J. appl. Physiol. *35*, 361–6.

Dempsey, J.A., Reddan, W., Balke, B., and Rankin, J. 1966. Work capacity determinants and physiologic cost of weight-supported work in obesity. J. appl. Physiol. *21*, 1815–20.

Dempsey, J.A., Rodriquez, J., Shahidi, N.T., Reddan, W.G., and MacDougall, J.D. 1971. Muscular exercise 2,3 DPG and oxyhaemoglobin affinity. Int. Z. angew. Physiol. *30*, 34–9.

Denning, H., Talbot, J.H., Edwards, H.T., and Dill, D.B. 1931. Effect of acidosis and alkalosis upon capacity for work. J. clin. Invest. *9*, 601–13.

– 1937. Über Steigerung der körperlichen Leistungsfähigkeit durch Eingriffe in den Saurebasenhaushalf. Dtsch. Med. Wschr. *63*, 733–6.

Deroanne, R., Juchmes, J., Hausman, A., Pirnay, F., and Petit, J.M. 1968. Resistance inspiratoire et tolerance à l'exercise musculaire chez l'homme normal. Arch. Int. Physiol. Biochim. *76*, 163–4.

de Schryver, C., Mertens-Strythagen, J., Becsei, I., and Lammerant, J. 1969. Effect of training on heart and skeletal muscle catecholamine concentration in rats. Amer. J. Physiol. *217*, 1589–92.

Detry, J.M., Brengelman, G.L., Rowell, L.B., and Wyss, C. 1972. Skin and muscle components of forearm flow in directly heated resting man. J. appl. Physiol. *32*, 506–11.

Devenney, H.M. 1974. Guest Editor. History of C.A.H.P.E.R. Commemorative Issue. C.A.H.P.E.R. J. *40* (5), 1–62.

de Vries, H.A. 1968. Immediate and long-term effects of exercise upon resting action potential level. J. Sports Med. *8*, 1–11.

– 1970. Physiological effects of an exercise training regimen upon men aged 52 to 88. J. Gerontol. *25*, 325–36.

de Wijn, J.F., de Jongste, J.L., Mosterd, W., and Willebrand, D. 1971. Haemoglobin, packed cell volume, serum iron and iron-binding capacity of selected athletes during training. J. Sports Med. Phys. Fitness *11*, 42–51.

Dickensen, S. 1929. The efficiency of bicycle pedaling as affected by speed and load. J. Physiol. *67*, 242–55.

Dickie, H.A., and Rankin, J. 1960. Interstitial disease of the lung: the alveolar-capillary block syndrome. In: Clinical Cardiopulmonary Physiology. Ed. B.L. Gordon. New York: Grune & Stratton.

Dill, D.B. 1942. Effects of physical strain and high altitudes on heart and circulation. Amer. Heart J. *23*, 441-54.

– 1967. The Harvard Fatigue Laboratory: Its development, contributions and demise. Circ. Res. *20*, Suppl. *I*, 161-70.

Dill, D.B., Edwards, H.T., and Talbott, J.H. 1932. Alkalosis and the capacity for work. J. biol. Chem. *97*, 58-9.

Dill, D.B., Robinson, S., and Ross, J.C. 1967. A longitudinal study of 16 champion runners. J. Sports Med. *7*, 4-32.

di Prampero, P.E. 1971. Anaerobic capacity and power. In: Frontiers of Fitness. Ed. R.J. Shephard. Springfield, Ill.: C.C. Thomas.

di Prampero, P.E., and Cerretelli, P. 1969. Maximal muscular power (aerobic and anaerobic) in African natives. Ergonomics *12*, 51-9.

di Prampero, P.E., Cerretelli, P., and Piiper, J. 1969. Capacita di diffusione del polmone per l'O_2 nel cane a riposo e durante il lavoro. Boll. del. Soc. Ital. di Biol. Sper. *45*, 375-7.

di Prampero, P.E., Cortili, G., Celentano, F., and Cerretelli, P. 1971. Physiological aspects of rowing. J. appl. Physiol. *31*, 853-7.

Dirix, A. 1973. Doping – théorie et pratique. Brit. J. Sports Med. *7*, 250-8.

Dittmer, D.S., and Grebe, R.M. 1958. Handbook of Respiration. USAF WADC Tech. Rept. *58*, 352. Dayton, Ohio: U.S. Air Force Wright Air Development Centre.

Doll, E. 1973. Oxygen pressure and content in the blood during physical exercise and hypoxia. In: Limiting Factors of Physical Performance. Ed. J. Keul. Stuttgart: Thieme.

Doll, E., Keul, J., and Maiwald, C. 1968. Oxygen tension and acid-base equilibria in venous blood of working muscle. Amer. J. Physiol. *215*, 23-9.

Donald, D.E., and Shepherd, J.T. 1964. Sustained capacity for exercise in dogs after complete cardiac denervation. Amer. J. Cardiol. *14*, 853-9.

Donald, K.W., Bishop, J.M., and Wade, O.L. 1954. A study of minute to minute changes of arterio-venous oxygen difference, oxygen uptake and cardiac output, and rate of achievement of a steady-state during exercise in rheumatic heart disease. J. clin. Invest. *33*, 1146-67.

Dorfman, R. 1965. Measuring Benefits of Government Investments. Washington, D.C.: The Brookings Institution.

Dosman, J., Bode, F., Urbanetti, J., Martin, R., and Macklem, P.T. 1975. The use of a helium-oxygen mixture during maximum expiratory flow to demonstrate obstruction in small airways in smokers. J. clin. Invest. *55*, 1090-9.

Douglas, F.G.V., and Becklake, M.R. 1968. Effect of seasonal training on maximal cardiac output. J. appl. Physiol. *25*, 600–5.

Drake, V., Jones, G., Brown, J.R., and Shephard, R.J. 1968. Fitness performance tests and their relationship to maximum oxygen uptake. Canad. Med. Assoc. J. *99*, 844–8.

Draper, H.H. 1976. Nutritional research in circumpolar populations. In: Circumpolar Health. Ed. R.J. Shephard and S. Itoh. Toronto: University of Toronto Press.

Dreyer, G. 1920. The Assessment of Physical Fitness. London: Cassell.

Drinkwater, B., and Horvath, S.M. 1972. Detraining effects on young women. Med. Sci. Sports *4*, 91–5.

Drinkwater, B.L. 1973. Physiological responses of women to exercise. Ex. Sport Sci. Rev. *1*, 126–53.

Dublin, L.L. 1932. College Honor Men Long-lived. Stat. Bull. Metrop. Life Ins. Co., New York *13*, 5–7.

Dubos, R. 1967. Individual morality and statistical morality. Ann. Int. Med. *67*, Suppl. 7, 57–60.

Dujardin, J., Deroanne, R., Pirnay, F., and Petit, J.M. 1967–68. Acide lactique et exercise musculaire. Trav. Soc. Med. Belge d'Ed. Phys. et de Sports *20*, 74–6.

Duling, B.R., and Pittman, R.N. 1975. Oxygen tension: dependent or independent variable in local control of blood flow? Fed. Proc. *34*, 2012–19.

Düner, H. 1959. Oxygen uptake and working capacity during work on the bicycle ergometer with one or both legs. Acta physiol. Scand. *46*, 55–61.

Durnin, J.V.G.A. 1966. Age, physical activity and energy expenditure. Proc. Nutr. Soc. *25*, 107–13.

– 1967a. The influence of nutrition. In: Proc. Int. Symp. on Physical Activity and Cardiovascular Health. Canad. Med. Assoc. J. *96*, 715–18.

– 1967b. Activity patterns in the community. In: Proc. Int. Symp. on Physical Activity and Cardiovascular Health. Canad. Med. Assoc. J. *96*, 882–6.

Durnin, J.V.G.A., Brockway, J.M., and Whitcher, H.W. 1960. Effects of a short period of training of varying severity on some measurements of physical fitness. J. appl. Physiol. *15*, 161–5.

Durnin, J.V.G.A., and Passmore, R. 1967. Energy, Work and Leisure. London: Heinemann.

Durnin, J.V.G.A., and Ramahan, M.M. 1967. The assessment of the amount of fat in the human body from measurement of skinfold thickness. Brit. J. Nutr. *21*, 681–9.

Durnin, J.V.G.A., and Womersley, J. 1971. The relationship of total body fat, 'fat-free mass' and total body weight in male and female human populations of varying ages. J. Physiol. *213*, 33p.

Durusoy, F., and Özgönül, H. 1971. Lung function studies on former athletes who are now football referees. J. Sports Med. Phys. Fitness *11*, 139–45.

Eaton, J.D. 1970. Arthur Stanley Lamb M.D. 1886-1958. His influence on Canadian Sport. Proc. 1st Canad. Symp. on the History of Sport and Physical Education, Edmonton, Alta.

Ebert, R.V., and Terracio, M.J. 1975. The bronchiolar epithelium in cigarette smokers. Amer. Rev. Resp. Dis. *111*, 4–11.

Eckstein, R.W. 1957. Effect of exercise and coronary artery narrowing on coronary collateral circulation. Circulation Res. *5*, 230–5.

Edgerton, R. 1975. Physiology of power endurance work. Annual Meeting, Canad. Assoc. Sports Sci., Ottawa. Published Can. J. Appl. Sport Sci., *1*, 49–58, 1976.

Edholm, O.G. 1966. The assessment of habitual activity. In: Physical Activity in Health and Disease. Ed. K. Evang and K.L. Andersen. Oslo: Oslo University Press.

– 1970. The changing pattern of human activity. Ergonomics *13*, 625–43.

Edholm, O.G., Adam, J.M., Healy, M.J.R., Wolff, H.S., Goldsmith, R., and Best, T.W. 1970. Food intake and energy expenditure of army recruits. Brit. J. Nutr. *24*, 1091-107.

Edholm, O.G., Fletcher, J.G., Widdowson, E.M., and McCance, R.A. 1955. Energy expenditure and food intake of individual men. Brit. J. Nutr. *9*, 286–300.

Edholm, O.G., Humphrey, S., Lourie, J.A., Tredre, B.E., and Brotherhood, J. 1973. VI. Energy expenditure and climatic exposure of Yemenite and Kurdish Jews in Israel. Phil. Trans. Roy. Soc. Lond. *B266*, 127–40.

Edwards, D.A.W., Hammond, W.H., Healy, M.J.R., Tanner, J.M., and Whitehouse, R.H. 1955. Design and accuracy of calipers for measuring subcutaneous tissue thickness. Brit. J. Nutr. *9*, 133–43.

Edwards, R.H.T., Ekelund, L.G., Harris, R.C., Hesser, C.M., Hultman, E., Melcher, A., and Wigertz, O. 1973. Cardio-respiratory and metabolic costs of continuous and intermittent exercise in man. J. Physiol. *234*, 481–97.

Edwards, R.H.T., Melcher, A., Hesser, C.M., Wigertz, O., and Ekelund, L.G. 1972. Physiological correlates of perceived exertion in continuous and intermittent exercise with the same average power output. Europ. J. clin. Invest. *2*, 108–14.

Eichna, L.W., Park, C.R., Nelson, N., Horvath, S.M., and Palmes, E.D. 1950. Thermal regulation during acclimatization in a hot, dry (desert-type) environment. Amer. J. Physiol. *163*, 585–97.

Ekblom, B. 1969a. Effect of physical training on adolescent boys. J. appl. Physiol. *27*, 350–5.

– 1969b. Effect of physical training on oxygen transport system in man. Acta physiol. Scand. Suppl. *328*, 1–45.

– 1971. Physical training in normal boys in adolescence. Acta Paediatr. Scand. *217*, 60-2.

Ekblom, B., Astrand, P.O., Saltin, B., Stenberg, J., and Wallstrom, B. 1968. Effect of training on circulatory response to exercise. J. appl. Physiol. *24*, 518–28.

Ekblom, B., and Gjessing, E. 1968. Maximal oxygen uptake of the Easter Island population. J. appl. Physiol. *25*, 124–9.

Ekblom, B., and Goldbarg, A.N. 1971. The influence of physical training and other factors on the subjective rating of perceived exertion. Acta physiol. Scand. *83*, 399–406.

Ekblom, B., Goldbarg, A.N., and Bullbring, B. 1972. Response to exercise after blood loss and reinfusion. J. appl. Physiol. *33*, 175–80.

Ekblom, B., and Hermansen, L. 1968. Cardiac output in athletes. J. appl. Physiol. *25*, 619–25.

Ekblom, B., and Huof, R. 1972. Response to sub-maximal and maximal exercise at different levels of carboxyhaemoglobin. Acta physiol. Scand. *86*, 474–82.

Ekelund, L.G. 1967a. Circulatory and respiratory adaptation during prolonged exercise of moderate intensity in the sitting position. Acta physiol. Scand. *69*, 327–40.

– 1967b. Circulatory and respiratory adaptation during prolonged exercise. Acta physiol. Scand. *70*, Suppl. *292*.

Ekelund, L.G., and Holmgren, A. 1964. Circulatory and respiratory adaptation during long-term, non-steady state exercise in the sitting position. Acta physiol. Scand. *62*, 240–55.

– 1967. Central haemodynamics during exercise. Circulation Res. *21*, Suppl. *1*, I33–I43.

Elbel, E.R., Ormond, D., and Close, D. 1961. Some effects of breathing oxygen before and after exercise. J. appl. Physiol. *16*, 48–52.

Ellis, F.R., and Nasser, S. 1973. A pilot study of vitamin B_{12} in the treatment of tiredness. Brit. J. Nutr. *30*, 277–83.

Ellis, G. 1971. Units, Symbols and Abbreviations. A Guide for Biological and Medical Editors and Authors. London: Royal Society of Medicine.

Elsner, R.F. 1959. Changes in peripheral circulation with exercise training. U.S.A.F. Arctic Aero-Med. Lab. Tech. Rept. *59*, 16.

Engel, L.A., Wood, L.D.H., Utz, G., and Macklem, P.T. 1973. Gas mixing during inspiration. J. appl. Physiol. *35*, 18–24.

Enghoff, H. 1938. Volumen Inefficax. Bemerkungen zur Frage des schädlichen Raümes. Uppsala Lakareforen Forhendl. *44*, 191–218.

Engström, I., Eriksson, B.O., Karlberg, P., Saltin, P., and Thoren, C. 1971. Preliminary report on the development of lung volumes in young girl swimmers. Acta Paediatr. Scand. Suppl. *217*, 73–6.

Engström, L-M. 1972. Idrott par fritid. En enkätstudie bland elever i årskurs 8. Stockholm: Pedagogiska Institutionen. Lärahogskolan.

Enos, W.F., Bayer, J.C., and Holmes, R.H. 1955. Pathogenesis of coronary disease in American soldiers killed in Korea. J. Amer. Med. Assoc. *158*, 912–14.

Epstein, F.H. 1968. Multiple risk factors and the prediction of coronary heart disease. Bull. N.Y. Acad. Med. *44*, 916–33.

Erb, B.D. (Chairman). 1970. Physician's Handbook for Evaluation of Cardiovascular and Physical Fitness. Nashville, Tenn.: Tennessee Heart Association Physical Exercise Committee.

Eriksson, B.O. 1972. Physical training, oxygen supply and muscle metabolism in 11–13 year old boys. Acta Physiol. Scand., Suppl. *384*, 1–48.

Ernsting, J., and Shephard, R.J. 1951. Respiratory adaptations in congenital heart disease. J. Physiol. *112*, 332–43.

Espenschade, A.S., and Meleney, H.E. 1961. Motor performance of adolescent boys and girls of today in comparison with those of 24 years ago. Res. Quart. *32*, 186–9.

Eysenck, H.J. 1959. Manual of the Maudsley Personality Inventory. London: University of London Press.

Fahey, T., and Brown, H. 1972. Effects of anabolic steroids plus weight training on normal males – a double blind study. Paper presented at 19th Annual Meeting, Amer. Coll. Sports Med., Philadelphia, May.

Falkenhahn, A., Hollmann, W., Kenter, H., Venrath, H., and Bouchard, C. 1967. Der Einfluss von digitalis auf die Leistungsfähigkeit gesunder Ratten im Schwimmerversuch. Arnzeim-Forsch. *17*, 551–3.

Fallis, N., Wilson, W.R., Tetreault, L.L., and LaSagna, L. 1963. Effect of potassium and magnesium aspartates on athletic performance. J. Amer. Med. Assoc. *185*, 129.

Falls, H.B., and Humphrey, L.D. 1973. A comparison of methods for eliciting maximum oxygen uptake from college women during treadmill walking. Med. Sci. Sports *5*, 239–41.

Falls, H.B., Ismail, A.H., and MacLeod, D.F. 1966. Estimation of maximum oxygen uptake in adults from AAHPER youth fitness test items. Res. Quart. *37*, 192–201.

Fardy, P.S. 1969. Effects of soccer training and detraining upon selected cardiac and metabolic measures. Res. Quart. *40*, 502–8.

Fardy, P.S., and Ilmarinen, J. 1975. Evaluating the effects and feasibility of an at work stairclimbing intervention program for men. Med. Sci. Sports *7*, 91–3.

Faria, I.E. 1970. Cardiovascular responses to exercise as influenced by training of various intensities. Res. Quart. *41*, 44–50.

Faulkner, J.A. 1966. Physiology of swimming. Res. Quart. *37*, 41–54.

– 1967. Training for maximum performance at altitude. In: The Effects of Attitude on Athletic Performance. Ed. R. Goddard. Chicago: Athletic Inst.

– 1973. Viewpoint – Exercise testing. Newsletter, Amer. Coll. Sports Med., Madison, Wis., July.

Faulkner, J.A., Roberts, D.E., Elk, R.L., and Conway, J. 1971. Cardiovascular responses to sub-maximum and maximum effort cycling and running. J. appl. Physiol. *30*, 457–61.

Faulkner, J.A., and Stoedfalke, K. 1975. Guidelines for graded exercise testing and exercise prescription and behavioural objectives for physicians, program directors, exercise leaders and exercise technicians. Madison, Wis.: Amer. Coll. Sports Med.

Ferro-Luzzi, A., Topi, G.C., and Caldarone, G. 1975. Consumi alimentari abituali di atleti italiani probabili olimpici (P.O. 1972). Med. dello Sport *28*, 109–25.

Fisher, H.K., Holton, P., St-J. Buxton, R., and Nadel, J.A. 1970. Resistance to breathing during exercise-induced asthma attacks. Amer. Rev. Resp. Dis. *101*, 885–96.

Fishman, A.P. 1963. Dynamics of the pulmonary circulation. In: Handbook of Physiology. Section 2: Circulation, Vol. II. Ed. W.F. Hamilton. Baltimore: Williams & Wilkins.

Fishman, A.P., and Richards, D.W. 1964. Circulation of the Blood. Men and Ideas. Oxford: Oxford University Press.

Fitch, K.D., and Morton, A.R. 1971. Specificity of exercise in exercise-induced asthma. Brit. Med. J. (ii), 577–88.

Fitts, R.H., Booth, F.W., Winder, W.W., and Holloszy, J.O. 1975. Skeletal muscle respiratory capacity, endurance and glycogen utilization. Amer. J. Physiol. *228*, 1029–33.

Fitts, R.H., Nagle, F.J., and Cassens, R.G. 1973. Characteristics of skeletal muscle fiber types in the miniature pig and the effect of training. Canad. J. Physiol. *51*, 825–31.

Flack, M. 1920. The Medical and Surgical Aspects of Aviation. Oxford: Oxford University Press.

Flandrois, R., and LaCour, J.R. 1971. The prediction of maximal oxygen intake in acute moderate hypoxia. Int. Z. angew. Physiol. *29*, 306–13.

Flenley, D.C., Fairweather, L.J., Cooke, N.J., and Kirby, B.J. 1973. The effects of variations in P_{50} on oxygen transport in chronic hypoxic lung disease. Proc. Med. Res. Soc., U.K., Dec. Clin. Sci. Mol. Biol. *46*, 18p, 1974.

Flook, V., and Kelman, G.R. 1973. Submaximal exercise with increased inspiratory resistance to breathing. J. appl. Physiol. *35*, 379–84.

Folkins, C.H., Lynch, S., and Gardner, M.M. 1973. Physiological fitness as a function of physical fitness. Arch. Phys. Med. Rehab. *53*, 503–8.

Folkow, B., Gaskell, P., and Waalen, B.A. 1970. Blood flow through limb muscles during heavy rhythmic exercise. Acta physiol. Scand. *80*, 61–72.

Folkow, B., Heymans, C., and Neil, E. 1965. Integrated aspects of cardiovascular regulation. In: Handbook of Physiology, Circulation. Vol. 3, pp.1787–823. Ed. W.F. Hamilton. Washington, D.C.: Amer. Physiol. Soc.

Forbes, G.B., and Reina, J.C. 1970. Adult lean mass declines with age: some longitudinal observations. Metabolism *19*, 653–63.

Fordtran, J.S., and Saltin, B. 1967. Gastric emptying and intestinal absorption during prolonged severe exercise. J. appl. Physiol. *23*, 331–5.

Forgraeus, L. 1973. Oxygen uptake in work at lowered and raised ambient air pressures. Acta physiol. Scand. *87*, 411–21.

Forster, R.E. 1964. Rate of gas uptake by red cells. In: Handbook of Physiology, Section 3: Respiration. Vol. 1. Ed. W.O. Fenn and H. Rahn. Washington, D.C.: Amer. Physiol. Soc.

Foster, W.L. 1914. A test of physical efficiency. Amer. Phys. Ed. Rev. *19*, Dec. (cited by Steinhaus, 1933).

Fowler, W.H., Gardner, G.H., and Egstrom, G.H. 1965. Effect of an anabolic steroid on physical performance of young men. J. appl. Physiol. *20*, 1038–40.

Fox, E.L., Bartels, R.L., Billings, C.E., O'Brien, R., Bason, R., and Mathews, D.K. 1975. Frequency and duration of interval training programs and changes in aerobic power. J. appl. Physiol. *38*, 481–4.

Fox, M., Minot, A.S., and Liddle, G.W. 1962. Oxandrolone: a potent anabolic steroid of novel chemical configuration. J. clin. Endocrinol. *22*, 921–4.

Fox, R.H., Goldsmith, R., Kidd, D.J., and Lewis, H.E. 1963. Acclimatization to heat in man by controlled elevation of body temperature. J. Physiol. *166*, 530–47.

Fox, S.M. 1969. Exercise and stress testing workshop report. J.S. Carol. Med. Assoc. Suppl. *1*, 77.

– 1974. Coronary Heart Disease. Prevention, Detection, Rehabilitation, with Emphasis on Exercise Testing. Denver: Int. Med. Corp.

Fox, S.M., and Haskell, W. 1968. The Exercise Stress Test: Needs for Standardization. 4th Asian/Pacific Congress of Cardiology, Tel Aviv. Cited in S. Fox: Exercise and stress testing workshop report, National Conference on Exercise in the Prevention, in the Evaluation and in the Treatment of Heart Disease. J.S. Carol. Med. Assoc. *65*, Suppl. *1*, 77.

Fox, S.M., and Skinner, J.S. 1964. Physical activity and cardiovascular health. Amer. J. Cardiol. *14*, 731–46.

Franks, B.D. 1969. Exercise and Fitness 1969. A Tribute to Thomas K. Cureton Jr. Chicago: Athletic Inst.

Franks, B.D., and Cureton, T.K. 1969. Effects of training on time components of the left ventricle. J. Sports Med. Phys. Fitness *9*, 80–8.

Frech, W.E., Schultehinrichs, D., Vogel, H.R., and Thews, G. 1968. Modelluntersuchungen zum Austausch der Atemgase. 1: Die O_2-Aufnahmezeiten des Erythrocyten unter den Bedingungen des Lungen capillarblutes. Pflüg. Archiv. *301*, 292–301.

Freedman, S. 1970. Sustained maximum voluntary ventilation. Resp. Physiol. *8*, 230–44.

Freyschuss, U., and Strandell, T. 1967. Limb circulation during arm and leg exercise in supine position. J. appl. Physiol. *23*, 163–70.

– 1968. Circulatory adaptation to one- and two-leg exercise in supine position. J. appl. Physiol. *25*, 511–15.

Frick, M.H., Konttinen, A., and Sarajas, H.S.S. 1963. Effects of physical training on circulation at rest and during exercise. Amer. J. Cardiol. *12*, 142–7.

Fried, T., and Shephard, R.J. 1969. Deterioration and restoration of physical fitness after training. Canad. Med. Assoc. J. *100*, 831–7.

– 1970. Assessment of a lower extremity training programme. Canad. Med. Assoc. J. *103*, 260–6.

Friedman, E.H., and Hellerstein, H.K. 1973. Influence of psycho-social factors on coronary risk and adaptation to a physical fitness evaluation program. In: Exercise Testing and Exercise Training in Coronary Heart Disease. Ed. J.P. Naughton and H.K. Hellerstein. New York: Academic Press.

Friedman, M., and Rosenman, R.H. 1974. Type A Behaviour and Your Heart. Greenwich, Conn.: Fawcett Publications.

Friedman, M., Rosenman, R.H., and Brown, A.E. 1963. The continuous heart rate in men exhibiting an overt behaviour pattern associated with an increased incidence of clinical coronary artery disease. Circulation *28*, 861–6.

Froelicher, V.F., Brammell, H., Davis, G., Noguera, I., Stewart, A., and Lancaster, M.C. 1974. A comparison of three maximal treadmill exercise protocols. Chest *65*, 512–17.

Froehlicher, V.F., Yanowitz, F., Thompson, A.J., and Lancaster, M.C. 1975. Physiological responses in aircrewmen and the detection of latent coronary artery disease. Neuilly-sur-Seine, France: N.A.T.O. Agardograph *210*, 1–60.

Frucht, A.H., and Jokl, E. 1964. The future of athletic records. In: International Research in Sport and Physical Education. Ed. E. Jokl and E. Simon. Springfield, Ill.: C.C. Thomas.

Fugelli, P. 1974. Health of arctic fishermen as related to occupational capacity. 3rd Int. Symp. on Circumpolar Health, Yellowknife, N.W.T. (See Shephard and Itoh, 1976)

Fulton, J.F. 1930. Selected Readings in Physiology. Springfield, Ill.: C.C. Thomas.

Gaesser, G.A., and Brooks, G.A. 1975. Muscular efficiency during steady-state exercise: effects of speed and work rate. J. appl. Physiol. 38, 1132-9.

Galen 1951. De Sanitate Tuenda (transl. by R.M. Green). Springfield, Ill.: C.C. Thomas (cited by Ryan, 1974).

Galevskaya, E.N. 1970. On the system and timing of gymnastic exercises for skilled industrial labourers at work. Theory and Practice of Physical Culture, Moscow. 7, 52-4. Cited by N. Schneidman, Soviet studies in the fitness of the aged. Canad. Fam. Phys. (Oct. 1972), 53-6.

Galton, D.J. 1966. An enzymatic defect in a group of obese patients. Brit. Med. J. (ii), 1498-500.

Ganslen, R.V., Balke, B., Nagle, F.J., and Phillips, E.E. 1963. Effects of some tranquilizing, analeptic, and vasodilating drugs on physical work capacity and orthostatic tolerance. U.S. Fed. Aviation Agency Rept. 63, 34.

Garlind, T., Goldberg, L., Graf, K., Perman, E.S., and Strandell, T. 1960. Effect of ethanol on circulatory, metabolic and neuro-hormonal function during muscular work in men. Acta pharmacol. toxicol. 17, 106-14.

Gaskell, W.H. 1877. On the vasomotor nerves of striated muscles. J. Anat. Lond. 11, 360-402.

Gayrard, P., Orehek, J., Grimaud, C.H., and Charpin, J. 1974. Bronchoconstriction due à l'inhalation de fumée de Tabac: effets comparés chez le sujet normal et l'asthmatique. Bull. Physio-Path. Resp. 10, 451-61.

Gedda, L. 1961. Sport and genetics. A study on twins (351 pairs). In: Health and Fitness in the Modern World. Washington, D.C.: Athletic Inst.

Geissler, H.J. 1960. Zu einigen Untersuchungsergebnissen auf dem Gebiete der Ausgleichsgymnastik wahrend der Arbeitszeit. Wiss. Zschr. DHFK, Leipzig, 3, 229-42.

Gemmill, C.L. 1942. Fuel for muscular exercise. Physiol. Rev. 22, 32-53.

Gerber, E.W. 1972. Critique of physical education and the reification of the human body. Proc. 2nd Canad. Symp. on the History of Sport and Physical Education, Windsor, Ont.

Gertler, M.M. 1967. Ischaemic heart disease, heredity and body build as affected by exercise. Canad. Med. Assoc. J. 96, 728-30.

Ghiringhelli, G., Bosisio, E., and Pasargiklian, M. 1957. L'influenza della frequenza respiratoria sui volumi di ventilazione polmonare massima. Riv. Med. Aeronaut. 20, 3-36.

Gillespie, J.A. 1967. Vasodilator properties of alcohol. Brit. Med. J. i, 274–7.

Gilligan, D.R., Altschule, M.D., and Katersky, E.M. 1943. Physiological intra-vascular hemolysis of exercise. Hemoglobinemia and haemoglobinuria following cross-country runs. J. clin. Invest. 22, 859–69.

Gilson, J.C. 1973. Asbestos cancer – past and future hazards. Proc. Roy. Soc. Med. 66, 395–403.

Gilson, J.C., and Hugh-Jones, P. 1955. Lung function in coal workers' pneumo-coniosis. MRC Special Rept. Ser. 290, 1–266. London: H.M.S.O.

Glagov, S., Rowley, D.A., Cramer, D.B., and Page, R.G. 1970. Heart rates during 24 hours of usual activity for 100 normal men. J. appl. Physiol. 29, 799–805.

Glaser, E.M. 1966. The Physiological Basis of Habituation. Oxford: University Press.

Glaser, E.M. McPherson, D., Prior, K., and Charles, E. 1954. Radiological investigations of the effects of haemorrhage on the lungs, liver and spleen, with special reference to the storage of blood in man. Clin. Sci. 13, 461–73.

Glassford, R.G. 1969. The Meso-American Rubber Ball Games. In: Proc. First Int. Seminar on the History of Physical Education and Sport, Natanya, Israel.

– 1970. Games of the traditional Canadian Eskimo. Proc. 1st Canad. Symp. on the History of Sport and Physical Education, Edmonton, Alta.

Glassford, R.G., Baycroft, G.H.Y., Sedgwick, A.W., and MacNab, R.B.J. 1965. Comparison of maximal oxygen uptake values determined by predicted and actual methods. J. appl. Physiol. 20, 509–13.

Glassford, R.G., and Howell, M.L. 1969. Smoking and physical fitness: a preliminary report. Canad. Fam. Phys. (Oct.).

Gledhill, N., and Eynon, R.B. 1972. The intensity of training. In: Training: Scientific Basis and Application. Ed. A.W. Taylor. Springfield, Ill.: C.C. Thomas.

Gleser, M., Horstman, D.H., and Mello, R.P. 1974. The effect on $\dot{V}_{O_2}$ max of adding arm work to maximal leg work. Med. Sci. Sports 6, 104–7.

Goddard, R. (Ed.) 1967. The Effects of Altitude on Athletic Performance. Chicago: Athletic Inst.

Godin, G., and Shephard, R.J. 1972. On the course of carbon monoxide uptake and release. Respiration 29, 317–29.

– 1973a. Activity patterns of the Canadian Eskimo. In: Human Polar Biology. Ed. O. Edholm and E.K.E. Gunderson. Cambridge, U.K.: Heinemann.

– 1973b. Body weight and the energy cost of activity. Arch. Env. Health 27, 289–93.

Godin, G., Wright, G., and Shephard, R.J. 1972. Urban exposure to carbon monoxide. A.M.A. Arch. Env. Health 25, 305–13.

Gold, A.J., Zornitzer, A., and Samueloff, S. 1969. Influence of season and heat on energy expenditure during rest and exercise. J. appl. Physiol. 27, 9–12.

Golding, L.A. 1972. Drugs and hormones. In: Ergogenic Aids and Muscular Performance. Ed. W.P. Morgan. New York: Academic Press.

Golding, L.A., and Barnard, R.J. 1963. The effect of d-amphetamine sulfate on physical performance. J. Sports Med. Phys. Fitness *3*, 221–4.

Goldsmith, R., and Hale, T. 1971. Relationship between habitual physical activity and physical fitness. Amer. J. clin. Nutr. *24*, 1489–93.

Goldsmith, J.R., Terzaghi, J., and Hackney, J.D. 1963. Evaluation of fluctuating carbon monoxide exposures. A.M.A. Arch. Env. Health *7*, 647–63.

Gollnick, P., and Hermansen, L. 1973. Biochemical adaptations to exercise. Anaerobic metabolism. Exercise and Sports Sci. Rev. *1*, 1–43.

Gollnick, P.D., Piehl, K., and Saltin, B. 1974. Selective glycogen depletion pattern in human muscle fibres after exercise of varying intensity and at varying pedalling rates. J. Physiol. *241*, 45–57.

Goode, R.C., Firstbrook, J.B., and Shephard, R.J. 1966. Effects of exercise and a cholesterol-free diet on human serum lipids. Canad. J. Physiol. Pharm. *44*, 575–80.

Goodman, R.F. 1968. The effects of football equipment on heat transfer. In: Physiological Aspects of Sports and Physical Fitness. Chicago: Athletic Inst.

Goodwin, J.E., and Levitt, P. 1962. Telemetering heart rate during exercise. Proc. Canad. Fed. Biol. Soc. *5*, 45.

Gordon, B. 1935. Cited by Ryan 1974. Ann. Med. Hist. *7*, 513–18.

Gould, L. 1970. Cardiac effects of alcohol. Amer. Heart J. *79*, 422–5.

Gould, L., Venkataraman, F.K., Goswami, M., and Gomprecht, R.F. 1973. The cardiac effects of coffee. Angiology *24*, 455–63.

Graeser, H.J., Kim, V.G., and Grandall, E.D. 1969. The effects of time-varying blood flow on diffusion resistance to oxygen transfer in the pulmonary capillaries. Biophys. J. *9*, 1100–14.

Graf, K., and Ström, G. 1960. Effect of ethanol ingestion on arm blood flow in healthy young men at rest and during leg work. Acta pharm. toxicol. *17*, 115–20.

Graf, O. 1930. Zur Frage der spezifischen Wirkung der Cola auf die körperliche Leistungsfähigkeit. Arbeitsphysiologie *2*, 474–506.

Granger, H.J., Goodman, A.H., and Cook, B.H. 1975. Metabolic models of microcirculatory regulation. Fed. Proc. *34*, 2025–30.

Green, H. 1967. Urban and rural differences in the work capacity of Alberta secondary school students as measured by the Åstrand predicted maximal oxygen intake test. Edmonton, Alta.: Unpublished Report, Fitness Research Unit.

Gregg, D.E., and Fisher, L.C. 1964. Blood supply to the heart. In: Handbook of Physiology, Section 2: Circulation, Vol. 1. Ed. W.F. Hamilton. Washington, D.C.: Amer. Physiol. Soc.

Grimby, G. 1965. Renal clearances during prolonged supine exercise at different loads. J. appl. Physiol. *20*, 1294–8.

Grollman, A. 1929. The determination of the cardiac output of man by the use of acetylene. Amer. J. Physiol. *88*, 432–45.

– 1931. Physiological variations in the cardiac output of man. Amer. J. Physiol. *98*, 8–15.

Gueli, D., and Shephard, R.J. 1976. Pedal frequency in bicycle ergometry. Can. J. appl. Sports Sci. *1*, 137–42.

Guillerm, R., Badré, R., Hée, J., and Masurel, G. 1972. Composition de la fumée de tabac. Analyse des facteurs de nuisance. Rev. Tuberc. Pneumol. *36*, 187–208.

Haddy, F.J., Overbeck, H.W., and Daugherty, R.M. 1968. Peripheral vascular resistance. Ann. Rev. Med. *19*, 167–94.

Haddy, F.J., and Scott, J.B. 1975. Metabolic factors in peripheral circulatory regulation. Fed. Proc. *34*, 2006–11.

Haekins, W.W., Speck, E., and Leonard, V.G. 1954. Variations of haemoglobin level with age and sex. Blood *9*, 999–1007.

Hagberg, J.M., Giese, M.D., and Mullin, J.P. 1975. Effect of different gear ratios on the metabolic responses of competitive cyclists to constant steady-state work. Med. Sci. Sports *7*, 74.

Hagerman, F.C., Bowers, R.W., Fox, E.L., and Ersing, W.W. 1968. The effects of breathing 100 percent oxygen during rest, heavy work and recovery. Res. Quart. *39*, 965–74.

Haines, R.F. 1974. Effect of bed rest and exercise on body balance. J. appl. Physiol. *36*, 323–7.

Haissly, J.C., Messin, R., Degré, S., Vandermoten, P., Demaret, B., and Denolin, H. 1974. Comparative response to isometric (static) and dynamic exercise tests in coronary disease. Amer. J. Cardiol. *33*, 791–6.

Halicka-Ambroziak, H.D., Eberhardt, A., Romanowski, W., and Klammer, M. 1975. Evaluation of the method of indirect determination of the maximum oxygen uptake after Åstrand and Ryhming in smokers and subjects in a state of emotional excitation. J. Sports Med. Phys. Fitness, *15*, 33–6.

Halle 1797. Cited by Sheldon et al. 1940.

Hammett, V.B.O. 1967. Physiological changes with physical training. In: Int. Symp. on Physical Activity and Cardiovascular Health. Canad. Med. Assoc. J. *96*, 764–8.

Hanke, D., Schlepper, M., Westermann, K., and Witzleb, E. 1969. Venentonus, Haut und Muskeldurchblutung an Unterarm und Hand bei Beinarbeit. Arch. Ges. Physiol. *309*, 115–27.

Hanna, J. 1970. The effects of coca chewing on exercise in Quechua of Peru. Human Biol. *42*, 1-11.

Hansen, J.E., and Ampaya, E.P. 1974. Lung morphometry: a fallacy in the use of the counting principle. J. appl. Physiol. *37*, 951-4.

Hanson, J.S. 1969. Physical training and the pulmonary diffusing capacity. Dis. Chest *56*, 488-93.

- 1973. Exercise responses following production of experimental obesity. J. appl. Physiol. *35*, 587-91.

Hanson, J.S., Tabakin, B.S., and Levy, A.M. 1968. Appendix by D.B. Hill. Comparative exercise-cardiorespiratory performance of normal men in the third, fourth, and fifth decades of life. Circulation *37*, 345-60.

Hardinge, M.G., and Peterson, D.I. 1964. The effect of forced exercise on body temperature and amphetamine toxicity. J. Pharm. exp. Ther. *145*, 47-51.

Harris, H.A. 1964. Greek Athletes and Athletics. London: Hutchinson.

- 1966. Nutrition and physical performances: the diet of Greek athletes. Proc. Nutr. Soc. *25*, 87-90.

- 1969. The Greek athletic programme. Proc. First Int. Seminar on the History of Physical Education and Sport, Natanya, Israel.

Harrison, T.R., and Reeves, T.J. 1968. Principles and Problems of Ischemic Heart Disease. Chicago: Year Book Medical Publishers.

Hartley, L.H. 1975. Growth hormone and catecholamine response to exercise in relation to physical training. Med. Sci. Sports *7*, 34-6.

Hartley, L.H., Pernow, B., Haggendal, H., LaCour, J., de Lattre, J., and Saltin, B. 1970. Central circulation during submaximal work preceeded by heavy exercise. J. appl. Physiol. *29*, 818-23.

Hartley, L.H., and Saltin, B. 1969. Blood gas tensions and pH in brachial artery, femoral vein and brachial vein during maximal exercise. Med. Sci. Sport *3*, 66-72.

Hartley, P.H.S., and Llewellyn, G.F. 1939. Longevity of oarsmen: study of those who rowed in Oxford and Cambridge boat race from 1829-1928. Brit. Med. J. (i), 657-62.

Hartung, M., Venrath, H., Hollmann, W., Isselhardt, W., and Jaenckner, D. 1966. Uber die Atmungsregulation unter Arbeit. Koln-Oplanden: Westdeutsch Verlag.

Harvey, W. 1628. Exercitatio Anatomica de motu cordis et sanguinis in animali. Frankfurt: W. Fitzeri. (Reprinted in: Founders of Experimental Physiology. Ed. W. Blasius, J. Boylan, and K. Kramer. Munich: Lehmanns, 1971.)

Haskell, W.L. 1966. The effect of three endurance training programs on energy metabolism. In: XVI Weltkongress für Sports Medizin. Hannover, Köln: Deutscher-Artzeverlag.

– 1968. Physical activity and cardiovascular disease. Paper presented at 15th Annual Meeting of Amer. Coll. Sports Med., Penn. State University, University Park, Pa.

Hatch, T., and Cook, K.M. 1955. Partitional respirometry. A.M.A. Arch. industr. Health *11*, 142–58.

Haymes, E.M., Buskirk, E.R., Hodgson, J.L., Lundegren, H.M., and Nicholas, W.C. 1974. Heat tolerance of exercising lean and heavy prepubertal girls. J. appl. Physiol. *36*, 566–71.

Hebbelinck, M. 1959. The effects of a moderate dose of alcohol on a series of functions of physical performance in man. Arch. Int. Pharm. Therap. *120*, 402–5.

– 1963. The effects of a small dose of ethyl alcohol on certain basic components of human physical performance. II. The effect on neuromuscular performance. Arch. int. Pharmacodyn. *143*, 247–57.

Hedman, R. 1957. The available glycogen in man and the connection between rise of oxygen intake and carbohydrate usage. Acta physiol. Scand. *40*, 305–21.

Heinrich, K.W., Ulmer, H.V., and Stegemann, J. 1968. Sauerstoffaufnahme, Pulsfrequenz und Ventilation bei Variation von Tretgeschwindigkeit und Tretkraft bei aerober Ergometer arbeit. Pflüg. Arch. Ges. Physiol. *298*, 191–6.

Heinzelmann, F., and Bagley, R. 1970. Response to physical activity programs and their effects on health behaviour. Publ. Health Rept. *85*, 905–11.

Helbing, G., and Nowacki, P.E. 1966. Die maximale Sauerstoffschuld als Leistungskriterium. In: XVI Weltkongress für Sports Medizin, Hannover, Köln: Deutscher-Artzeverlag.

Hellerstein, H.K., and Friedman, E.H. 1969. Sexual activity and the post-coronary patient. Medical Aspects of Human Sexuality, *3*, 70.

Hellerstein, H.K., Hornsten, T.R., Goldberg, A., Burlando, A.G., Friedman, E.G., Hirsch, E.Z., and Marik, S. 1967. The influence of active conditioning upon subjects with coronary artery disease: cardio-respiratory changes during training on 67 patients. In: Proc. Int. Symp. on Physical Activity and Cardiovascular Health. Canad. Med. Assoc. J. *96*, 758–9.

Henry, F.M., and Fitzhenry, J.R. 1950. Oxygen metabolism of moderate exercise with some observations on effects of tobacco smoking. J. appl. Physiol. *2*, 464–8.

Henschel, A., Taylor, H.L., and Keys, A. 1950. Experimental malaria in man. 1. Physical deterioration and recovery. J. clin. Invest. *29*, 52–9.

Herbert, W.G., and Ribisl, P.M. 1972. Effect of dehydration upon physical working capacity of wrestlers under competitive conditions. Res. Quart. *43*, 416–22.

Herbert, W.H. 1975. Cigarette smoking and arteriographically demonstrable coronary artery disease. Chest 67, 49–52.

Hermannsen, J. 1933. Untersuchungen über die maximale Ventilationsgrösse (Atemgrenzwert). Z. Ges. exp. Med. 90, 130–7.

Hermansen, L., and Oseid, S. 1971. Direct and indirect estimation of maximal oxygen uptake in pre-pubertal boys. Acta Paed. Scand. Suppl. 217.

Hermansen, L., and Saltin, B. 1969. Oxygen uptake during maximal treadmill and bicycle exercise. J. appl. Physiol. 26, 31–7.

Hermansen, L., and Wachtlová, M. 1971. Capillary density of skeletal muscle in well-trained and untrained men. J. appl. Physiol. 30, 860–3.

Herrlich, H.C., Raab, W., and Gigee, W. 1960. Influence of muscular training and of catecholamines on cardiac acetylcholine and cholinesterase. Arch. Intern. Pharmacodyn. 129, 201–15.

Herxheimer, H. 1929. Untersuchungen über die Änderung der Herzgrösse unter dem Einfluss bestimmter Sportarten. Z. klin. Med. 3, 376–93.

Hettinger, T. 1961. Physiology of Strength. Springfield, Ill.: C.C. Thomas.

Hill, A.V. 1925. The physiological basis of athletic records. Sci. Monthly 21, 409–28.

Hill, A.V., Long, C.N., and Lupton, H. 1924–25. Muscular exercise, lactic acid and the supply and utilization of oxygen. Proc. Roy. Soc. (Biol.) 96, 438–; 97, 84–, 155–.

Hill, E.P., Power, G.G., and Longo, L.D. 1973. Mathematical simulation of pulmonary O_2 and CO_2 exchange. Amer. J. Physiol. 224, 904–17.

Hill, J.S., Wearring, G.A., and Eynon, R.B. 1971. Effect of frequency of exercise on adult fitness. Med. Sci. Sports 3, k.

Hill, L. 1895. The influence of the force of gravity on the circulation of the blood. J. Physiol. 18, 15–53.

Hill, L., and Flack, M. 1910. The influence of oxygen inhalations on muscular work. J. Physiol. 40, 347–72.

Hinckle, L.E., Carver, S.T., and Stevens, M. 1969. The frequency of asymptomatic disturbances of cardiac rhythm and conduction in middle-aged men. Amer. J. Cardiol. 24, 629–50.

Hirsch, C. 1899. Über die Beziehungen zwischen dem Herzmuskel und der Körpermuskulatur und über sein Verhalten bei Herzhypertrophie. Dtsch. Arch. klin. Med. 64, 597–634.

His Majesty's Stationery Office 1919. Syllabus of physical training for schools. London, U.K.: H.M.S.O.

Hjalmarson, A., and Isaksson, O. 1972. In vitro work load and rat heart metabolism. I. Effect on protein synthesis. Acta physiol. Scand. 86, 126–44.

Hlastala, M.P. 1972. A model of fluctuating alveolar gas exchange during the respiratory cycle. Resp. Physiol. *15*, 214–32.

Ho, K-J., Taylor, C.B., and Biss, K. 1970. Overall control of sterol synthesis in animals and man. In: Atherosclerosis: Proc. 2nd Int. Symp. Ed. R.J. Jones. New York: Springer-Verlag.

Hoes, M., Binkhorst, R.A., Smeekes-Kuyl, A., and Vissurs, A.C. 1968. Measurement of forces exerted on a pedal crank during work on the bicycle ergometer at different loads. Int. Z. angew. Physiol. *26*, 33–42.

Hofer, H.W., and Pette, D. 1968. Wirkungen und Wechselwirkungen von Substraten und Effektoren an der Phosphofructokinase des Kaninchen-skeletmuskeln. Z. Physiol. Chem. *349*, 1378–92.

Holbrook, L. 1970. George Catlin 1796–1872. Proc. 1st Canad. Symp. on the History of Sport and Physical Education, Edmonton, Alta.

Hollmann, D. 1972. Lungenfunktion, Atmung und Stoffwechsel im Sport. In: Zentrale Themem der Sportmedizin. Ed. W. Hollmann. Berlin: Springer Verlag.

Hollmann, W. 1965. Körperliches Training als Prävention von Herzkreislauf Krankheiten. Stuttgart: Hippokrates-Verlag.

– 1966. Diminution of cardiopulmonary capacity in the course of life and its prevention by participation in sports. In: Proc. Int. Congress of Sports Sciences, Tokyo, 3–8 Oct. 1964. Ed. K. Kato. Tokyo, Japan: Japanese Union of Sports Sciences.

Hollmann, W., Herkenrath, G., Grunewald, B., Budinger, H., Jonath, U., Russmann, H., and Hain, D. 1966. Untersuchungen über Möglichkeiten zur Steigerung des körperlichen Leistungsvermögens von Rekruten. Sportarzt und Sportmedizin *12*, 582–92.

Holloszy, J.O. 1967. Biochemical adaptations in muscle – effects of exercise on mitochondrial oxygen uptake and respiratory enzyme activity in skeletal muscle. J. biol. Chem. *242*, 2278–82.

– 1973. Biochemical adaptations to exercise: aerobic metabolism. Exercise and Sports Sci. Rev. *1*, 45–71.

Holloszy, J.O., Oscai, L.B., Molé, P.A., and Don, I.J. 1971. Biochemical adaptations to endurance exercise in skeletal muscle. In: Muscle Metabolism during Exercise. Ed. B. Pernow and B. Saltin. New York: Plenum Press.

Holmberg, S., Serzysko, W., and Varnauskas, E. 1971. Coronary circulation during heavy exercise in control subjects and patients with coronary heart disease. Acta med. Scand. *190*, 465–80.

Holmer, I. 1972. Oxygen uptake during swimming in man. J. appl. Physiol. *33*, 502–9.

Holmgren, A. 1965. On the variation of $D_{L,CO}$ with increasing oxygen uptake during exercise in healthy trained young men and women. Acta physiol. Scand. *65*, 207–20.

- 1967a. Vaso-regulatory asthenia. In: Proc. Int. Symp. on Physical Activity and Cardiovascular Health. Canad. Med. Assoc. J. *96*, 853.
- 1967b. Cardio-respiratory determinants of cardiovascular fitness. In: Proc. Int. Symp. on Physical Activity and Cardiovascular Health. Canad. Med. Assoc. J. *96*, 697–702.
- 1967c. Commentary. In: Proc. Int. Symp. on Physical Activity and Cardiovascular Health. Canad. Med. Assoc. J. *96*, 794.

Holmgren, A., and McIlroy, M.B. 1964. Effect of temperature on arterial blood gas tensions and pH during exercise. J. appl. Physiol. *19*, 243–5.

Holmgren, A., Mossfeldt, F., Sjöstrand, T., and Ström, G. 1964. Effect of training on work capacity, total haemoglobin, blood volume, heart volume, and pulse rate in recumbent and upright positions. In: International Research in Sport and Physical Education. Ed. E. Jokl and E. Simon. Springfield, Ill.: C.C. Thomas.

Holmgren, A., and Svanborg, N. 1966. On the influence of body position on the steady-state diffusion capacity during exercise – studies in patients with pulmonary sarcoidosis. Acta med. Scand. *179* (6), 703–14.

Holter, N.J. 1961. New method for heart studies. Science *134*, 1214–20.

Holtz, P., Bachmann, F., Englehardt, A., and Greeff, K. 1952. Die Milzwirkung des Adrenalins und Arterenols. Pflüg. Arch. Ges. Physiol. *255*, 232–50.

Hoogerwerf, S. 1929. Elektrokardiographische Untersuchungen der Amsterdamer Olympiadekampfer. Arbeitsphysiol. *2*, 61–75.

Horsfield, K., Dart, G., Olson, D.E., Filley, G.F., and Cumming, G. 1971. Models of the human bronchial tree. J. appl. Physiol. *31*, 207–17.

Horvath, S.M. 1967. The physiological stimuli to training in a normal climate. In: Proc. Int. Symp. on Physical Activity and Cardiovascular Health. Canad. Med. Assoc. J. *96*, 791–3.

Horvath, S.M., and Michael, E.D. 1970. Responses of young women to gradually increasing and constant load maximal exercise. Med. Sci. Sports *2*, 128–31.

Houston, C.S., and Riley, R.L. 1947. Respiratory and circulatory changes during acclimatization to high altitude. Amer. J. Physiol. *149*, 565–88.

Howald, H. 1975. Ultrastructural adaptation of skeletal muscle to prolonged physical exercise. In: Metabolic Adaptations to Prolonged Physical Exercise. Ed. H. Howald and J.R. Poortmans. Basel: Birkhauser Verlag.

Howe, B.L., Collis, M.L., and Docherty, D. 1973. Validation of the U-Vic step test as a practical measure of cardiovascular efficiency. J. Sports Med. *13*, 226–30.

Howell, M.L. 1971. Archaeological evidence of sports and games in ancient civilizations: interpretive comments. Proc. 2nd World Symp. on the History of Sport and Physical Education, Banff, Alta.

Howell, M.L., and Palmer, D. 1970. Sports and games in the Minoan period. Proc. 1st Int. Seminar on the History of Physical Education and Sport, Natanya, Israel.

Howell, N., and Howell, M.L. 1969. Sports and Games in Canadian Life. 1700 to the Present. Toronto: Macmillan.

Howitt, J.S., Balkwill, J.S., Whiteside, T.C.D., and Whittingham, P.D.G. 1966. A preliminary study of flight deck work loads in civil air transport aircraft. U.K. Ministry of Defence, F.P.R.C. *1240*.

Hueting, J., and Poulus, A. 1970. Amphetamine, performance, effort and fatigue. Pflüg. Arch. *318*, 260.

Hughes, A.L., and Goldman, R.F. 1970. Energy cost of hard work. J. appl. Physiol. *29*, 570-2.

Hultman, E. 1967. Studies on muscle metabolism of glycogen and active phosphate in man with special reference to exercise and diet. Scand. J. clin. Lab. Invest. *19*, Suppl. *94*, 1-63.

– 1971. Muscle glycogen stores and prolonged exercise. In: Frontiers of Fitness. Ed. R.J. Shephard. Springfield, Ill.: C.C. Thomas.

Hultman, E., Bergström, J., and McLennan Anderson, N. 1967. Breakdown and resynthesis of phosphorylcreatine and adenosine-triphosphate in connection with muscular work in man. Scand. J. Lab. Invest. *19*, 56-66.

Hunt, G.H., and Pembrey, M.S. 1921. Tests for physical efficiency. Guy's Hosp. Rept. *71*, 415-28.

Hurst, P.M., Radlow, R., and Bagley, S.K. 1968. The effects of d-amphetamine and chlordiazepoxide upon strength and estimated strength. Ergonomics *11*, 47-52.

Husain, K. 1962. The History of the Development of Our Knowledge Regarding the Circulatory System. Hyderabad.

Hyatt, R.E. 1972. Reaction to Dr. Shephard's paper. Ventilatory mechanics during exercise in health and disease. In: Exercise and the Lungs. Ed. J.F. Alexander, R.C. Serfass, and C.M. Tipton. Chicago: Athletic Inst.

Ikai, M., Ishii, K., Miyamura, M., Kusano, K., Bar-Or, O., Kollias, J., and Buskirk, E.R. 1971. Aerobic capacity of Ainu and other Japanese on Hokkaido. Med. Sci. Sports *3*, 6-11.

Iliev, I.B., and Velev, V. 1976. Physical performance and non-organic cardiovascular murmurs by young athletes 11-14 years of age. In: VIIth Int. Symp. of Paediatric Work Physiology. Ed. H. Lavallée and R.J. Shephard. Quebec: Pelican Press.

Innes, J.A., Campbell, I.W., Campbell, C.J., Needle, A.L., and Munroe, J.F. 1974. Long-term follow-up of therapeutic starvation. Brit. Med. J. (ii), 357-9.

International Committee for Standardization in Haematology. 1965. Brit. Med. J. (i), 645.

– 1967. Brit. J. Haematol. Suppl. *13*, 71.

International Committee on the Standardization of Physical Fitness Tests 1969. Physical Fitness Measurements Standards. Tel Aviv.

Irving, D.W., and Yamomoto, T. 1963. Cigarette smoking and cardiac output. Brit. Heart J. *25*, 126–32.

Ishiko, T. 1967. Aerobic capacity and external criteria of performance. Canad. Med. Assoc. J. *96*, 746–9.

Ishiko, T., Ikeda, N., and Enomoto, Y. 1968. Obese children in Japan. Res. J. Phys. Educ. *12*, 168–74.

Issekutz, B., Birkhead, N.C., and Rodahl, K. 1962. Use of respiratory quotients in assessment of aerobic work capacity. J. appl. Physiol. *17*, 47–50.

Jaffé, D., and Manning, M. 1971. Coronary arteries in early life. Proc. 13th Annual Congress of Pediatrics, Vienna.

Jebavy, P., and Widimsky, J. 1973. Lung-transfer factor at maximal effort in healthy men. Respiration *30*, 297–310.

Jetté, M. 1971. Primitive Indian Lacrosse – skill or slaughter? Proc. 2nd World Symp. on the History of Sport and Physical Education, Banff, Alta.

Jetté, M., Campbell, J., Mongeon, J., and Routhier, R. 1975. The energy requirements of the Canadian Home Fitness Test. Annual Meeting, Canadian Assoc. Sports Sci. Published Canad. Med. Assoc. J. *114*, 680–2, 1976.

Jick, H., Miettinen, O.S. Neff, R.K., Shapiro, S., Heinonen, O.P., and Slone, D. 1973. Coffee and myocardial infarction. New Engl. J. Med. *289*, 63–7.

Johnson, H.E. 1946. Applied physiology. Ann. Rev. Physiol. *8*, 535–58.

Johnson, J.M., Rowell, L.B., and Brengelmann, G.L. 1974. Modification of the blood flow–body temperature relationship by upright exercise. J. appl. Physiol. *37*, 880–6.

Johnson, L.C., Fisher, G., Silvester, L.J., and Hofheins, C.C. 1972. Anabolic steroid: effects on strength, body weight, oxygen uptake and spermatogenesis upon mature males. Med. Sci. Sports *4*, 43–5.

Johnson, L.R., and Van Liew, H.D. 1974. Use of arterial P_{O_2} to study convective and diffusive gas mixing in the lungs. J. appl. Physiol. *36*, 91–7.

Johnson, P.C., Leach, C.S., and Rambant, P.C. 1973. Estimates of fluid and energy balance of Apollo 17. Aerospace Med. *44*, 1227–30.

Johnson, R.H., and Rennie, M.J. 1973. The effect of diet upon the metabolic changes with exercise in long distance runners. J. Physiol. *232*, 73–4p.

Johnson, R.L. 1967. Pulmonary diffusion as a limiting factor in exercise stress. Circulation Res. *21*, Suppl. *I*, I-154–I-160.

Johnson, R.L., Spicer, W.S., Bishop, J.M., and Forster, R.E. 1960. Pulmonary capillary blood volume, flow, and diffusing capacity during exercise. J. appl. Physiol. *15*, 893–902.

Johnson, W., and Black, D. 1953. Comparison of effects of certain blood alkalinizers and glucose upon competitive endurance performance. J. appl. Physiol. *5*, 577–8.

Jokl, E. 1958. The Clinical Physiology of Physical Fitness and Rehabilitation. Springfield, Ill.: C.C. Thomas.

– 1967. The future of athletic records. Paper presented at Annual Meeting of Ont. Med. Assoc., Toronto.

– 1971. What Is Sports Medicine? Springfield, Ill.: C.C. Thomas.

Jokl, E., and Jokl, P. 1968. The Physiological Basis of Athletic Records. Springfield, Ill.: C.C. Thomas.

Jokl, E., Jokl-Ball, M., Jokl, B., and Frankel, L. 1968. Notation of exercise. Work-Environment-Health *5*, 24–33.

Joliffe, N., Rinzler, S.N., and Archer, M. 1959. The anti-coronary club, including a discussion of the effects of a prudent diet on the serum cholesterol of middle-aged men. Amer. J. clin. Nutr. *7*, 451–62.

Jones, N.L., Campbell, E.J.M., McHardy, G.J.R., Higgs, B., and Clode, M. 1967. The estimation of carbon dioxide pressure of mixed venous blood during exercise. Clin. Sci. *32*, 311–27.

Jones, N.L., and Haddon, R.W.T. 1973. Effect of a meal on cardio-pulmonary and metabolic changes during exercise. Canad. J. Physiol. Pharm. *51*, 445–50.

Jones, N.L., McHardy, G.J.R., Naimark, A., and Campbell, E.J.M. 1966. Physiological dead space and alveolar-arterial gas pressure differences during exercise. Clin. Sci. *31*, 19–29.

Jorgensen, C.R. 1972. Coronary blood flow and myocardial oxygen consumption in man. In: Fitness and Exercise. Ed. J.F. Alexander, R.C. Serfass, and C.M. Tipton. Chicago: Athletic Inst.

José, A.D., Stitt, F., and Collison, D. 1970. The effects of exercise and changes in body temperature on the intrinsic heart rate in man. Amer. Heart J. *79*, 488–97.

Josenhans, W.T. 1967. Muscular factors. In: Proc. Int. Symp. on Physical Activity and Cardiovascular Health. Canad. Med. Assoc. J. *96*, 761–3.

Kaijser, L. 1970. Limiting factors for aerobic muscle performance. Acta physiol. Scand. Suppl. *346*, 1–96.

Kallfelz, I. 1962. Die apnoische Pause. Untersuchungen über ihre Beziehungen zum Sauerstoffmangel-Belastungstest. Zentrale für wissenschaftliches Berichtowesen der Deutschen Versuchanstalt für Luft- und Raumfahrt e.V. Porz-Wahn, Rheinland, Germany.

Kamon, E., and Pandolf, K.B. 1972. Maximal aerobic power during ladder-mill climbing, uphill running and cycling. J. appl. Physiol. *32*, 467–73.

Kamper, E. 1972. Encyclopaedia of the Olympic Games. New York: McGraw-Hill.

Kannel, W.B. 1967. Habitual level of physical activity and risk of coronary heart disease. The Framingham Study. In: Proc. Int. Symp. on Physical Activity and Cardiovascular Health. Canad. Med. Assoc. J. *96*, 811–12.

Karlsson, H., and Wigertz, O. 1971. Ventilation and heart rate responses to ramp function changes in work load. Acta physiol. Scand. *81*, 215–24.

Karlsson, J., Hermansen, L., Agnevik, G., and Saltin, B. 1967. Energikraven vid Löpning. Idrottsfysiologi *4*, Framtiden, Stockholm.

Karlsson, J., Nordesjo, L.O., Jorfeldt, L., and Saltin, B. 1972. Muscle lactate, ATP and CP levels during exercise after physical training in man. J. appl. Physiol. *33*, 199–203.

Karpovich, P.V. 1934. The effect of oxygen inhalation on swimming performance. Res. Quart. *5*, 24–30.

– 1959. Physiology of Muscular Activity, 5th ed. Philadelphia: Saunders.

Karpovich, P.V., and Hale, C.J. 1951. Tobacco smoking and physical performance. J. appl. Physiol. *3*, 616–21.

Karpovich, P.V., and Sinning, W.E. 1971. Physiology of Muscular Activity, 7th ed. Philadelphia: Saunders.

Karpovich, P.V., Starr, M.P., Kimbra, R.W., Stoll, C.G., and Weiss, R.A. 1946. Physical reconditioning after rheumatic fever. J. Amer. Med. Assoc. *130*, 1198–203.

Karvinen, E., Miettinen, M., and Ahlman, K. 1962. Physical performance during hangover. Quart. J. Studies on Alcohol *23*, 208–15.

Karvonen, M.J. 1959. Effects of vigorous exercise on the heart. In: Work and the Heart. Ed. F.F. Rosenbaum and E.L. Belknap. New York: Hoeber.

Karvonen, M.J., Kentala, E., and Mustala, O. 1957. The effects of training on heart rate. A 'longitudinal' study. Ann. Med. Exp. Fenn. *35*, 307–15.

Kasch, F.W., Phillips, W.H., Ross, W.D., and Carter, J.E.L. 1965. A step test for inducing maximal work. J. Assoc. Phys. Ment. Rehab. *19*, 84–6.

Kasch, F.W., Phillips, W.H., Ross, W.D., Carter, J.E.L., and Boyer, J.L. 1966. A comparison of maximal oxygen uptake by treadmill and step-test procedures. J. appl. Physiol. *21*, 1387–8.

Kasser, I.S., and Bruce, R.A. 1969. Comparative effects of aging and coronary heart disease on sub-maximal and maximal exercise. Circulation *39*, 759–74.

Katch, F.I., Girandola, R.N., and Henry, F.M. 1972. The influence of the estimated oxygen cost of ventilation on oxygen deficit and recovery oxygen intake for moderately heavy bicycle ergometer exercise. Med. Sci. Sports *4*, 71–6.

Katch, F.I., Girandola, F.N., and Katch, V.L. 1971. The relationship of body weight on maximum oxygen uptake and heavy work endurance capacity on the bicycle ergometer. Med. Sci. Sports *3*, 101-6.

Katch, F.I., McArdle, W.D., and Pechar, G.S. 1974. Relationship of maximal leg force and leg composition to treadmill and bicycle ergometer maximum oxygen uptake. Med. Sci. Sports *6*, 38-43.

Katch, V.L. 1972. The role of maximal oxygen debt in endurance performance. Paper presented at the National Convention of AAHPER, Houston, Texas.

Kattus, A.A. (Chairman). 1972. Exercise Testing and Training of Apparently Healthy Individuals: A Handbook for Physicians. New York: American Heart Assoc.

Kattus, A., and Grollman, J. 1972. Patterns of coronary collateral circulation in angina pectoris: relation to exercise training. In: Changing Concepts in Cardiovascular Disease. Ed. H.I. Russek and B.L. Zohman. Baltimore: Williams & Wilkins.

Kavanagh, T., Pandit, V., and Shephard, R.J. 1973. The application of exercise testing to the elderly amputee. Canad. Med. Assoc. J. *108*, 314-17.

Kavanagh, T., and Shephard, R.J. 1973. Special Review: Importance of physical activity in post-coronary rehabilitation. Amer. J. Phys. Med. *52*, 304-13.

– 1975a. Conditioning of post-coronary patients: comparison of continuous and interval training. Arch. Phys. Med. Rehabil. *56*, 72-6.

– 1975b. Maintenance of hydration in post-coronary marathon runners. Brit. J. Sports Med. *9*, 130-5.

– 1975c. On the choice of fluid for the hydration of middle-aged marathon runners. Brit. J. Sports Med. (in press).

– 1976a. Maximum exercise tests on 'post-coronary' patients. J. appl. Physiol. *40*, 611-18.

– 1976b. Characteristics of the Master Athlete. Med. Sci. Sports *8*, 76.

Kavanagh, T., Shephard, R.J., Doney, H., and Pandit, V. 1973. Intensive exercise in coronary rehabilitation. Med. Sci. Sports *5*, 34-9.

Kavanagh, T., Shephard, R.J., and Pandit, V. 1974. Marathon running after myocardial infarction. J. Amer. Med. Assoc. *229*, 1602-5.

Kavanagh, T., Shephard, R.J., Pandit, V., and Doney, H. 1970. Exercise versus hypnotherapy in the rehabilitation of the coronary patient. A preliminary report. Arch. Phys. Med. Rehab. *51*, 578-87.

Kavanagh, T., Shephard, R.J., and Tuck, J.A. 1975. Depression following myocardial infarction. Canad. Med. Assoc. J. *113*, 23-7.

Kay, C., and Shephard, R.J. 1969. On muscle strength and the threshold of anaerobic work. Int. Z. angew. Physiol. *27*, 311-28.

Kearney, J.T., and Byrnes, W.C. 1974. The relationship between running performance and predicted maximum oxygen uptake among divergent ability groups. Res. Quart. *45*, 9–15.

Kemper, H.C.G., Ras, J.G.A., Snel, J., Splinter, P.G., Tavecchio, L.W.C., and Verschuur, R. 1974. Investigation to the effects of two extra lessons in physical education a week during one school year upon the physical development of 12 and 13 years old boys. In: 6th International Cong. of Pediatric Work Physiology, Seč, Czechoslovakia.

Kemper, H.C.G., and Verschuur, R. 1976. Validity and reliability of pedometers in research on habitual physical activity. In: VIIth Int. Symp. of Pediatric Work Physiology. Ed. R.J. Shephard. Quebec: Pelican Press.

Kemsley, W.F.F. 1952. Body-weight at different ages and heights. Ann. Eugen. *16*, 316–34.

Kemsley, W.F.F., Billewicz, W.Z., and Thomson, A.M. 1962. A new weight-for-height standard based on British Anthropometric Data. Brit. J. prev. Soc. Med. *16*, 189–95.

Kendrick, Z.B., Pollock, M.L., Hickman, T.N., and Miller, H.S. 1971. Effects of training and detraining on cardiovascular efficiency. Amer. Corr. Ther. J. *25*, 79–83.

Kenyon, G.S. 1965. Assessing attitudes toward sport and physical activity. Paper presented at 1st Int. Cong. of Physiology of Sport, Rome, Italy.

Keroes, J., Ecker, R.R., and Rapaport, E. 1969. Ventricular function curves in the exercising dog: effects of rapid intravenous infusions and of propranolol. Circulation Res. *25*, 557–67.

Keul, J. 1973. Limiting Factors of Physical Performance. Stuttgart: Thieme.

Keul, J., and Doll, E. 1973. Intermittent exercise: metabolites, P_{O_2} and acid-base equilibrium in the blood. J. appl. Physiol. *34*, 220–5.

Keys, A. 1970. Coronary heart disease in seven countries. Circulation *41*, Suppl. *1*.

Keys, A., Aravanis, C., Blackburn, H., Van Buchem, F.S.P., Buzina, R., Djordjevic, B.S., Fidanza, F., Karvonen, M.J., Menotti, A., Puddu, V., and Taylor, H.L. 1972. Coronary heart disease: overweight and obesity. Ann. Int. Med. *77*, 15–27.

Keys, A., Brozek, J., Henschel, A., Mickelsen, O., and Taylor, H.L. 1950. Biology of Human Starvation. Minneapolis: University of Minnesota Press.

Khosla, T., and Lowe, C.R. 1967. Indices of obesity derived from body weight and height. Brit. J. prev. Soc. Med. *21*, 122–8.

– 1972. Obesity and smoking habits by social class. Brit. J. prev. Soc. Med. *26*, 249–56.

Kiessling, K.H., Pilstrom, L., Karlsson, J., and Piehl, K. 1973. Mitochondrial volume in skeletal muscle from young and old physically untrained and trained healthy men and from alcoholics. Clin. Sci. 44, 547–54.

Kiiskinen, A., and Heikkinen, E. 1975. Effect of prolonged physical training on the development of connective tissues in growing mice. In: Metabolic Adaptation to Prolonged Physical Exercise. Ed. H. Howald and J.R. Poortmans. Basel: Birkhauser Verlag.

Kiiskinen, A., Kemppinen, L., and Hasan, J. 1975. Is the anemia following repeated sessions of heavy physical exercise caused by a decreased rate of production of red cells? In: Metabolic Adaptation to Prolonged Physical Exercise. Ed. H. Howald and J.R. Poortmans. Basel: Birkhauser Verlag.

Kilbom, Å. 1971a. Physical training with submaximal intensities in women. I. Reaction to exercise and orthostasis. Scand. J. clin. Lab. Invest. 28, 141–61.

– 1971b. Physical training with sub-maximal intensities in women. 3. Effect on adaptation to professional work. Scand. J. clin. Lab. Invest. 28, 331–43.

Kilbom, Å., and Åstrand, I. 1971. Physical training with sub-maximal intensities in women. II. Effect on cardiac output. Scand. J. clin. Lab. Invest. 28, 163–75.

Kilbom, Å., Hartley, L.H., Saltin, B., Bjure, J., Grimby, G., and Åstrand, I. 1969. Physical training in sedentary middle-aged and older men. I. Medical evaluation. Scand. J. clin. Lab. Invest. 24, 315–22.

Kinne, F.L., and Seagrave, R.C. 1974. Effects of mixing patterns on respiratory gas exchange. J. appl. Physiol. 36, 698–705.

Kirschner, H. 1972. Physical capacity after moderate blood loss in dogs. Acta physiol. Pol. 23, 597–608.

Kissling, G., and Jacob, R. 1973. Limitation of the stroke volume during increased myocardial performance. In: Limiting Factors of Physical Performance. Ed. J. Keul. Stuttgart: Thieme.

Klarman, H.E. 1964. Socio-economic impact of heart disease. In: The Heart and Circulation. Second National Conference on Cardiovascular Diseases: Vol. 2. Community Services and Education. Ed. E.C. Andrus. Washington, D.C.: U.S. Public Health Service.

Klausen, K., Dill, D.B., Phillips, E.E., and McGregor, D. 1967. Metabolic reactions to work in the desert. J. appl. Physiol. 22, 292–6.

Klausen, K., Rasmussen, B., Clausen, J.P., and Trap-Jensen, J. 1974. Blood lactate from exercising extremities before and after arm or leg training. Amer. J. Physiol. 227, 67–72.

Klein, K.E., Wegmann, H.M., and Bruner, H. 1968. Circadian rhythms in indices of human performance, physical fitness and stress resistance. Aerospace Med. 39, 512–18.

Klein, K.K. 1959. A preliminary study of the dynamics of force as applied to knee injury in athletics. Medicina Sportiva *13*, 327-34.

Klein, K.K., and Allman, F.L. 1969. The Knee in Sports. Austin, Texas: Pemberton Press.

Kleinhauss, G., and Franke, W. 1971. Zum Aussagewert indirekter Blutdruckbestimmungen in Ruhe und bei Kreislaufbelastung durch Ergometerarbeit. Z. f. Kreislauff. *60*, 588-99.

Klimt, F. 1966. Telemotorische Herzschlagfrequenzregistrierungen bei Kleinkindern wahrend einer körperlichen Tätigkeit. Deutsches Gesundheitwesen *21*, 599.

Klimt, F., and Voigt, G.B. 1971. Investigations on the standardization of ergometry in children. Acta Paediatr. Scand. Suppl. *217*, 35-6.

– 1974. Untersuchungen zur Standardisierung der Drehzahl und Kurbellange bei Arbeit am Fahrradergometer um Kindern im Alter von 6 bis 10 Jahren. Europ. J. appl. Physiol. *33*, 315-26.

Klissouras, V. 1971. Heritability of adaptive variation. J. appl. Physiol. *31*, 338-44.

– 1972. Genetic limit of functional adaptability. Int. Z. angew. Physiol. *30*, 85-94.

Klissouras, V., and Weber, G. 1973. Training: growth and heredity. In: Proc. 4th Int. Symp. of Pediatric Work Physiology, Natanya, Israel. Ed. O. Bar-Or.

Knehr, C.A., Dill, D.B., and Neufeld, W. 1942. Training and its effects on man at rest and at work. Amer. J. Physiol. *136*, 148-56.

Knibbs, A.V. 1971. Some physiological effects of intensity and frequency of exercise on young non-athletic females. J. Physiol. *216*, 25-6p.

Knuttgen, H.G. 1961. Comparison of fitness of Danish and American school children. Res. Quart. *32*, 190-6.

Knuttgen, H.G., Bonde-Petersen, F., and Klausen, K. 1971. Oxygen uptake and heart rate responses to exercise performed with concentric and eccentric muscle contractions. Med. Sci. Sports *3*, 1-5.

Knuttgen, H.G., Nordesjo, L.O., Ollander, B., and Saltin, B. 1973. Physical conditioning through interval training with young adults. Med. Sci. Sports *5*, 220-6.

Knuttgen, H.G., and Steendahl, K. 1963. Fitness of Danish school children during the course of one academic year. Res. Quart. *34*, 34-40.

Kofranyi, E., and Michaelis, H.F. 1949. Ein tragbarer Apparat zur Bestimmung des Gasstoffwechsels. Arbeitsphysiologie *11*, 148-50.

Kohn, R.M., Ibrahim, M.A., and Feldman, J.G. 1971. Premature ventricular beats and coronary heart disease risk factors. Amer. J. Epidemiol. *94*, 556-63.

Kollias, J., and Buskirk, E.R. 1974. Exercise and altitude. In: Science and Medicine of Exercise and Sport, 2nd ed. Ed. W.R. Johnson and E.R. Buskirk. New York: Harper & Row.

Komi, P.V., Klissouras, V., and Karvinen, E. 1973. Genetic variation in neuromuscular performance. Int. Z. angew. Physiol. *31*, 289–304.

Koroxenidis, G.T., Shepherd, J.T., and Marshall, R.J. 1961. Cardiovascular response to acute heat stress. J. appl. Physiol. *16*, 869–72.

Kramer, J.D., and Lurie, P.R. 1964. Maximal exercise tests in children. Amer. J. Dis. Childh. *108*, 283–97.

Kreitler, H., and Kreitler, S. 1970. Movement and aging: a psychological approach. In: Physical Activity and Aging. Ed. D. Brunner and E. Jokl. Basel: Karger.

Kretschmer, E., and Enke, W. 1936. Die Personlichkeit der Athletiker. Leipzig: Thieme.

Kreuzer, F. 1970. Facilitated diffusion of oxygen and its possible significance; a review. Resp. Physiol. *9*, 1–30.

Kruger, H.C. 1962. Avicenna's Poem on Medicine (transl.). Springfield, Ill.: C.C. Thomas.

Külbs, F. 1912. Ueber den Einfluss der Bewegung auf den wachsenden und erwachsenen Organismus. Dtsch. med. Wschr. *38*, 1916–20.

Kuo, P.T. 1972. Plasma lipids and atherosclerosis. In: Atherosclerosis and Coronary Heart Disease. Ed. W. Likoff, B.L. Segal, and W. Insull. New York: Grune & Stratton.

Lacquet, L.M., Olson, D.E., and Filley, G.F. 1967. The series conductors of the lung in controlled breathing. In: Proc. 10th Aspen Emphysema Conf. Ed. R.S. Mitchell. Washington, D.C.: U.S. Public Health Service, Publication *1787*.

LaForce, R.C., and Lewis, B.M. 1970. Diffusional transport in the human lung. J. appl. Physiol. *28*, 291–8.

Lalonde, M. 1974. A new perspective on the health of Canadians – a working document. Ottawa: Dept. of National Health and Welfare, Government of Canada.

Lamb, D.R. 1975. Androgens and exercise. Med. Sci. Sports *7*, 1–5.

Lammert, O. 1972. Maximal aerobic power and energy expenditure of Eskimo hunters in Greenland. J. appl. Physiol. *33*, 184–8.

Landis, E.M., and Pappenheimer, J.R. 1963. Exchange of substances through the capillary walls. In: Handbook of Physiology. Section 2, Circulation. Vol. 2. Ed. W.F. Hamilton. Washington, D.C.: Amer. Physiol. Soc.

Laporte, W. 1966. The influence of a gymnastic pause upon recovery following post-office work. Ergonomics *9*, 501–6.

Larson, L.A. 1974. Fitness, Health and Work Capacity: International Standards for Assessment. New York: Macmillan.

Lavallée, H., Larivière, G., and Shephard, R.J. 1974. Correlations between field tests of performance and laboratory measurements of fitness. Results in the ten year old school child. Acta Paed. Belg. *28*, Suppl., 19–28.

Lawson, W.H. 1970. Rebreathing measurements of pulmonary diffusing capacity for CO during exercise. J. appl. Physiol. *29*, 896–900.

Lawther, P.J. 1967. Human responses to air pollutants. Lecture at Gas Club, Toronto.

Layman, E.M. 1970. Aggression in relation to play and sports. In: Contemporary Psychology of Sport. Ed. G.S. Kenyon. Chicago: Athletic Inst.

Leake, C.D. 1964. The historical development of cardiovascular physiology. In: Handbook of Physiology, Section 2: Circulation, Vol. 1. Ed. W.F. Hamilton. Washington, D.C.: Amer. Physiol. Soc.

Lee, R.B. 1969. !Kung Bushman subsistence: an input-output analysis. In: Environment and Cultural Behaviour. Ed. A.P. Vayda. New York: Natural History Press.

– 1972a. Population growth and the beginning of sedentary life among the !Kung Bushmen. In: Population Growth: Anthropological Implications. Ed. B. Spooner. Cambridge, Mass.: M.I.T. Press.

– 1972b. !Kung spatial organization: an ecological and historical perspective. Human Ecol. *1*, 125–47.

Lefcoe, N.M., Carter, R.P., and Ahmad, D. 1971. Post-exercise bronchoconstriction in normal subjects. Amer. Rev. Resp. Dis. *104*, 562–7.

Leithead, C.S., and Lind, A.R. 1964. Heat Stress and Heat Disorders. Philadelphia: Davis.

Lepkovsky, S. 1973. Newer concepts in the regulation of food intake. Amer. J. clin. Nutr. *26*, 271–84.

Lester, M., Sheffield, L.T., Trammell, P., and Reeves, T.J. 1968. The effect of age and athletic training on the maximal heart rate during muscular exercise. Amer. Heart. J. *76*, 370–6.

Leveille, G.A., and Romsos, D.R. 1974. Meal eating and obesity. Nutr. Today, Nov./Dec.

Levison, H., and Cherniak, R.M. 1968. Ventilatory cost of exercise in chronic obstructive pulmonary disease. J. appl. Physiol. *25*, 21–7.

Lewis, S.M., and Burgess, B.J. 1969. Quality control in haematology: report of inter-laboratory trials in Britain. Brit. Med. J. *4*, 253–6.

L'Huillier, J.P., Varena, P., and Jacquemin, Ch. 1969. Exercise musculaire maximale en milieu hyperbare. J. Physiol. (Paris) *61*, 147.

Lind, A.R., and McNicol, G.W. 1967. Muscular factors which determine the cardiovascular responses to sustained and rhythmic exercise. In: Proc. Int. Symp. on Physical Activity and Cardiovascular Health. Canad. Med. Assoc. J. *96*, 706-12.

Lindemann, H., Rutenfranz, J., Mocellin, R., and Sbresney, W. 1973. Methodische Untersuchung zur indirekten Bestimmung der maximalen O_2-aufnahme. Europ. J. appl. Physiol. *32*, 25-53.

Lindén, V. 1969. Absence from work and physical fitness. Brit. J. industr. Med. *26*, 47-53.

Linderholm, H. 1959. Diffusing capacity of the lungs as a limiting factor for physical working capacity. Acta med. Scand. *163*, 61-84.

Lindhard, J. 1915. Ueber das Minutenvolum des Herzens bei Ruhe und die Muskelarbeit. Pflüg. Arch. Ges. Physiol. *161*, 233-383.

Lindsay, P. 1970. Sport in Canada 1807-1867. Proc. 1st Canad. Symp. on the History of Sport and Physical Education, Edmonton, Alta.

Littler, W.A., Honour, A.J., and Sleight, P. 1973. Direct arterial pressure and electrocardiogram during motor car driving. Brit. Med. J. (2), 273-7.

Lombardo, T.A., Rose, L., Taeschler, M., Tuluy, S., and Bing, R.J. 1953. The effect of exercise on coronary blood flow myocardial oxygen consumption and cardiac efficiency in man. Circulation *7*, 71-8.

Lonne, E., Lonne, C.H., Fahrenberg, J., and Roskamm, H. 1968. Pulsfrequenzmessungen und EKG Registrierung bei Autorenne. Sportarzt und Sportmedizin *19*, 103-11.

Luft, U.C., Cardus, D., Lim, T.P.K., Anderson, E.C., and Howarth, J.L. 1963. Physical performance in relation to body size and composition. Ann. N.Y. Acad. Sci. *110*, 795-808.

Luft, U.C., Finkelstein, S., and Elliott, J.C. 1972. Respiratory gas exchange, acid-base balance and electrolytes during and after maximal work breathing 15 mm Hg P_{I,CO_2}. In: CO_2 and Metabolic Regulation. In press.

Luijomba-Sengero, J.M. 1963. Venous thrombosis and pulmonary embolism. Makere Med. J. *12*, 20.

MacDiarmid, J.A. 1970. The Strathcona Trust – its influence on physical education. Proc. 1st Canad. Symp. on the History of Sport and Physical Education, Edmonton, Alta.

MacIntosh, D.L., Skrien, T., and Shephard, R.J. 1972. Physical activity and injury. A study of sports injuries at the University of Toronto, 1951-1968. J. Sports Med. *12*, 224-37.

Macklem, P.T., and Mead, J. 1967. The physiological basis of common pulmonary function tests. Arch. Env. Health *14*, 5-9.

MacNab, R.B.J., and Conger, P. 1966. Observations on the use of the Åstrand-Ryhming nomogram in university women. Paper presented to Amer. Coll. Sports Med., Madison, Wis.

Magel, J.R. 1971. Comparison of the physiological response to varying intensities of submaximal work in tethered swimming and treadmill running. J. Sports Med. Fitness *11*, 203–12.

Magnussen, H., and Scheid, P. 1974. Gas transport between dead space and alveolar space during breath-holding in man. Bull. Physiol. Pathol. Resp. *10*, 608–9.

Magora, A., and Taustein, I. 1969. An investigation of the problem of sick-leave in the patient suffering from low back pain. Industr. Med. *38*, 80–90.

Maksud, M.G., and Coutts, K.D. 1971. Application of the Cooper Twelve Minute Run-Walk Test to young males. Res. Quart. *42*, 54–9.

Malhotra, M.S., Ramaswamy, S.S., and Ray, S.N. 1962. Influence of body weight on energy expenditure. J. appl. Physiol. *17*, 433–5.

Malhotra, M.S., Sen Gupta, J., and Joseph, N.T. 1973. Comparative evaluation of different training programmes on physical fitness. Ind. J. Physiol. Pharm. *17*, 356–64.

Manguroff, J., Channe, N., and Georgieff, N. 1960. Tempo, Dosierung, Anzahl und Charakter der Ubungen für Berufsgymnastik. Vuprosi na F. z. Kult. Sofia *5*, 161 (Bulgarian). Quoted by Laporte (1966).

Mann, G.V., Shaffer, R.D., Anderson, R.S., and Sandstead, H.H. 1964. Cardiovascular disease in the Masai. J. Atherosclerosis Res. *4*, 289–312.

Mann, G.V., Teel, K., Hayes, O., McNally, A., and Bruno, D. 1955. Exercise in the disposition of dietary calories. New Engl. J. Med. *253*, 349–55.

Marcus, P. 1972. Heat acclimatization by exercise-induced elevation of body temperature. J. appl. Physiol. *33*, 283–8.

Margaria, R. 1966. An outline for setting significant tests of muscular performance. In: Human Adaptability and Its Methodology. Ed. H. Yoshimura and J.S. Weiner. Tokyo: Society for the Promotion of Sciences.

– 1967a. Anaerobic metabolism in muscle. In: Proc. Int. Symp. Physical Activity and Cardiovascular Health. Canad. Med. Assoc. J. *96*, 770–4.

– 1967b. Aerobic and anaerobic energy sources in muscular exercise. In: Exercise at Altitude. Ed. R. Margaria. Amsterdam: Excerpta Medica Fdn.

Margaria, R., Aghemo, P., and Rovelli, E. 1964. The effect of some drugs on the maximal capacity of athletic performance in man. Int. Z. angew. Physiol. *20*, 281–7.

– 1965. Indirect determination of maximal O_2 consumption in man. J. appl. Physiol. *20*, 1070–3.

Margaria, R., Aghemo, P., and Sassi, G. 1971. Effect of alkalosis on performance and lactate formation in supramaximal exercise. Int. Z. angew. Physiol. 29, 215–23.

Margaria, R., Cerretelli, P., Aghemo, P., and Sassi, G. 1963. Energy cost of running. J. appl. Physiol. 18, 367–70.

Margaria, R., Cerretelli, P., Marchi, S., and Rossi, L. 1961. Maximum exercise in oxygen. Int. Z. angew. Physiol. 18, 465–7.

Margaria, R., di Prampero, P.E., Aghemo, P., Derevenco, P., and Mariani, M. 1971. Effect of a steady state exercise on maximal anaerobic power in man. J. appl. Physiol. 30, 885–9.

Maritz, J.S., Morrison, J.F., Peter, J., Strydom, N.B., and Wyndham, C.H. 1961. A practical method of estimating an individual's maximum oxygen intake. Ergonomics 4, 97–122.

Martin, B.J., Robinson, S., Wiegman, D.L., and Aulick, L.H. 1975. Effect of warm-up on metabolic responses to strenuous exercise. Med. Sci. Sports 7, 146–9.

Martin, R.R., Lindsay, D., Despas, P., Bruce, D., Leroux, M., Anthonisen, N.R., and Macklem, P.T. 1975. The early detection of airway obstruction. Amer. Rev. Resp. Dis. 111, 119–25.

Masironi, R. 1971. Development of a multi-dial wrist-watch pulse counter. Personal communication to author.

– 1974. Determination of habitual physical activity in WHO study. I.S.C. Symp. on Daily Energy Expenditure, Bad Kissingen, April.

Massie, J., Rode, A., Skrien, T., and Shephard, R.J. 1970. A critical review of the 'Aerobics' points system. Med. Sci. Sports 2, 1–6.

Massie, J., and Shephard, R.J. 1971. Physiological and psychological effects of training. Med. Sci. Sports 3, 110–17.

Master, A.M. 1969. The Master Two-Step Test. Some historical highlights and current concepts. J. S. Carol. Med. Assoc., Suppl. (Dec.), 12–17.

Masters, E.H., and Johnson, V.E. 1966. Human Sexual Response. Boston: Little, Brown & Co. Inc.

Mayer, J. 1960. Exercise and weight control. In: Science and Medicine of Exercise and Sports, 1st ed. Ed. W.E. Johnson. New York: Harper.

– 1972. Human Nutrition. Its Physiological, Medical and Social Aspects. A Series of Eighty-two Essays. Springfield, Ill.: C.C. Thomas.

Maynard, J.E. 1976. Coronary heart disease risk factors in relation to urbanization in Alaskan Eskimo men. In: Circumpolar Health. Ed. R.J. Shephard and S. Itoh. Toronto: University of Toronto Press.

McArdle, W.D., Glaser, R.M., and Magel, J.R. 1971. Metabolic and cardiorespiratory responses during free swimming and treadmill walking. J. appl. Physiol. 30, 733–8.

McArdle, W.D., Katch, F.I., and Pechar, G.S. 1973. Comparison of continuous and discontinuous treadmill and bicycle tests for max $\dot{V}_{O_2}$. Med. Sci. Sports 5, 156-60.

McArdle, W.D., Zwiren, L., and Magel, J.R. 1969. Validity of the post-exercise heart rate as a means of estimating heart rate during work of varying intensities. Res. Quart. 40, 523-8.

McCurdy, J.H. 1928. The Physiology of Exercise. Philadelphia: Lea & Febiger.

McCurdy, J.H., and Larson, L.A. 1939. The Physiology of Exercise, 2nd ed. Philadelphia: Lea & Febiger.

McDermott, M.G. 1962. Acute respiratory effects of the inhalation of coal dust particles. J. Physiol. 162, 53p.

McDonald, G.A., and Fullerton, H.W. 1958. Effect of physical activity on increased coagulability of blood after ingestion of high-fat meal. Lancet (ii), 600-1.

McDonough, J.R., and Bruce, R.A. 1969. Maximal exercise testing in assessing cardiovascular function. In: Proc. National Conf. on Exercise in the Prevention, in the Evaluation and in the Treatment of Heart Disease. J. S. Carol. Med. Assoc. 65, Suppl. 1, 26-33.

McFarland, E.M. 1970. A historical analysis of the development of public recreation in Canadian communities. Proc. 1st Canad. Symp. on the History of Sport and Physical Education, Edmonton, Alta.

McHenry, P.L., Fisch, C., Jordan, J.W., and Corya, B.R. 1972. Cardiac arrhythmias observed during maximal treadmill exercise testing in clinically normal men. Amer. J. Cardiol. 29, 331-6.

McIntosh, P.C. 1963. Sport in Society. London: C.A. Watts.

– 1970. An historical view of sport and culture. Proc. 1st Canad. Symp. on the History of Sport and Physical Education, Edmonton, Alta.

McKee, W.P., and Bolinger, R.E. 1960. Calorie expenditure of normal and obese subjects during standard work test. J. appl. Physiol. 15, 197-200.

McKeever, W.P., Gregg, D.E., and Canney, P.C. 1958. Oxygen uptake of the non-working left ventricle. Circulation Res. 6, 612-23.

McKenzie, R.T. 1909. Exercise in Education and Medicine. Philadelphia: Saunders.

– 1916. Treatment of convalescent soldiers by physical means. Proc. Roy. Soc. Med. (Surg. Sect.) 9, 31-70.

Medalie, J.H. 1970. Current developments in the epidemiology of atherosclerosis in Israel. In: Atherosclerosis: Proc. 2nd Int. Symp. Ed. R.J. Jones. New York: Springer-Verlag.

Mellerowicz, H. 1962. Ergometrie. Munich: Von Urban & Schwarzenburg.

– 1966. Bericht über die Sitzung der Internationales Ergometrie-Standardisierungskommission. Sportarzt und Sportmedizin 8, 405-8.

– 1968. Standardisierung in der Ergometrie. In: Proc. 2nd Int. Seminar for Ergometry, Berlin.

Mellerowicz, H., Meller, W., Woweries, J., Zerdick, J., Ketusinh, O., Kral, B., and Heepe, W. 1970. Vergleichende Untersuchungen über Wirkung von Hohentraining auf die Dauerleistung in Meereshohe. Sportarzt. Sportmed. *10*, 240–.

Mendryk, S., and Dickau, G.W. 1968. The incidence of injury in athletic and physical education activities in the Edmonton school system. Paper presented at First Annual Meeting, Canad. Assoc. Sports Sciences.

Menke, F.G. 1947. The New Encyclopaedia of Sports, p. 314. New York: A.S. Barnes.

Merchant, J.A., Lumsden, J.C., Kilburn, K.H., O'Fallon, W.M., Ujda, J.R., Germino, U.H., and Hamilton, J.F. 1973. An industrial study of the biological effects of cotton dust and cigarette smoke exposure. J. occup. Med. *15*, 212–21.

Merriman, J.E. 1967. Canadian Association of Sports Sciences: historical review. Canad. Med. Assoc. J. *96*, 1340–2.

Mertens, D.J., Kavanagh, T., and Shephard, R.J. 1976. Exercise rehabilitation for chronic obstructive lung disease. Respiration (in press).

Métivier, G., and Orban, W.A.R. 1971. The physical fitness performance and work capacity of Canadian adults. Aged 18 to 44 years. Ottawa: Canad. Assoc. Physical Health Education and Recreation.

Meurman, L.O., Kiviluoto, R., and Hakama, M. 1974. Mortality and morbidity among the working population of anthophyllite asbestos miners. Brit. J. industr. Med. *31*, 105–12.

Meyer, M.B., Tonascia, J.A., and Buck, C. 1974. The inter-relationship of maternal smoking and increase of perinatal mortality with other risk factors. Further analysis of the Ontario perinatal mortality study 1960–61. Amer. J. Epidemiol. *100*, 443–52.

Meylan, G.L. 1904. Harvard University oarsmen. Harvard Grad. Mag. *9*, 362–76.

Milic-Emili, G., Cerretelli, P., Petit, J.M., and Falconi, C. 1959. La consommation d'oxygène en fonction de l'intensité de l'exercise musculaire. Arch. Int. Physiol. Biochim. *67*, 10–14.

Milic-Emili, G., Petit, J.M., and Deroanne, R. 1962. Mechanical work of breathing during exercise in trained and untrained subjects. J. appl. Physiol. *17*, 43–6.

Millahn, H.P., and Helke, H. 1968. Uber Beziehungen zwischen der Herzfrequenz während Arbeitsleistung und in der Erholungsphase in Abhängigkeit von der Leistung und der Erholungsdauer. Int. Z. angew. Physiol. *26*, 245–57.

Miller, A.T. 1952. The influence of oxygen administration on cardiovascular function during exercise and recovery. J. appl. Physiol. *5*, 165–8.

Miller, G.J., Cotes, J.E., Hall, A.M., Salvosa, C.B., and Ashworth, A. 1972. Lung function and exercise performance of healthy Caribbean men and women of African ethnic origin. Quart. J. exp. Physiol. *57*, 325–41.

Miller, W.F. 1967. Rehabilitation of patients with chronic obstructive lung disease. Med. Clin. N. America *51*, 349–61.

Millikan, G.A. 1937. Experiments on muscle haemoglobin *in vivo*; the instantaneous measurement of muscle metabolism. Proc. Roy. Soc. (Biol.) *123*, 218–41.

Mitchell, J.H., Sproule, B.J., and Chapman, C.B. 1958. The physiological meaning of the maximum oxygen intake test. J. Clin. Invest. *37*, 538–47.

Miyamoto, Y. 1972. A morphological study of flowing red cells in the capillaries. II. Red cell density and blood volume inside the capillaries of the rapidly frozen lungs in situ. Hokkaido: Monograph Ser. Res. Inst. Appl. Electricity *20*, 24–31.

Miyamoto, Y., and Moll, W. 1971. Measurement of dimension and pathway of red cells in rapidly frozen lungs in situ. Resp. Physiol. *12*, 141–56.

Mocellin, R., and Bastanier, C. 1976. Aerobic capacity and stroke volume in children with Fallot's Tetralogy after corrective surgery. In: Proc. Int. Symp. Pediatric Work Physiology. Ed. R.J. Shephard, Quebec: Pelican Press.

Mocellin, R., and Wasmund, U. 1973. Investigations on the influence of a running-training programme on the cardiovascular and motor performance capacity in 53 boys and girls of a second and third primary school class. In: Pediatric Work Physiology. Ed. O. Bar-Or. Natanya, Israel: Wingate Inst.

Mohme-Lundholm, E., Svedmyr, N., and Vamos, N. 1965. Enzymatic micromethod for determining the lactic acid content of finger-tip blood. Scand. J. clin. Lab. Invest. *17*, 501–2.

Molnar, S., Milesis, C.A. and Massey, B. 1974. Comparison of maximal oxygen consumption elicited at different treadmill grades. J. Sports Med. Phys. Fitness *14*, 85–92.

Monod, H. 1967. La validité des mesures de fréquence cardiaque en ergonomie. Ergonomics *10*, 485–537.

Montoye, H.J. 1960. Summary of research on the relationship of exercise to heart disease. Paper presented at 7th Annual Meeting, Amer. Coll. Sports Med., Miami Beach, Fla. J. Sports Med. Fitness *2*, 35–43.

– 1971. Estimation of habitual activity by questionnaire and interview. Amer. J. clin. Nutr. *24*, 1113–18.

– 1975. Physical activity and health: an epidemiologic study of an entire community. Englewood Cliffs, N.J.: Prentice-Hall.

Montoye, H.J., Van Huss, W.D., Olson, H., Hudec, A., and Mahoney, E. 1956. Study of the longevity and morbidity of college athletes. J. Amer. Med. Assoc. *162*, 1132–4.

Montoye, H.J., Van Huss, W.D., Olson, H.W., Pierson, W.O., and Hudec, A.J. 1957. The longevity and morbidity of college athletes. Michigan State University, Phi Epsilon Kappa Fraternity.

Montpetit, R.R., Montoye, H.J., and Laeding, L. 1967. Grip strength of school children, Saginaw, Michigan: 1899 and 1964. Res. Quart. *38*, 231–40.

Moody, D.L., Kollias, J., and Buskirk, E.R. 1969. Evaluation of aerobic capacity in lean and obese women with four test procedures. J. Sports Med. Fitness *9*, 1–9.

Morgan, A.D. 1968. Some forms of undiagnosed coronary disease in nineteenth century England. Med. Hist. *12*, 344–58.

Morgan, D.C., Smyth, J.T., Lister, R.W., Pethybridge, R.J., Gilson, J.C., Callaghan, P., and Thomas, G.O. 1975. Chest symptoms in farming communities with special reference to farmer's lung. Brit. J. industr. Med. *32*, 228–34.

Morgan, J.E. 1873. Critical enquiry into the after-health of the men who rowed in the Oxford and Cambridge boat race from the year 1829–1859. University Oars, cited by Hartley & Llewellyn (1939).

Morgan, R.E., and Adamson, G.T. 1965. Circuit Training, 2nd Ed. London: G. Bell & Sons.

Morgan, W.P. 1972. Ergogenic Aids and Muscular Performance. New York: Academic Press.

Morgan, W.P., Roberts, J.A., Brand, F.R., and Feinerman, A.D. 1970. Psychological effect of chronic physical activity. Med. Sci. Sports *2*, 213–17.

Morgan, W.P., Roberts, J.A., and Feinerman, A.D. 1971. Psychological effects of acute physical activity. Arch. Phys. Med. Rehab. *52*, 422–5.

Morpugo, B. 1897. Uber Aktivität-Hypertrophie der willkurlichen Muskeln. Virchows Arch. Pathol. Anat. *150*, 522–44.

Morris, J.N. 1951. Recent history of coronary disease. Lancet (i), 1–7.

Morris, J.N., Chave, S.P., Adam, C., Sirey, C., and Epstein, L. 1973. Vigorous exercise in leisure-time and the incidence of coronary heart-disease. Lancet (i), 333–9.

Morris, J.N., and Crawford, M.D. 1958. Coronary heart disease and physical activity of work; evidence of a national necropsy survey. Brit. Med. J. (ii), 1485–96.

Morris, J.N., Heady, J., and Raffle, P. 1956. Physique of London busmen. Lancet (ii), 569–70.

Morris, J.N., Heady, J., Raffle, P., Roberts, C., and Parks, J. 1953. Coronary heart disease and physical activity of work. Lancet (ii), 1053–7, 1111–20.

Morris, J.N., Kagan, A., Pattison, D.C., Gardner, M.J., and Raffle, P.A.B. 1966. Incidence and prediction of ischaemic heart disease in London busmen. Lancet (ii), 553–9.

Morris, W.H.M. 1967. Heart disease in farm workers. In: Proc. Int. Symp. on Physical Activity and Cardiovascular Health. Canad. Med. Assoc. J. *96*, 821–4.

Mostyn, E.M., Helle, S., Gee, J.B.L., Bentivoglio, L.G., and Bates, D.V. 1963. Pulmonary diffusing capacity of athletes. J. appl. Physiol. *18*, 687–95.

Muir, D.C.F. 1967. Distribution of aerosol particles in exhaled air. J. appl. Physiol. *23*, 210–14.

Mulder, G. and Mulder-Hajonides van der Meulen, W.R.E.H. 1973. Mental load and the measurement of heart rate variability. Ergonomics *16*, 69–83.

Müller, E.A. 1950. Ein Leistungs-Pulsindex als Mass der Leistungsfähigkeit. Arbeitsphysiologie *14*, 271–84.

– 1953. Physiological basis of rest pauses in heavy work. Quart. J. exp. Physiol. *38*, 205–15.

– 1963. How to keep fit during a voyage in space. New Scientist *17*, 187–9.

Müller, E.A., and Franz, H. 1952. Energieverbrauchmessungen bei beruflicher Arbeit mit einer verbesserten Respirations Gesuhr. Int. Z. angew. Physiol. *14*, 499–504.

Müller, E.A., and Himmelmann, W. 1957. Gerate zur kontinuierlichen fotoelektrischen Pulszahlung. Int. Z. angew. Physiol. *16*, 400–8.

Munro, I. 1965. The early years. In: Physical Education in Canada. Ed. M.L. Van Vliet. Scarborough, Ont.: Prentice-Hall.

Murphy, J., and Eagan, C. 1971. Effects of exercise and anabolic steroids on body and organ weights of mature rats. Nutr. Rept. Int. *4*, 65–76.

Murphy, R.J., and Ashe, W.F. 1965. Prevention of heat illness in football players. J. Amer. Med. Assoc. *194*, 650–4.

Musshoff, K., and Reindell, H. 1956. Zur Röntgenuntersuchung des Herzens in horizontal und vertikler Körperstellung; der Einfluss der Korperstellung auf das Herzvolumen. Dtsch. med. Wschr. *81*, 1001–8.

Mutimer, B.T.P. 1970. Play forms of the ancient Egyptians. Proc. 1st Canad. Symp. on the History of Sport and Physical Education, Edmonton, Alta.

Nagle, F.J., Balke, B., and Naughton, J.P. 1965. Gradational step tests for assessing work capacity. J. appl. Physiol. *20*, 745–8.

Nagle, F.J., and Irwin, L.W. 1960. Effects of two systems of weight training on circulo-respiratory endurance and related physiological factors. Res. Quart. *31*, 607–15.

Nahas, G.G. 1962. The pharmacology of tris (hydroxymethyl) amino methane (THAM). Pharmacol. Rev. *14*, 447–72.

National Health and Welfare, Canada 1964. Smoking and Health. Ottawa: Queen's Printer.

Needham, C.D., Rogan, M.C., and McDonald, I. 1954. Normal standards for lung volumes, intra-pulmonary gas mixing and maximum breathing capacity. Thorax *9*, 313–25.

Newman, F., Smalley, B.F., and Thomson, M.L. 1962. Effect of exercise, body and lung size on CO diffusion in athletes and non-athletes. J. appl. Physiol. *17*, 649–55.

Nicholas, J.J., Gilbert, R., Gabe, R., and Auchincloss, J.H. 1970. Evaluation of an exercise therapy program for patients with chronic obstructive pulmonary disease. Amer. Rev. Resp. Dis. *102*, 1–9.

Nielsen, M., and Hansen, O. 1937. Maximale körperlich Arbeit bei O_2-reicher Luft. Skand. Arch. Physiol. *76*, 37–59.

Niinimaa, V. 1976. Oxygen transport in the elderly before and after training. M.Sc. Thesis, University of Toronto.

Niinimaa, V.M.J., Wright, G., Clarke, A.J., Clapp, J., and Shephard, R.J. 1974. Physiological profile of competitive dinghy sailing. Proc. Canad. Assoc. Sports Sci., Edmonton.

Nordstrom-Ohrberg, G. 1964. Effect of digitalis glucosides on electrocardiogram and exercise test in healthy subjects. Acta med. Scand. Suppl. *420*, 1–75.

Norris, A.H., Lundy, T., and Shock, N.W. 1963. Trends in selected indices of body composition in men between the ages 30 and 80 years. Ann. N.Y. Acad. Sci. *110*, 623–39.

Nowacki, P.E. 1966. Die bedeutung des Ventilations-RQ bei ergometrischer Leistung. In: Proc. First Int. Seminar für Ergometrie, Berlin. Ed. G. Hansen. West Berlin: Inst. Sports Med.

O'Hara, W., Allen, C., and Shephard, R.J. 1976. The energy expenditure of arctic patrols. In: Circumpolar Health. Ed. R.J. Shephard and S. Itoh. Toronto: University of Toronto Press.

Olafsson, S., and Hyatt, R.E. 1969. Ventilatory mechanics and expiratory flow limitation during exercise in normal subjects. J. clin. Invest. *48*, 564–73.

Orban, W.R. (Ed.). 1972. Proc. National Conf. on Fitness and Health. Ottawa: Health and Welfare Canada.

Oscai, L.B., Molé, P.A., and Holloszy, J.O. 1971. Effects of exercise on cardiac weight and mitochondria in male and female rats. Amer. J. Physiol. *220*, 1944–8.

Oseid, S., Hövde, R., Osnes, J-B., and Hermansen, L. 1969. Circulatory responses to prolonged exercise in pre-pubertal boys. Acta physiol. Scand. Suppl. *330*.

Oseid, S., and Hermansen, L. 1973. Evaluation of physical work capacity in Norwegian female gymnasts. Brit. J. Sports Med. *7*, 38.

O'Shea, J., and Winkler, W. 1970. Biochemical and physical effects of an anabolic steroid in competitive swimmers and weightlifters. Nutr. Rept. Int. *2*, 351–62.

Otis, A.B. 1964. The work of breathing. In: Handbook of Physiology, Section 3: Respiration, Vol. 1. Ed. W.O. Fenn and H. Rahn. Washington, D.C.: Amer. Physiol. Soc.

Paez, P.N., Phillipson, E.A., Masangkay, M., and Sproule, B.J. 1967. The physiological basis of training patients with emphysema. Amer. Rev. Resp. Dis. *95*, 944–53.

Paffenbarger, R.S., and Hale, W.E. 1975. Work activity and coronary heart mortality. New Engl. J. Med. *292*, 545–50.

Paiva, M. 1973. Gas transport in the human lung. J. appl. Physiol. *35*, 401–10.

Paiva, M., and Paiva-Veretennicoff, I. 1972. Stochastic simulation of the gas diffusion in the air phase of the human lung. Bull. Math. Biophys. *34*, 457–66.

Paivio, A. 1967. Commentary. In: Int. Symp. on Physical Activity and Cardiovascular Health. Canad. Med. Assoc. J. *96*, 768.

Palmore, E. 1970. Health practices and illness among the aged. Gerontologist *10*, 313–16.

Pandolf, K.B., and Noble, B.J. 1973. The effect of pedalling speed and resistance changes on perceived exertion for equivalent power outputs on the bicycle ergometer. Med. Sci. Sports *5*, 132–6.

Panksepp, J. 1974. Hypothalamic regulation of energy balance and feeding behaviour. Fed. Proc. *33*, 1150–65.

Pappenheimer, J.C. 1950. Chairman of Committee on Standardization of Definitions and Symbols in Respiratory Physiology. Fed. Proc. *9*, 602–5.

Parizkova, J. 1964. Impact of age, diet, and exercise on man's body composition. In: International Research in Sport and Physical Education. Ed. E. Jokl and E. Simon. Springfield, Ill.: C.C. Thomas.

Parker, J.O., diGiorgi, S., and West, R.O. 1966. A hemodynamic study of acute coronary insufficiency precipitated by exercise. With observations on the effects of nitroglycerin. Amer. J. Med. *17*, 470.

Pasquis, P., Cevaer, A.M., Denis, Ph., Hellot, M.F., Pietrini, C., and Lefrancois, R. 1973. Valeurs normales du coefficient de transfert pulmonaire du CO en état stable. Bull. Physio-pathol. Resp. *9*, 553–68.

Passmore, R., and Durnin, J.V.G.A. 1955. Human energy expenditure. Physiol. Rev. *35*, 801.

Patterson, S.W., and Starling, E.H. 1914. On the mechanical factors which determine the output of the ventricles. J. Physiol. *48*, 357.

Paul, P. 1970. F.F.A. metabolism of normal dogs during steady state exercise at different work loads. J. appl. Physiol. *28*, 127–32.

Pechar, G.S., McArdle, W.D., Katch, F.I., Magel, J.R., and deLuca, J. 1974. Specificity of cardio-respiratory adaptation to bicycle and treadmill training. J. appl. Physiol. *36*, 753–6.

Perkins, J.F. 1964. Historical development of respiratory physiology. In: Handbook of Physiology, Section 3: Respiration, Vol. 1. Ed. W.O. Fenn and H. Rahn. Washington, D.C.: Amer. Physiol. Soc.

Petersen, B. 1962. The effect of training with varying work intensities on muscular strength and circulatory adaptation to work. Comm. Test. and Obs. Inst., Hellerup, Denmark *12*, 1.

Petow, H., and Siebert, W. 1925. Studien über Arbeitshypertrophie des Muskels. Z. klin. Med. *102*, 427–33.

Petty, T.L., Brink, G.A., Miller, M.W., and Corsello, P.R. 1970. Objective functional improvement in chronic airway obstruction. Chest *57*, 216–23.

Phillips, W.H., and Ross, W.D. 1967. Timing error in determining maximal oxygen uptake. Res. Quart. *38*, 315–16.

Pierce, A.K., Luterman, D., Loudermilk, J., Blomqvist, G., and Johnson, R.L. 1968. Exercise ventilatory patterns in normal subjects and patients with airway obstruction. J. appl. Physiol. *25*, 249–54.

Piiper, J., Dejours, P., Haab, P., and Rahn, H. 1971. Concepts and basic quantities in gas exchange physiology. Resp. Physiol. *13*, 292–304.

Pimm, P., and Shephard, R.J. 1976. Some physiological effects of passive exposure to cigarette smoke. A.M.A. Arch. Env. Health (in press).

Pirnay, F., Deroanne, R., and Petit, J.M. 1970. Maximal oxygen consumption in a hot environment. J. appl. Physiol. *28*, 642–5.

Pirnay, F., Deroanne, R., Marechal, R., Dujardin, J., and Petit, J.M. 1971. Consommation maximum d'oxygène dans differents types d'exercise musculaire. Arch. Int. Physiol. Biochim. *79*, 319–26.

Pirnay, F., Dujardin, J., Deroanne, R., and Petit, J.M. 1972a. Muscular exercise during intoxication by carbon monoxide. J. appl. Physiol. *31*, 573–5.

Pirnay, F., Dujardin, J., Lamy, M., Degaeque, C., Deroanne, R., and Petit, J.M. 1972b. Débit cardiaque mésuré per catheterisme au cours d'exercices musculaires intenses. Med. du Sport *46*.

Pirnay, F., Fassotte, A., Gazon, J., Deroanne, R., and Petit, J.M. 1969. Diffusion pulmonaire au cours de l'exercise musculaire. Int. Z. angew. Physiol. *28*, 31–7.

Pirnay, F., Lamy, M., Dujardin, J., Deroanne, R., and Petit, J.M. 1971. Utilisation de l'oxygène par les muscles de la jambe pendant une exercise musculaire maximum. J. Physiol. (Paris) *63*, 266–7.

Pirnay, F., Petit, J.M., Bottin, R., Deroanne, R., Juchmes, J., and Belge, G. 1966. Comparison de deux méthodes de mésure de la consommation maximum d'oxygène. Int. Z. angew. Physiol. *23*, 203–11.

Pirnay, F., Petit, J.M., and Deroanne, R. 1969. Consommation maximum d'oxygène et temperature corporelle. J. Physiol. (Paris) Suppl. *2*, 376.

Pirnay, F., Petit, J.M., Deroanne, R., and Hausman, A. 1968a. Aptitude à l'exercise musculaire sous contrainte thermique. Arch. Int. Physiol. Biochim. *76*, 867–92.

Pirnay, F., Petit, J.M., Dujardin, J., Deroanne, R., Juchmers, J., and Bottin, R. 1968b. Influence de l'amphétamine sur quelques exercises musculaires effectués par l'individu normal. Int. Z. angew. Physiol. 25, 121–9.

Piwonka, R.W., Robinson, S., Gay, V.L., and Manalis, R.S. 1965. Preacclimatization of men to heat by training. J. appl. Physiol. 20, 379–84.

Plato 1960. The Laws. Transl. by A.E. Taylor. New York: E.P. Dutton (cited by Gerber, 1972).

Pollock, M.L. 1973. The quantification of endurance training. Exercise Sport Sci. Rev. 1, 155–88.

Pollock, M.L., Cureton, T.K., and Greninger, L. 1969. Effects of frequency of training on working capacity, cardiovascular function, and body composition of adult men. Med. Sci. Sports 1, 70–4.

Poortmans, J.R. 1975. Effects of long lasting physical exercise and training on protein metabolism. In: Metabolic Adaptation to Prolonged Physical Exercise. Eds. H. Howald and J.R. Poortmans. Basel: Birkhauser Verlag.

Popejoy, D.I. 1967. The effects of a physical fitness program on selected psychological and physiological measures of anxiety. Ph.D. dissertation in Phys. Ed., Urbana, Ill.

Powles, A.C.P., Sutton, J.R., and Jones, N.L. 1974. The prediction of maximal working capacity from sub-maximal exercise testing in persons with ischaemic heart disease. Med. Sci. Sports 6, 70.

President's Council on Physical Fitness and Sports (U.S.A.). 1973. National adult physical fitness survey. Newsletter – Special Edition (May), 1–27.

Price-Jones, C. 1931. Concentration of haemoglobin in normal human blood. J. Path. Bact. 34, 779.

Pruett, E.D.R. 1970. Glucose and insulin during prolonged work stress in men living on different diets. J. appl. Physiol. 28, 199–208.

Pugh, L.G.C.E. 1962. Physiological and medical aspects of the Himalayan Scientific and Mountaineering Expedition 1960–1961. Brit. Med. J. ii, 621.

Pugh, L.G.C.E., Corbett, J.L., and Johnson, R.H. 1967. Rectal temperatures, weight losses and sweat rates in marathon runners. J. appl. Physiol. 23, 347–52.

Pugh, L.G.C.E., Edholm, O.G., Fox, R.H., Wolff, H.S., Harvey, G.R., Hammond, W.H., Tanner, J.M., and Whitehouse, R.H. 1960. A physiological study of channel swimming. Clin. Sci. 19, 257–73.

Queen's Printer 1969. Report of Task Force on Sports for Canadians. Ottawa: Queen's Printer.

Raab, W. 1964. Loafer's heart. In: International Research in Sport and Physical Education. Ed. E. Jokl and E. Simon. Springfield, Ill.: C.C. Thomas.

Raab, W., and Krzywanek, H.J. 1966. Cardiac sympathetic tone and stress response related to personality patterns and exercise habits. In: Prevention of Ischemic Heart Disease. Principles and Practice. Ed. W. Raab. Springfield, Ill.: C.C. Thomas.

Rakusan, K., Ost'adal, B., and Wachtlová, M. 1971. The influence of muscular work on the capillary density in the heart and skeletal muscle of pigeon. Canad. J. Physiol. Pharm. *49*, 167–70.

Ramanathan, N.L., and Kamon, E. 1974. The application of stair-climbing to ergometry. Ergonomics *17*, 13–22.

Ramsey, J.M. 1967. Carboxyhemoglobinemia in parking garage employees. A.M.A. Arch. Env. Health *15*, 580.

Rasch, P.J. 1964. Isometric Exercise. In: International Research in Sport and Physical Education. Ed. E. Jokl and E. Simon. Springfield, Ill.: C.C. Thomas.

– 1971. Isometric exercise and gains of muscle strength. In: Frontiers of Fitness. Ed. R.J. Shephard. Springfield, Ill.: C.C. Thomas.

Rautaharju, P.M., Friedrich, H., and Wolf, H. 1971. Measurement and interpretation of exercise electrocardiograms. In: Frontiers of Fitness. Ed. R.J. Shephard. Springfield, Ill.: C.C. Thomas.

Read, J., and Williams, R.S. 1959. Pulmonary ventilation. Blood flow relationships in interstitial disease of the lungs. Amer. J. Med. *27*, 545–50.

Rechnitzer, P.A., Paivio, A., Pickard, H.A., and Yuhasz, M.S. 1971. Long-term follow-up study of survival and recurrence rates following myocardial infarction in exercising subjects and matched controls. Med. Sci. Sports *3*, c.

Rechnitzer, P.A., Sangal, S., Cunningham, D.A., Andrew, G., Buck, C., Jones, N.L., Kavanagh, T., Parker, J.O., Shephard, R.J., and Yuhasz, M.S. 1975. A controlled prospective study of the effect of endurance training on the recurrence rate of myocardial infarction – a description of the experimental design. Amer. J. Epidemiol. *102*, 358–65.

Regan, T.J., Frank, M.J., McGinty, J.F., Zobl, E., Hellems, H.K., and Bing, R.J. 1961. Myocardial response to cigarette smoking in normal subjects and patients with coronary disease. Circulation *23*, 365–9.

Reid, L. 1960. Chronic bronchitis and hypersecretion of mucus. In: Lectures on the Scientific Basis of Medicine, *8*. London: Butterworth Scientific Publications.

Reindell, H., Klepzig, H., Steim, H., Musshoff, K., Roskamm, H., and Schildge, E. 1960. Herz Kreislaufkrankheiten und Sport. Munich: J.A. Barth.

Reindell, H., König, K., and Roskamm, H. 1966. Funktionsdiagnostik des gesunden und kranken Herzens. Stuttgart: Thieme.

Reville, P. 1970. Sport for All. Physical Activity and the Prevention of Disease. Council of Europe: Council for Cultural Cooperation.

Ribisl, P.M., and Kachadorian, W. 1969. Maximal oxygen intake prediction in young and middle-aged males. J. Sports Med. Phys. Fitness *9*, 17–22.

Rice, D.P. 1967. Estimating the cost of illness. Amer. J. Publ. Health *57*, 424–40.

Richardson, J.F., and Pincherle, G. 1969. Heights and weights of British businessmen. Brit. J. Prev. Soc. Med. *23*, 267–70.

Richardson, M. 1966. Physiological responses and energy expenditures of women using stairs of 3 designs. J. appl. Physiol. *21*, 1078-82.

Riley, R.L. 1974. Pulmonary function in relation to exercise. In: Science and Medicine of Exercise and Sport, 2nd ed. New York: Harper & Row.

Rinzler, S.H. 1968. Primary prevention of coronary heart disease by diet. Bull. N.Y. Acad. Med. *44*, 936-49.

Roberts, J., and Alspaugh, J. 1972. Specificity of training effects resulting from programs of treadmill running and bicycle ergometer riding. Med. Sci. Sports *4*, 6-10.

Roberts, M., Pirnay, F., Donea, B., André, A., and Petit, J.M. 1972. Tolerance à l'exercise musculaire après soustraction d'hématies. Arch. Int. Physiol. Biochim. *80*, 741-7.

Robinson, B.F., Epstein, S.E., Kahler, R.L., and Braunwald, E. 1966. Circulatory effects of acute expansion of blood volume: studies during maximal exercise and at rest. Circulation Res. *19*, 26-32.

Robinson, S. 1938. Experimental studies of physical fitness in relation to age. Arbeitsphysiol. *4*, 251-323.

Rochelle, R.H., Stumpner, R.L., Robinson, S., Dill, D.B., and Horvath, S.M. 1971. Peripheral blood flow response to exercise consequent to physical training. Med. Sci. Sports *3*, 122-9.

Rochmis, P., and Blackburn, H. 1971. Exercise tests. A survey of procedures, safety, and litigation experience in approximately 170,000 tests. J. Amer. Med. Assoc. *217*, 1061-6.

Rodahl, L., Åstrand, P.O., Birkhead, N.C., Hettinger, T., Issekutz, B., Jones, D.M., and Weaver, R. 1961. Physical work capacity. A study of some children and young adults in the United States. A.M.A. Arch. Env. Health *2*, 499-510.

Rode, A., and Shephard, R.J. 1971a. Cardiorespiratory fitness of an arctic community. J. appl. Physiol. *31*, 519-26.

– 1971b. The influence of cigarette smoking upon the work of breathing in near maximal exercise. Med. Sci. Sports *3*, 51-5.

– 1973a. Pulmonary function of Canadian Eskimos. Scand. J. Resp. Dis. *54*, 191-205.

– 1973b. On the mode of exercise appropriate to an arctic community. Int. Z. angew. Physiol. *31*, 187-96.

– 1973c. Fitness of the Canadian Eskimo – the influence of season. Med. Sci. Sports *5*, 170-3.

– 1973d. Growth, development and fitness of the Canadian Eskimo. Med. Sci. Sports *5*, 161-9.

– 1973e. The cardiac output, blood volume and total haemoglobin of the Canadian Eskimo. J. appl. Physiol. *34*, 91-6.

Rode, A., Ross, R., and Shephard, R.J. 1972. Smoking withdrawal program. A.M.A. Arch. Env. Health *24*, 27–36.

Röhmert, W. 1960. Ermittlung von Erholungspausen für statische Arbeit des Menschen. Int. Z. angew. Physiol. *18*, 123.

– 1968. Die Beziehung zwischen Kraft und Ausdauer bei statischer Muskelarbeit. In: Muskelarbeit und Muskel Training. Ed. W. Rohmert. Stuttgart: Gentner Verlag.

Rook, A. 1954. Investigation into longevity of Combridge sportsmen. Brit. J. Med. (i), 773–7.

Roos, A., Dahlstrom, H., and Murphy, J.P. 1955. Distribution of inspired air in the lungs. J. appl. Physiol. *7*, 645–59.

Rose, G. 1970. Current developments in Europe. In: Atherosclerosis. Proc. 2nd Int. Symp. Ed. R.J. Jones. Berlin: Springer.

Rose, G.A., and Blackburn, H. 1968. Cardiovascular survey methods. Geneva: W.H.O.

Rosen, H., Blumenthal, A., and Agersborg, H.P.K. 1962. Effects of the potassium and magnesium salts of aspartic acid on metabolic exhaustion. J. Pharm. Sci. *51*, 592.

Rosenhamer, G.J., Friesen, W.O., and McIlroy, M.B. 1971. A bloodless method for measurement of diffusing capacity of the lungs for oxygen. J. appl. Physiol. *30*, 603–10.

Roskamm, H. 1967. Optimum patterns of exercise for healthy adults. Canad. Med. Assoc. J. *96*, 895–9.

– 1973. Limits and age dependency in the adaptation of the heart to physical stress. In: Sport in the Modern World – Chances and Problems. Ed. O. Grupe, D. Kurz, and J.M. Teipel. Berlin: Springer-Verlag.

Roskamm, H. König, K., Guttel, W., Weidemann, H., Thomae, R., Lönne, E., Blumchen, G., Friedrichsen, A., and Reindell, H. 1966. Systematische Trainingsversuche auf dem Ergometer bei 80 Rekruten. Sportarzt und Sportmedizin *12*, 569.

Roskamm, H., and Reindell, H. 1972. The heart and circulation of the superior athlete. In: Training – Scientific Basis and Application. Ed. A.W. Taylor. Springfield, Ill.: C.C. Thomas.

Ross, J.C., Ley, G.D., Krumholz, R.A., and Rahbari, H. 1967. A technique for evaluation of gas mixing in the lung: Studies in cigarette smokers and non-smokers. Amer. Rev. Resp. Dis. *95*, 447–53.

Rossier, P.H., and Bühlmann, A. 1955. The respiratory dead space. Physiol. Rev. *35*, 860–76.

Rothschuh, K.E. 1973. History of Physiology. Huntington, N.Y.: Krieger.

Rottenstein, H., Peirce, G., Russ, E., Felder, O., and Montgomery, H. 1960. Influence of nicotine on the blood flow of resting skeletal muscle and of the digits in normal subjects. Ann. N.Y. Acad. Sci. *90*, 102–13.

Roughton, F.J.W. 1945. The average time spent by the blood in the human lung capillary and its relation to the rates of CO uptake and elimination in man. Amer. J. Physiol. *143*, 621–33.

Rowe, G.G., Castillo, C.A., Afonso, S., and Crumpton, C.W. 1964. Coronary flow measured by the nitrous oxide method. Amer. Heart J. *67*, 457–68.

Rowell, L.B. 1971. Visceral blood flow and metabolism during exercise. In: Frontiers of Fitness. Ed. R.J. Shephard. Springfield, Ill.: C.C. Thomas.

– 1974. Human cardiovascular adjustments to exercise and thermal stress. Physiol. Rev. *54*, 75–159.

Rowell, L.B., Blackmon, J.R., Martin, R.H., Mazzarella, J.A., and Bruce, R.A. 1967. Effects of strenuous exercise and heat stress on estimated hepatic blood flow in normal man. In: Physical Activity and the Heart. Ed. M.J. Karvonen and A.J. Barry. Springfield, Ill.: C.C. Thomas.

Rowell, L.B., Brengelmann, G.L., Blackmon, J.R., Bruce, R.A., and Murray, J.A. 1968. Disparities between aortic and peripheral pulse pressures induced by upright exercise and vasomotor changes in man. Circulation *37*, 954–64.

Rowell, L.B., Brengelmann, G.L., and Murray, J.A. 1969a. Cardiovascular responses to sustained high skin temperature in resting man. J. appl. Physiol. *27*, 673–80.

Rowell, L.B., Brengelmann, G.L., Murray, J.A., Kraning, K.K., and Kusumi, F. 1969b. Human metabolic responses to hyperthermia during mild to maximal exercise. J. appl. Physiol. *26*, 395–402.

Rowell, L.B., Marx, H.J., Bruce, R.A., Conn, R.D., and Kusumi, F. 1966. Reductions in cardiac output, central blood volume and stroke volume with thermal stress in normal men during exercise. J. clin. Invest. *45*, 1801–16.

Rowell, L.B., Taylor, H.L., and Wang, Y. 1964. Limitations to prediction of maximal oxygen intake. J. appl. Physiol. *19*, 919–27.

Royal Canadian Air Force 1962. 5BX Plan, rev. ed. Ottawa: Queen's Printer.

Royal College of Physicians 1971. Smoking and Health Now. London: Pitman.

Royce, J. 1959. Isometric fatigue curves in human muscle with normal and occluded circulation. Res. Quart. *29*, 204–12.

Rummel, J.A., Michel, E.L., and Berry, C.A. 1973. Physiological response to exercise after space flight – Apollo 7 to Apollo 11. Aerospace Med. *44*, 235–8.

Rummel, J.A., Sawin, C.F., Buderer, M.C., Mauldin, G., and Michel, E.L. 1975. Physiological response to exercise after space flight – Apollo 14 through Apollo 17. Aviat. Space Env. Med. *46*, 679–83.

Rushmer, R.F. 1959. Constancy of stroke volume in ventricular response to exertion. Amer. J. Physiol. *196*, 745–50.

Rusk, H.A. 1943. Convalescent Training Program in the Army Air Forces Hospitals. Washington, D.C.: U.S. Army Air Force Rept. (cited by Cureton, 1945).

Russell, M.A.H., Wilson, C., Patel, V.A., Feyerband, C., and Cole, P.V. 1975. Plasma nicotine levels after smoking cigarettes with high, medium and low nicotine yields. Brit. Med. J. (ii), 414–16.

Rutenfranz, J. 1964. Entwicklung und Beurteilung der Körperlichen Leistungs-fähigkeit bei Kindern und Jugendlichen. Basel: Karger.

Rutenfranz, J., Berndt, L., Frost, H., Mocellin, R., Singer, R., and Sbresny, W. 1973. Physical performance capacity determined as W_{170} in youth. In: Proc. 4th Int. Symp. on Pediatric Work Physiology, pp.245–50. Ed. O. Bar-Or. Natanya, Israel: Wingate Inst.

Ryan, A.J. 1960. The role of training and conditioning in the prevention of athletic injuries. In: Health and Fitness in the Modern World. Ed. L.A. Larson. Chicago: Athletic Inst.

– 1968. A medical history of the Olympic Games. J. Amer. Med. Assoc. *205* (11), 715–20.

– 1974. The history of sports medicine. In: Sports Medicine. Ed. A.J. Ryan and F.L. Allman. New York: Academic Press.

– 1974. Role of skills and rules in the prevention of sports injuries. In: Sports Medicine. Ed. A.J. Ryan and F.L. Allman. New York: Academic Press.

– 1974. The limits of human performance. In: Sports Medicine. Ed. A.J. Ryan and F.L. Allman. New York: Academic Press.

Ryhming, I. 1954. A modified Harvard step test for the evaluation of physical fitness. Arbeitsphysiol. *15*, 235–50.

Rylander, R. 1968. Pulmonary defence mechanisms to airborne bacteria. Acta physiol. Scand. Suppl. *306*.

Sabry, Z.I. 1973. Nutrition Canada – National Survey. Ottawa: Dept. of National Health and Welfare.

Sadoul, P., Heran, J., Arouette, A., and Grieco, B. 1966. Valeur de la puissance maximale supportée, determinée par des exercises musculaires de 20 minutes pour évaluer la capacité fonctionelle des handicapés respiratoires. Bull. Physio-pathol. Resp. *2*, 209–22.

Salter, M.A. 1971. The relationship of Lacrosse to physical survival among primitive tribes. Proc. 2nd World Symp. on the History of Sport and Physical Education, Banff, Alta.

– 1972. Mortuary games of the Eastern Culture Area. Proc. 2nd Canad. Symp. on the History of Sport and Physical Education, Windsor, Ont.

Saltin, B. 1964. Circulatory response to submaximal and maximal exercise after thermal dehydration. J. appl. Physiol. *19*, 1125–32.

– 1966. Aerobic and anaerobic work capacity at 2300 metres. Schweiz. Z. Sportmed. *14*, 81–7.

– 1972. The effect of physical training on the O_2 transporting system in man. Proc. 5th Pan-American Cong. on Sports Medicine. In: Environmental Effects on Work Performance. Ed. G.R. Cumming, A.W. Taylor, and D. Snidal. Ottawa: Canad. Assoc. Sports Sci.

– 1973. Oxygen transport by the circulatory system during exercise. In: Limiting Factors of Physical Performance. Ed. J. Keul. Stuttgart: G. Thieme.

– 1974. Energy metabolism in skeletal muscle fibres of man with exercise. Melbourne, Australia: 20th World Cong. in Sports Med.

Saltin, B., and Åstrand, P.O. 1967. Maximal oxygen uptake in athletes. J. appl. Physiol. *23*, 353–8.

Saltin, B., Blomqvist, G., Mitchell, J.H., Johnson, R.L., Wildenthal, K., and Chapman, C.B. 1968. Response to exercise after bed rest and after training. Amer. Heart Assoc. Monograph *23*, 1–68 (Circulation: 37–8, Suppl. 7).

Saltin, B., Gagge, A.P., Bergh, V., and Stolwijk, J.A.J. 1972. Body temperature and sweating during exhaustive exercise. J. appl. Physiol. *32*, 635–43.

Saltin, B., and Grimby, G. 1968. Physiological analysis of middle-aged and old former athletes: comparison with still active athletes of the same ages. Circulation *38*, 1104–15.

Saltin, B., Hartley, L.H., Kilbom, Å., and Åstrand, I. 1969. Physical training in sedentary middle-aged and older men. II. Oxygen uptake, heart rate, and blood lactate concentration at submaximal and maximal exercise. Scand. J. clin. Lab. Invest. *24*, 323–34.

Saltin, B., and Hermansen, L. 1967. Glycogen stores and prolonged severe exercise. In: Nutrition and Physical Activity. Ed. G. Blix. Uppsala: Almqvist & Wiksell.

Saltin, B., and Karlsson, J. 1971. Muscle ATP, CP, and lactate during exercise after physical conditioning. In: Muscle Metabolism during Exercise, pp.395–9. Ed. B. Pernow and B. Saltin. New York: Plenum.

– 1973. Muscle glycogen utilization during work of different intensities. In: Muscle Metabolism during Exercise. Ed. B. Pernow and B. Saltin. New York: Plenum Press.

Sargent, D.A. 1921. The physical test of a man. Amer. Phys. Ed. Rev. *26*, 188–94.

Sasajima, K. 1971. Ancient Chinese sports and games brought into Japan in ancient times and their Japanization. Proc. 2nd World Symp. on the History of Sport and Physical Education, Banff, Alta.

Sayed, J., Schaefer, O., Hildes, J.A., and Lobban, M.A. 1976. Biochemical indices of nutrient intake by Eskimos of Northern Foxe basin, NWT. In: Circumpolar Health. Ed. R.J. Shephard and S. Itoh. Toronto: University of Toronto Press.

Sawula, L.W. 1970. Etruscan dominance upon Roman physical activity. Proc. 1st Canad. Symp. on the History of Sport and Physical Education, Edmonton, Alta.

Schellberg, R. 1970. Physical feats of the Voyageurs. Proc. 1st Canad. Symp. on the History of Sport and Physical Education, Edmonton, Alta.

Scherrer, M., and Bitterli, J. 1970. Repeated estimates of D_{L,O_2} in men at different work levels. Experientia 26, 677.

Schieffer, K. 1907. Uber Herzvergrösserung infolg Redfahren. Dtsch. Arch. Klin. Med. 89, 604–25.

Schilling, J.A., Harvey, R.R., Becker, E.L., Velasquez, T., Wells, G., and Balke, B. 1956. Work performance at altitude after adaptation in man and dog. J. appl. Physiol. 8, 381–7.

Schmidt, C.F., and Comroe, J.H. 1944. Dyspnea. Mod. Concepts Cardiovasc. Dis. 13 (3).

Schnackenberg, R.C. 1973. Caffeine as a substitute for Schedule II stimulants in hyperkinetic children. Amer. J. Psychiatry 130, 796–8.

Schneider, E.C. 1920. A cardiovascular rating as a measure of physical fatigue and efficiency. J. Amer. Med. Assoc. 74, 1507–10.

Schöbel, H. 1966. The Ancient Olympic Games. London: Studio Vista.

Schreiber, S.S., Oratz, M., Evans, C.D., Gueyikian, I., and Rothschild, M.A. 1970. Myosin, myoglobin and collagen synthesis in acute cardiac overload. Amer. J. Physiol. 219, 481–6.

Schreiber, S.S., Rothschild, M.A., Evans, C., Reff, F., and Oratz, M. 1975. The effect of pressure or flow stress on right ventricular protein synthesis in the face of constant and restricted coronary perfusion. J. clin. Invest. 55, 1–11.

Scott, J.P. 1970. Sport and aggression. In: Contemporary Psychology of Sport. Ed. G.S. Kenyon. Chicago: Athletic Inst.

Scott, V.T. 1924. Study of effects of daily exercise. Military Surgeon 55, 334–6.

Scrimshire, D.A., Tomlin, P.J., and Ethridge, R.A. 1973. Computer simulation of gas exchange in human lungs. J. appl. Physiol. 34, 687–96.

Sebben, J., Pimm, P., and Shephard, R.J. 1976. Cigarette smoke in enclosed public facilities. A.M.A. Arch. Env. Health (in press).

Secher, N.H., Ruberg-Larsen, N., Binkhorst, R.A., and Bonde-Petersen, F. 1974. Maximal oxygen uptake during arm cranking and combined arm plus leg exercise. J. appl. Physiol. 36, 515–18.

Seliger, V. 1967. Energetický metabolismus u Vybraných telesných cuiceni. Fakulta Telesné Vychovy a Sportu, Charles University, Prague, Czechoslovakia.

- 1970. Physical fitness of Czechoslovak children at 12 and 15 years of age. International Biological Programme, results of investigations 1968-1969. Acta Univ. Carol. Gymnica (Prague) 5, 6-169.

Seliger, V., Bartuněk, Zd., and Trefný, Zd. 1974. Comparison of the habitual activity in two groups of boys. Int. Cong. of Pediatric Work Physiology, Seč, Czechoslovakia.

Seliger, V., Horak, J., Cermak, V., Handzo, P., Jirka, Z., Macek, M., and Skranc, O. 1973. Physical fitness of Czechoslovak populations at 12, 15, and 18 years of age. In: Physical Fitness. Ed. V. Seliger. Prague: Charles University.

Seltzer, C.C. 1966. Some re-evaluations of the build and blood pressure study, 1959, as related to ponderal index, somatotype, and mortality. New Engl. J. Med. 274, 254-9.

Sharkey, B.J. 1970. Intensity and duration of training and the development of cardio-respiratory endurance. Med. Sci. Sports 2, 197-202.

Sharkey, B.J., and Holleman, J.P. 1967. Cardio-respiratory adaptations to training at specified intensities. Res. Quart. 38, 698-704.

Sharma, S.D., Ballantyne, F., and Goldstein, S. 1974. The relationship of ventricular asynergy in coronary artery disease to ventricular premature beats. Chest 66, 358-62.

Sharman, I.M., Down, M.G., and Sen, R.N. 1971. The effect of vitamin E and training on physiological function and athletic performance in adolescent swimmers. Brit. J. Nutr. 26, 265-76.

Sharrock, N., Garrett, H.L., and Mann, G.V. 1972. Practical exercise test for physical fitness and cardiovascular performance. Amer. J. Cardiol. 30, 727-32.

Shaw, D.L., Chesney, M.A., Tullis, I.F., and Agersborg, H.P.K. 1962. Management of fatigue: A physiologic approach. Amer. J. Med. Sci. 243, 758-69.

Shaw, J.H., and Cordts, H.J. 1960. Athletic participation and academic performance. In: Science and Medicine of Sports. Ed. W.R. Johnson. New York: Harper.

Sheffield, L.T. 1974. The meaning of exercise test findings. In: Coronary Heart Disease. Prevention, Detection, Rehabilitation with Emphasis on Exercise Testing. Ed. S. Fox. Denver: Int. Med. Corp.

Sheldon, W.H., Stevens, S.S., and Tucker, W.B. 1940. The Varieties of Human Physique. New York: Harper & Row.

Shepard, R.H. 1958. Effect of pulmonary diffusing capacity on exercise tolerance. J. appl. Physiol. 12, 487-8.

Shephard, R.J. 1955. A critical examination of the Douglas bag technique. J. Physiol. 127, 515-24.

- 1956. Assessment of ventilatory efficiency by the single-breath technique. J. Physiol. 134, 630-49.

- 1957. Some factors affecting the open-circuit determination of maximum breathing capacity. J. Physiol. *135*, 98–113.
- 1959. Partitional respirometry in human subjects. J. appl. Physiol. *13*, 357–67.
- 1962. The ergonomics of the respirator. In: Design and Use of Respirators. New York: Macmillan.
- 1965. The development of cardio-respiratory fitness. Med. Services J., Canada *21*, 533–44.
- 1966a. The relative merits of the step test, bicycle ergometer, and treadmill in the assessment of cardiorespiratory fitness. Int. Z. angew. Physiol. *23*, 219–30.
- 1966b. A comparison of paramagnetic and chemical methods for the determination of oxygen. Int. Z. angew. Physiol. *22*, 279–84.
- 1966c. World standards of cardio-respiratory performance. A.M.A. Arch. Env. Health *13*, 664–72.
- 1966d. Initial 'fitness' and personality as determinants of the response to a training regime. Ergonomics *9*, 3–16.
- 1966e. Oxygen cost of breathing during vigorous exercise. Quart. J. exp. Physiol. *51*, 336–50.
- 1966f. On the timing of post-exercise pulse readings. J. Sports Med. Fitness *6*, 23–7.
- 1967a. Commentary. In: Proc. Int. Symp. on Physical Activity and Cardio-vascular Health. Canad. Med. Assoc. J. *96*, 702–3.
- 1967b. Pulse rate and ventilation as indices of metabolic load. A.M.A. Arch. Env. Health *15*, 562–7.
- 1967c. Normal levels of activity in Canadian city dwellers. Canad. Med. Assoc. J. *96*, 912–14.
- 1967d. Glossary of specialized terms and units. Canad. Med. Assoc. J. *96*, 912–14.
- 1967e. Ethical considerations in human experimentation. J. Canad. Assoc. Health, Phys. Ed., Recr. *33*, 13–16.
- 1967f. Physical performance of unacclimatized men in Mexico City. Res. Quart. *38*, 291–9.
- 1967g. The prediction of maximum oxygen intake from post-exercise pulse readings. Int. Z. angew. Physiol. *24*, 31–8.
- 1967h. The maximum sustained voluntary ventilation in exercise. Clin. Sci. *32*, 167–76.
- 1967i. The prediction of 'maximal' oxygen consumption using a new progressive step test. Ergonomics *10*, 1–15.
- 1968a. Rapporteur: Meeting of investigators on exercise tests in relation to cardiovascular function. W.H.O. Tech. Rept. *388*, Geneva, Switzerland.

- 1968b. Exercise and physical fitness. Ont. Med. Rev. *35*, 77–82.
- 1968c. A nomogram to calculate the oxygen cost of running at slow speeds. J. Sports Med. Phys. Fitness *9*, 10–16.
- 1968d. Practical indices of metabolic activity. An experimental comparison of pulse rate and ventilation. Int. Z. angew. Physiol. *25*, 13–24.
- 1968e. The heart and circulation under stress of Olympic conditions. J. Amer. Med. Assoc. *205*, 150–5.
- 1968f. Intensity, duration and frequency of exercise as determinants of the response to a training regime. Int. Z. angew. Physiol. *26*, 272–8.
- 1969a. Endurance Fitness, 1st ed. Toronto: University of Toronto Press.
- 1969b. Learning, habituation, and training. Int. Z. angew. Physiol. *28*, 38–48.
- 1969c. The validity of the oxygen conductance equation. Int. Z. angew. Physiol. *28*, 61–75.
- 1970a. For exercise testing, please. A review of procedures available to the clinician. Bull. Physio-path. Resp. *6*, 425–74.
- 1970b. The validity of the oxygen conductance equation. Int. Z. angew. Physiol. *28*, 61–75.
- 1970c. Comments on 'cardiac frequency in relation to aerobic capacity for work.' Ergonomics *13*, 509–13.
- 1970d. Computer programmes for solution of the Åstrand nomogram. J. Sports Med. Phys. Fitness *10*, 206–10.
- 1970e. Human endurance and the heart at altitude. J. Sports Med. Phys. Fitness *10*, 72–83.
- 1971a. The oxygen conductance equation. In: Frontiers of Fitness. Ed. R.J. Shephard. Springfield, Ill.: C.C. Thomas.
- 1971b. Standard tests of aerobic power. In: Frontiers of Fitness. Ed. R.J. Shephard. Springfield, Ill.: C.C. Thomas.
- 1971c. The working capacity of schoolchildren. In: Frontiers of Fitness. Ed. R.J. Shephard. Springfield, Ill.: C.C. Thomas.
- 1972a. Exercise and the lungs. In: Fitness and Exercise. Ed. J.F. Alexander, R.C. Serfass, and C.M. Tipton. Chicago: Athletic Inst.
- 1972b. Alive, Man – The Physiology of Physical Activity. Springfield, Ill.: C.C. Thomas.
- 1972c. An integrated approach to cardio-respiratory performance at sea level and at an altitude of 7350 ft. In: Environmental Effects on Work Performance. Ed. G.R. Cumming, A.W. Taylor, and D. Snidal. Ottawa: Canad. Assoc. Sports Sci.
- 1974a. A new look at aerobic power. Satellite Symp. on Exercise Physiology, Int. Union Physiol. Sci., Patiala, India, Oct.
- 1974b. What causes second wind? Physician and Sports Med., *2* (11), 36–42.

354 References

- 1974c. Work physiology and activity patterns of circumpolar Eskimos and Ainu. A synthesis of I.B.P. data. Human Biol. *46*, 263–94.
- 1974d. Sport for Youth - The Eskimo Approach. Brit. J. Sports Med. *7*, 315–16.
- 1974e. Some determinants of continuous and intermittent isometric endurance. Spor Hekimligi Dergisi *9*, 89–103.
- 1974f. Physical fitness from the viewpoint of the physiologist. Keynote address: Int. Comm. on Physical Fitness Research, Jerusalem, Israel, Aug.
- 1974 g. The dimensions of sports medicine. Canad. Med. Assoc. J. *110*, 1167–9.
- 1974h. Fitness and recreation - cost to a nation. In: Recreation for the Handicapped, pp.7–12. Ed. J. Yeo. Melbourne: Australian Council for Rehabilitation of Disabled.
- 1974i. The phenomenon of the 'second wind.' Bull. Post-grad. Comm. in Med., University of Sydney, Australia *30*, 71–83.
- 1974j. Altitude training camps. Brit. J. Sports Med. *8*, 38–45.
- 1974k. Sudden death - a significant hazard of exercise? Brit. J. Sports Med. *8*, 101–10.
- 1974l. Men at Work. Applications of Ergonomics to Performance and Design. Springfield, Ill.: C.C. Thomas.
- 1975a. Work physiology and activity patterns. In: I.B.P. Synthesis Volume: Circumpolar Peoples. Ed. F. Milan. London: Cambridge University Press.
- 1975b. Specificity versus generality: the training of the swimmer. Med. del. Sport *28*, 89–98.
- 1975c. On the prediction of athletic performance. Proc. Pan Amer. Cong. Sports Med., San Paõlo.
- 1975d. Respiratory gas exchange ratio and the prediction of aerobic power. J. appl. Physiol. *38*, 402–6.
- 1975e. Future research on the quantifying of endurance training. J. Human Ergol. *3*, 163–81.
- 1976a. For discussion - the risks of exercise. Physician and Sports Med. (in press).
- 1976b. The prediction of athletic performance. Proc. Pan Amer. Sports Cong., Porto Allegre, Brazil.
- 1976c. The Fit Athlete. Oxford: University Press.
- 1976d. Environment and sports medicine. In: Sports Medicine, 2nd ed. Ed. J. Williams and P. Sperryn. London: Arnold.
- 1976e. The working capacity of selected populations. In: International Biological Programme, Synthesis Volume *4*. Ed. J. Weiner. Cambridge, U.K.: University Press.
- 1976f. Exercise and training in chronic obstructive lung disease. Exercise Sports Sci. Rev. *5* (in press).

Shephard, R.J., Allen, C., Bar-Or, O., Davies, C.T.M., Degré, S., Hedman, R., Ishii, K., Kaneko, M., LaCour, J.R., di Prampero, P.E., and Seliger, V. 1968a. The working capacity of Toronto schoolchildren. Canad. Med. Assoc. J. *100*, 560–6, 705–14.

Shephard, R.J., Allen, C., Benade, A.J.S., Davies, C.T.M., dePrampero, P.E., Hedman, R., Merriman, J.E., Myhre, K., and Simmons, R. 1968b. The maximum oxygen intake – an international reference standard of cardio-respiratory fitness. Bull. W.H.O. *38*, 757–64.

– 1968c. Standardization of sub-maximal exercise test. Bull. W.H.O. *38*, 765–76.

Shephard, R.J., and Bar-Or, O. 1970. Alveolar ventilation in near maximum exercise. Data on pre-adolescent children and young adults. Med. Sci. Sports *2*, 83–92.

Shephard, R.J., and Callaway, S. 1966. Principal component analysis of the responses to standard exercise training. Ergonomics *9*, 141–54.

Shephard, R.J., Campbell, R., Pimm, P., Stuart, D., and Wright, G.R. 1974. Vitamin E and the recovery from physical activity. Int. Z. angew. Physiol. *33*, 119–26.

Shephard, R.J., Godin, G., and Campbell, R. 1973. Characteristics of sprint, medium and middle distance swimmers. Int. Z. angew. Physiol. *32*, 1–19.

Shephard, R.J., Hatcher, J., and Rode, A. 1973. On the body composition of the Eskimo. Europ. J. appl. Physiol. *30*, 1–13.

Shephard, R.J., and Itoh, S. 1976. Circumpolar Health. Toronto: University of Toronto Press.

Shephard, R.J., Jones, G., and Brown, J.R. 1968. Some observations on the fitness of a Canadian population. Canad. Med. Assoc. J. *98*, 977–84.

Shephard, R.J., Jones, G., Ishii, K., Kaneko, M., and Olbrecht, A.J. 1969. Factors affecting body density and the thickness of subcutaneous fat. Data on 518 Canadian city-dwellers. Amer. J. clin. Nutr. *22*, 1175–89.

Shephard, R.J., and Kavanagh, T. 1975a. Mild or intensive exercise in post-coronary rehabilitation? Proc. 20th World Cong. Sports Med., Melbourne.

– 1975b. What exercise to prescribe for the post M.I. patient. Physician and Sports Med. *3*, 56–63.

Shephard, R.J., Kavanagh, T., Conway, S., Thomson, M., and Anderson, G.H. 1976. Nutritional demands of sub-maximal work: marathon and trans Canadian events. In: Proc. Symp. on Athletic Nutrition, Warsaw (in preparation).

Shephard, R.J., Lavallée, H., Beaucage, C., Perusse, M., Rajic, M., Brisson, G., Jequier, J.C., Larivière, G., and LaBarre, R. 1975. La capacité physique des enfants canadiens: une comparaison entre les enfants canadiens-francais, canadiens-anglais et esquimaux. III. Psychologie et sociologie des enfants canadiens-français. Union Med. *104*, 1131–6.

Shephard, R.J., Lavallée, H., Larivière, G., Rajic, M., Brisson, G., Beaucage, C., Jequier, J.C., and LaBarre, R. 1974. La capacité physique des enfants canadiens:

une comparaison entre les enfants canadiens-français, canadiens-anglais et esquimaux. I. Consommation maximale d'oxygène et debit cardiaque. Union Med. *103*, 1767–77.

Shephard, R.J., Lavallée, H., Rajic, M., Jecquier, C., Beaucage, C., and LaBarre, R. 1976. Influence of added activity classes upon the working capacity of Quebec schoolchildren. Proc. VIth Int. Symp. of Pediatric Work Physiology. Québec: Pelican Press.

Shephard, R.J., and McClure, R.L. 1965. The prediction of cardiorespiratory fitness. Int. Z. angew. Physiol. *21*, 212–23.

Shephard, R.J., and Olbrecht, A.J. 1970. Body weight and the estimation of working capacity. S. Afr. Med. J. *44*, 296–8.

Shephard, R.J., and Pelzer, A.M. 1966. The working capacity of an exhibition crowd. Canad. Med. Assoc. J. *94*, 171–4.

Shephard, R.J., and Pimm, P. 1976. Physical fitness of Canadian physical education students with a note on international differences. Brit. J. Sports Med. *9*, 165–74.

Shephard, R.J., and Rode, A. 1973. Fitness for arctic life: the cardiorespiratory status of the Canadian Eskimo. In: Polar Human Biology. Ed. O.G. Edholm and E.K.E. Gunderson. Cambridge, U.K.: Heinemann.

Shephard, R.J., Rode, A., and Ross, R. 1973. Reinforcement of a smoking withdrawal program: the role of the physiologist and the psychologist. Can. J. Publ. Health *64* (Suppl.), 542–51.

Shephard, R.J., and Sidney, K.H. 1975. Effects of physical exercise on plasma growth hormone and cortisol levels in human subjects. Exercise Sport Sci. Rev. *3*, 1–30.

Shephard, R.J., Weese, C.H., and Merriman, J.E. 1971. Prediction of maximal oxygen intake from anthropometric data – some observations on pre-adolescent schoolchildren. Int. Z. angew. Physiol. *29*, 119–30.

Shepherd, J.T. 1951. Effect of cigarette smoking on blood flow through the hand. Brit. Med. J. (ii), 1007–10.

– 1963. Physiology of the Circulation in Human Limbs in Health and Disease. Philadelphia: Saunders.

Shock, N.W. 1967. Physical activity and the rate of ageing. In: Proc. Int. Symp. on Physical Activity and Cardiovascular Health. Canad. Med. Assoc. J. *96*, 836–40.

Sidney, K. 1973. Effects of frequency of training on the fitness of elderly men and women. Med. Sci. Sports *5*, 63.

Sidney, K.H. 1975. Responses of elderly subjects to a program of progressive exercise training. Ph.D. Thesis, University of Toronto.

Sidney, K.H., Eynon, R.B., and Cunningham, D.A. 1972. The effect of frequency of exercise upon physical work performance and selected variables representative of cardio-respiratory fitness. In: Training, Scientific Basis and Application, pp.144–8. Ed. A.W. Taylor. Springfield, Ill.: C.C. Thomas.

Sidney, K.H., and Shephard, R.J. 1973. Physiological characteristics and performance of the whitewater paddler. Int. Z. angew. Physiol. *32*, 55–70.

– 1975. Patterns of habitual activity in elderly city dwellers. J. Gerontol. (in press).

Siegel, W., Blomqvist, G., and Mitchell, J.H. 1970. Effects of a quantitated physical training program on middle-aged sedentary men. Circulation *41*, 19–29.

Simmons, R.C.G. 1969. Some effects of training upon cardiac output and its distribution. M.Sc. Thesis, University of Toronto.

Simmons, R., and Shephard, R.J. 1971a. Measurement of cardiac output in maximum exercise. Application of an acetylene rebreathing method to arm and leg exercise. Int. Z. angew. Physiol. *29*, 159–72.

– 1971b. Effects of physical conditioning upon the central and peripheral circulatory responses to arm work. Int. Z. angew. Physiol. *30*, 73–84.

Simonson, E. 1971. The Physiology of Work Capacity and Fatigue. Springfield, Ill.: C.C. Thomas.

Simri, V. 1969. The religious and magical function of ball games in various cultures. In: Proc. 1st Int. Seminar on the History of Physical Education and Sport, Natanya, Israel.

Sjöstrand, T. 1947. Changes in respiratory organs of workmen at ore smelting works. Acta med. Scand. *128*, Suppl. *196*, 687–99.

– 1960. Functional capacity and exercise tolerance in patients with impaired cardiovascular function. In: Clinical Cardiopulmonary Physiology. New York: Grune & Stratton.

Skinner, J.S., Holloszy, J.O., and Cureton, T.K. 1964. Effects of a program of endurance exercises on physical work capacity and anthropometric measurements of fifteen middle-aged men. Amer. J. Cardiol. *14*, 747–52.

Skinner, J.S., Hutsler, R., Bergsteinova, V., and Buskirk, E.R. 1973. The validity and reliability of a rating scale of perceived exertion. Med. Sci. Sports *5*, 94–6.

Sloan, A.W. 1963. Human physical fitness. S. Afr. J. Sci. *59*, 3–11.

– 1966. Physical fitness tests of Cape Town high-school children. S. Afr. Med. J. *40*, 682–7.

Sloan, A.W., and Hansen, J.D.L. 1969. Nutrition and physical fitness of white, coloured, and Bantu high-school children. S. Afr. Med. J. *43*, 508–11.

Smit, C.M. 1961. J. Soc. Res. *12*, 1. Quoted by Sloan 1966.

Society of Actuaries 1959. Build and Blood Pressure Study. Chicago: Society of Actuaries.

Sohar, E., and Sneh, E. 1973. Follow-up of obese patients: 14 years after a successful reducing diet. Amer. J. clin. Nutr. *26*, 845–8.

Sonnenblick, E.H., Ross, J., and Braunwald, E. 1968. Oxygen consumption of the heart. Newer concepts of its multifactoral determination. Amer. J. Cardiol. *22*, 328–36.

Southgate, D.A.T., and Shirling, D. 1970. The energy expenditure and food intake of the ship's company of a submarine. Ergonomics *13*, 777–82.

Spickard, A. 1968. Heat stroke in college football and suggestions for its prevention. South. Med. J. *61*, 791–6.

Special Committee on Aging 1966. Report of the Sub-committee on Health of the Elderly. 89th U.S. Congress. Washington, D.C.: U.S. Government Printing Office.

Spier, D.L. 1970. The influences of warfare on the recreational activities of the ancient Assyrians. Proc. 1st Canad. Symp. on the History of Sport and Physical Education, Edmonton, Alta.

Spiro, S.G., Juniper, E., Bowman, P., and Edwards, R.H.T. 1974. An increasing work rate test for assessing the physiological strain of submaximal exercise. Clin. Sci. *46*, 191–206.

Sproule, B.J., Mitchell, J.H., and Miller, W.F. 1960. Cardio-pulmonary responses to heavy exercise in patients with anemia. J. clin. Invest. *39*, 378–88.

Stainsby, W.N. 1966. Some critical oxygen tensions and their significance. In: Proc. Int. Symp. on Cardiovascular and Respiratory Effects of Hypoxia. Ed. I.D. Hatcher and D.B. Jennings. Basel: Karger.

Stainsby, W.N., and Barclay, J.K. 1970. Exercise metabolism: O_2 deficit, steady level O_2 uptake and O_2 uptake for recovery. Med. Sci. Sports *2*, 177–81.

Stainsby, W.N., Cain, S.M., and Otis, A.B. 1960. Oxygen use by dog skeletal muscle during progressive hypoxia. Fed. Proc. *19*, 380.

Stamler, J. 1971. Acute myocardial infarction – progress in primary prevention. Brit. Heart J. *33* (Suppl.), 145–64.

Staub, N.C., and Schultz, E.L. 1968. Pulmonary capillary length in dog, cat and rabbit. Resp. Physiol. *5*, 371–8.

Stefanik, P.A., Heald, F.P., and Mayer, J. 1959. Caloric intake in relation to energy output of obese and non-obese adolescent boys. Amer. J. clin. Nutr. *7*, 55–62.

Stein, E.S., Rothstein, M.S., and Clements, C.J. 1967. Calibration of two bicycle ergometers used by the health examination survey. Washington, D.C.: U.S. Dept. of Health, Education and Welfare, National Center for Health Statistics *2*, 21.

Steinhaus, A. 1933. Chronic effects of exercise. Physiol. Rev. *13*, 103–47.

– 1961. Physical education in the United States. In: L'Education physique dans le Monde. Ed. P. Seurin. Bordeaux: Editions Bière.

– 1963. Strength from Morpugo to Müller – a half century of research. In: Towards an Understanding of Health and Physical Education, pp.132–6. Dubuque, Iowa: W.C. Brown.

Steinhaus, A.H., Hoyt, L.A., and Rice, H.A. 1932. Studies in the physiology of exercise. X. The effects of running and swimming on the organ weight of growing dogs. Amer. J. Physiol. *99*, 512–20.

Stenberg, J., Åstrand, P.O. Ekblom, B., Royce, J., and Saltin, B. 1967. Hemodynamic response to work with different muscle groups sitting and supine. J. appl. Physiol. *22*, 61–70.

Stenberg, J., Ekblom, B., and Messin, R. 1966. Hemodynamic response to work at simulated altitude, 4000 m. J. appl. Physiol. *21*, 1589–94.

Steplock, D.A., Veicsteinas, A., and Mariani, M. 1971. Maximal aerobic and anaerobic power and stroke volume of the heart in a sub-alpine population. Int. Z. angew. Physiol. *29*, 203–14.

Sterling, G.M. 1967. Mechanism of bronchoconstriction caused by cigarette smoking. Brit. Med. J. (ii), 275–6.

Stevenson, J.A.F. 1967. Exercise, food intake and health in experimental animals. Canad. Med. Assoc. J. *96*, 862–6.

Stewart, W.K. 1941. Influence of drugs on ability to withstand centrifugal force. Report dated August 11th, 1941. Farnborough, U.K.: R.A.F. Physiological Laboratories.

Stibitz, G.R. 1969. Calculating diffusion in biological systems by random walks with special reference to gaseous diffusion in the lung. Resp. Physiol. 7, 230–62.

– 1973. A model of diffusion in the respiratory unit. Resp. Physiol. *18*, 249–57.

Stiles, M.H. 1967. Motivation for sports participation in the community. In: Int. Symp. on Physical Activity and Cardiovascular Health. Canad. Med. Assoc. J. *96*, 889–92.

Stoddard, G. 1974. Protective equipment. In: Sports Medicine. Ed. A.J. Ryan and F.L. Allman. New York: Academic Press.

Suzuki, S. 1970. Experimental studies on factors in growth. Soc. Res. Child Develop., Washington, Monograph *35*, 6–11.

Symposium on Nutrition, Ageing and Longevity 1965. Amer. Inst. Nutr. and Nutr. Soc. Canad. Canad. Med. Assoc. J. *93*, 893–919.

Tabakin, B.S., Hanson, J.S., and Levy, A.M. 1965. Effects of physical training on the cardiovascular response to graded upright exercise in distance runners. Brit. Heart J. *27*, 205–10.

Taguchi, S., Raven, P.B., and Horvath, S.M. 1971. Comparisons between bicycle ergometry and treadmill walking maximum capacity tests. Jap. J. Physiol. *21*, 681-90.

Tanner, J.M. 1962. Growth at Adolescence, 2nd ed., Oxford: Blackwell.

Taunton, J.E., Banister, E.W., Patrick, T.R., Oforsagd, P., and Duncan, W.R. 1970. Physical work capacity in hyperbaric environments and conditions of hyperoxia. J. appl. Physiol. *28*, 421-7.

Taylor, A. 1975. The effects of exercise and training on the activities of human glycogen cycle enzymes. In: Metabolic Adaptation to Prolonged Physical Exercise. Ed. H. Howald and J.R. Poortmans. Basel: Birkhauser Verlag.

Taylor, A.W., Stothart, J., Thayer, R., Booth, M., and Rao, S. 1974. Human skeletal muscle debranching enzyme activities with exercise and training. Europ. J. appl. Physiol. *33*, 327-30.

Taylor, H.L., Buskirk, E.R., and Henschel, A. 1955. Maximal oxygen intake as an objective measure of cardio-respiratory performance. J. appl. Physiol. *8*, 73-80.

Taylor, H.L., Haskell, W.L., Fox, S.M., and Blackburn, H. 1969. Exercise tests: a summary of procedures and concepts of stress testing for cardiovascular diagnosis and function evaluation. In: Measurement in Exercise Electrocardiography. Ed. H. Blackburn. Springfield, Ill.: C.C. Thomas.

Taylor, H.L., Henschel, A., Brozek, J., and Keys, A. 1949. The effect of bed rest on cardiovascular function and work performance. J. appl. Physiol. *2*, 223-39.

Terry, L.L. 1967. World Conference on Smoking and Health. New York: National Interagency Council on Smoking and Health.

– 1970. National Conference on Smoking and Health. New York: National Interagency Council on Smoking and Health.

Thinkaran, T., Chan, O.L., Duncan, M.T., and Klissouras, V. 1975. Absence of the influence of ethnic origin on the maximal aerobic power of Malaysians. World Cong. Sports Med., Melbourne, Australia.

Thomas, B.M., and Miller, A.T. 1958. Adaptation to forced exercise in the rat. Amer. J. Physiol. *193*, 350-4.

Thomas, C.B., Bateman, J.L., and Lindberg, E.F. 1956. Observations on the individual effects of smoking on the blood pressure, heart rate, stroke volume, and cardiac output of healthy young adults. Ann. Int. Med. *44*, 874-92.

Thomson, M.L., and Pavia, D. 1973. Long-term tobacco smoking and muco-ciliary clearance. A.M.A. Arch. Env. Health *26*, 86-90.

Thorndike, A. 1942. Athletic Injuries, Prevention, Diagnosis and Treatment. Philadelphia: Lea & Febiger.

Tillman, K. 1965. The relation between physical fitness and selected personality traits. Res. Quart. *36*, 483–9.

Tipton, C.M. 1965. Training and bradycardia in rats. Amer. J. Physiol. *209*, 1089–94.

Tipton, C.M., Martin, R.K., Matthes, R.D., and Carey, R.A. 1975. Hydroxyproline concentrations in ligaments from trained and non-trained rats. In: Metabolic Adaptation to Prolonged Physical Exercise. Ed. H. Howald and J.R. Poortmans. Basel: Birkhauser Verlag.

Tomanek, R.J. 1970. Effects of age and exercise on the extent of the mycardial capillary bed. Anat. Rec. *167*, 55–62.

Treumann, F., and Schroeder, W. 1968. Trainingseinfluss auf Muskeldurchblutung und Herzfrequenz. Z. f. Kreislauff. *57*, 1024–33.

Trivedi, B., and Danforth, W.H. 1966. Effect of pH on the kinetics of frog muscle phosphofructokinase. J. biol. Chem. *241*, 4110–12.

Turpeinen, O., Miettinen, M., Karvonen, M.J., Roine, P., Pekkarinen, M., Lehtosuo, E.J., and Alivirta, P. 1968. Dietary prevention of coronary heart disease: long term experiment. I. Observations on male subjects. Amer. J. clin. Nutr. *21*, 255–76.

Turrell, D.J., Austin, R.C., and Alexander, J.K. 1964. Cardio-respiratory response of very obese subjects to treadmill exercise. J. Lab. clin. Med. *64*, 107–16.

Tuttle, W.W. 1931. The use of the pulse-rate for rating physical efficiency. Res. Quart. *2*, 5–17.

U.S. Dept. Health, Education and Welfare 1964–68. National Centre for Health Statistics, Ser. *10*, Nos. 5, 13, 25, 37 and 43. Current Estimates from the Health Interview Survey. Washington, D.C.: Superintendent of Documents, U.S. Government Printing Office.

– 1969. Chartbook on Smoking, Tobacco and Health. Arlington, Va.: U.S. Public Health Service Pub. 1937.

U.S. Public Health Service 1964. Smoking and Health. Report of the Advisory Committee to the Surgeon General of the Public Health Service. Washington, D.C.: U.S. Public Health Service Pub. *1103*.

– 1966. Obesity and Health; a Source Book of Current Information for Professional Health Personnel. Washington, D.C.: U.S. Public Health Service Pub. *1485*.

– 1967. The Health Consequences of Smoking. A Public Health Service Review. Washington, D.C.

– 1972. The Health Consequences of Smoking. Washington: U.S. Department of Health, Education and Welfare.

Vahlquist, B. 1950. Cause of sexual differences in erythrocyte, haemoglobin, and serum iron levels in human adults. Blood *5*, 874–5.

Vale, J.R. 1970. Pulmonary gas exchange and venous-arterial shunt in normal subjects breathing oxygen at rest and during exercise. Scand. J. resp. Dis. *51*, 305–15.

Van Citters, R.L., and Franklin, D.L. 1969. Cardiovascular performance of Alaska sled dogs during exercise. Circ. Res. *24*, 33–42.

Van Dalen, D.B., and Bennett, B.L. 1971. A World History of Physical Education. Englewood Cliffs, N.J.: Prentice-Hall.

Van de Woestyne, K.P., and Zapletal, A. 1970. The maximum expiratory flow-volume curve: peak flow and effort-independent portion. In: Airway Dynamics – Physiology and Pharmacology. Ed. A. Bouhuys. Springfield, Ill.: C.C. Thomas.

Van Graan, C.H., and Greyson, J.S. 1970. A comparison between the bicycle ergometer and the step-test for determining maximum oxygen intake on Kalahari bushmen. Int. Z. angew. Physiol. *28*, 344–8.

Van Itallie, T.B., and Hashim, S.A. 1965. Avenues of control of serum cholesterol. In: Metabolism of Lipids as Related to Atherosclerosis. Ed. F.A. Kummerow. Springfield, Ill.: C.C. Thomas.

Van Itallie, T.B., Sinisterra, L., and Stare, F.J. 1960. Nutrition and athletic performance. In: Science and Medicine of Exercise and Sports. Ed. W.E. Johnson. New York: Harper.

Vannotti, A., and Magiday, M. 1934. Untersuchungen zum Studium des Capillarisierung der Trainierten Muskulatur. Arbeitsphysiol. *7*, 615–22.

Van Uytvanck, P., and Vrijens, J. 1971. Der Einfluss dynamischen und statischen Trainings auf die Entwicklung der Muskel-hypertrophie und Muskelkraft. Sportarzt und Sportmedizin *7*, 149–52.

Vejby-Christensen, H., and Petersen, E.S. 1973. Effect of body temperature on ventilatory transients at start and end of exercise. Resp. Physiol. *17*, 315–24.

Vellar, O.D., and Hermansen, L. 1971. Physical performance and hematological parameters with special reference to hemoglobin and maximal oxygen uptake. Acta med. Scand. *190*, Suppl. *522*, 1–40.

Vilnay, Z. 1969. Sport in Ancient Israel. Proc. 1st Int. Seminar on the History of Physical Education and Sport, Natanya, Israel.

Viteri, F.E., Torun, B., Galicia, J.C., and Herrera, E. 1971. Determining energy costs of agricultural activities by respirometer and energy balance techniques. Amer. J. clin. Nutr. *24*, 1418–30.

Vogel, J.A., and Gleser, M.A. 1972. Effect of carbon monoxide on oxygen transport during exercise. J. appl. Physiol. *32*, 234–9.

Voigt, E.D., Engel, P., and Klein, H. 1967. Tages rhythmische Schwankungen des Leistungspulsindex (Daily fluctuations of the performance-pulse index). German Med. Monthly *12*, 394–5.

Von Döbeln, W. 1954. A simple bicycle ergometer. J. appl. Physiol. 7, 222-4.

– 1966. Kroppsstorlek, Energiomsättning och Kondition. In: Handbok i Ergonomi. Ed. G. Luthman, U. Åberg, and N. Lundgren. Stockholm: Almqvist & Wiksell.

Von Euler, U.S. 1974. Sympatho-adrenal activity in physical exercise. Med. Sci. Sports 6, 165-73.

Von Euler, U.S., and Hellner, S. 1952. Excretion of noradrenaline and adrenaline in muscular work. Acta physiol. Scand. 26, 183-91.

Vranic, M., Kawamori, R., and Wrenshall, G.A. 1975. The role of insulin and glucagon in regulating glucose turnover in dogs during exercise. Med. Sci. Sports 7, 27-33.

Vuori, I. 1974. Studies in the feasibility of long-distance (20-90 km) ski-hikes as a mass sport. 20th World Cong. Sports Med., Melbourne, Australia.

Vyas, M.N., Banister, E.W., Morton, J.W., and Grzybowski, S. 1971. Response to exercise in patients with chronic airway obstruction. 1. Effects of exercise training. Amer. Rev. Resp. Dis. 103, 390-400.

Wade, O.L., and Bishop, J.M. 1962. Cardiac Output and Regional Blood Flow. Oxford: Blackwell.

Wade, O.L., Combes, B., Childs, A.W., Wheeler, H.O., Cournand, A., and Bradley, S.E. 1956. The effect of exercise on the splanchnic blood flow and splanchnic blood volume in normal man. Clin. Sci. 15, 457-63.

Wagner, P.D., and West, J.R. 1972. Effects of diffusion impairment on O_2 and CO_2 time courses in pulmonary capillaries. J. appl. Physiol. 33, 62-71.

Wagner, W.W., Latham, L.P., Brinkman, P.D., and Filley, G.F. 1969. Pulmonary gas transport time: larynx to alveolus. Science 163, 1210-11.

Wahlund, H. 1948. Determination of physical working capacity. Acta med. Scand. 215, Suppl. 9, 1-127.

Wald, N., Howard, S., Smith, P.G., and Kjeldsen, K. 1973. Association between atherosclerotic diseases and carboxyhaemoglobin levels in smokers. Brit. Med. J. (i), 761-5.

Wanner, A., Hirsch, J.A., Greeneltch, E., and Swenson, W. 1973. Tracheal mucous velocity after chronic exposure to cigarette smoke. Arch. Env. Health 27, 370-2.

Weibel, E.R. 1963. Morphometry of the Human Lung. New York: Academic Press; Berlin: Springer Verlag.

– 1970. Morphometric estimation of pulmonary diffusing capacity. I. Model and method. Resp. Physiol. 11, 54-75.

– 1973. A simplified morphometric method for estimating diffusing capacity in normal and emphysematous human lungs. Amer. Rev. Resp. Dis. 107, 579-88.

Weiner, J.S., and Lourie, J.A. 1969. Human Biology. A Guide to Field Methods. Oxford: Blackwell.

Weiser, P.C., Kinsman, R.A., and Stamper, D.A. 1973. Task-specific symptomatology changes resulting from prolonged submaximal bicycle riding. Med. Sci. Sports 5, 79–85.

Weiss, B., and Laties, V. 1962. Enhancement of human performance by caffeine and the amphetamines. Pharmacol. Rev. 14, 1–36.

Wen, C.P., and Gershoff, S.N. 1973. Changes in serum cholesterol and coronary heart disease mortality associated with changes in the post-war Japanese diet. Amer. J. clin. Nutr. 26, 616–19.

Wendt, V., Ajluni, R., Bruce, T.A., Prasad, A.S., and Bing, R.J. 1966. Acute effects of alcohol on the human myocardium. Amer. J. Cardiol. 17, 804–12.

Wenger, H.A., and MacNab, R.B.J. 1972. Total work intensity and duration of a training program as determinants of endurance fitness. Proc. Canad. Assoc. Sports Sci., Vancouver (in press). In: Application of Science and Medicine to Sport. Ed. A.W. Taylor. Springfield, Ill.: C.C. Thomas.

Werner, A.C., and Gottheil, E. 1966. Personality development and participation in college athletics. Res. Quart. 37, 126–31.

Wessel, J.A., Ufer, A., Van Huss, D., and Cederquist, D. 1963. Age trends of various components of body composition and functional characteristics in women aged 20–69 years. Ann. N.Y. Acad. Sci. 110, 608–22.

Wezler, K., and Böger, A. 1937. Über einen neuen Weg zur Bestimmung des absoluten Schlagvolumens des Herzens beim Menschen auf Grund der Windkesseltheorie und seine experimentelle Prüfung. Arch. exp. Path. Pharm. 184, 482–505.

Whalen, W.J., and Nair, P. 1967. Intracellular P_{O_2} and its regulation in resting skeletal muscle of the guinea pig. Circ. Res. 21, 251–61.

– 1970. Skeletal muscle pO_2: effect of inhaled and topically applied O_2 and CO_2. Amer. J. Physiol. 218, 973–80.

Wheeler, E.F., el Neil, H., Wilson, J.O., and Weiner, J.S. 1973. The effect of work level and dietary intake on water balance and the excretion of sodium, potassium and iron in a hot climate. Brit. J. Nutr. 30, 127–37.

Whipp, B.J. 1972. Oxygen uptake kinetics for various intensities of constant work load. J. appl. Physiol. 33, 351–6.

Whipp, B.J., and Wasserman, K. 1969. Alveolar-arterial gas tension differences during graded exercise. J. appl. Physiol. 27, 361–5.

White, K.L., and Ibrahim, M.A. 1963. The distribution of cardiovascular disease in the community. Ann. Int. Med. 58, 627–36.

White, N.M., Parker, W.S., Binning, R.A., Kimber, E.R., Ead, H.W., and Chamberlain, D.A. 1973. Mobile coronary care provided by ambulance personnel. Brit. Med. J. (3), 618–22.

Whitney, R.J. 1954. Circulatory changes in the forearm and hand of man with repeated exposure to heat. J. Physiol. 125, 1–24.

Wildt, K. 1971. Physical education and sports in the federal republic of Germany. A review of their development and present status. Proc. 2nd World Symp. on the History of Sport and Physical Education, Banff, Alta.

Wiley, J.F. 1971. Effects of 10 weeks of endurance training on left ventricular intervals. J. Sports Med. Phys. Fitness *11*, 104–11.

Wiley, J.F., and Shaver, L.G. 1972. Prediction of maximum oxygen intake from running performances of untrained young men. Res. Quart. *43*, 89–93.

Williams, C.G., Bredell, G.A.G., Wyndham, C.H., Strydom, N.B., Morrison, J.F., Peter, J., Fleming, P.W., and Ward, J.S. 1962. Circulatory and metabolic reactions to work in heat. J. appl. Physiol. *17*, 625–38.

Williams, C.G., Viljoen, J.H., Van Graan, C.H., and Munro, A. 1966. The influence of lubrication on the energy cost of pushing a mine car. Int. Z. angew. Physiol. *22*, 311–16.

Williams, M.H. 1974. Drugs and Athletic Performance. Springfield, Ill.: C.C. Thomas.

Williams, M.H., and Edwards, R.L. 1971. Effect of varient training regimens upon submaximal and maximal cardiovascular performance. Amer. Corr. Therapy J. *25*, 11–15.

Wilson, R.H., Meador, R.S., Jay, B.E., and Higgins, E. 1960. The pulmonary pathologic physiology of persons who smoke cigarettes. New Engl. J. Med. *262*, 956–61.

Wojtczak-Jaroszowa, J., and Banaszkiewicz, A. 1974. Physical work capacity during the day and at night. Ergonomics *17*, 193–8.

Wolf, E., Tzivani, D., and Stern, S. 1974. Comparison of exercise tests and 24-hour ambulatory electrocardiographic monitoring in detection of ST-T changes. Brit. Heart J. *36*, 90–5.

Wolff, H.S. 1958. The integrating pneumotachograph: a new instrument for the measurement of energy expenditures by indirect calorimetry. Quart. J. exp. Physiol. *43*, 270–83.

Wolff, H. 1966. Physiological measurement on human subjects in the field, with special reference to a new approach to data storage. In: Human Adaptability and Its Methodology. Ed. H. Yoshimura and J.S. Weiner. Tokyo: Japanese Society for the Promotion of Sciences.

Wood, J.E., and Bass, D.E. 1960. Responses of the veins and arterioles of the forearm to walking during acclimatization to heat in man. J. clin. Invest. *39*, 825–33.

Wood, T.D., and Cassidy, R.F. 1927. The New Physical Education. New York: Macmillan.

Woolf, C., and Suero, J.T. 1969. Alterations in lung mechanics following training in chronic obstructive lung disease. Dis. Chest *55*, 37–44.

Workman, J.M., and Armstrong, B.W. 1964. A nomogram for predicting treadmill-walking oxygen consumption. J. appl. Physiol. *19*, 150-1.

Wright, G.R., Bompa, T., and Shephard, R.J. 1975. Physiological evaluation of a winter training programme for oarsmen. J. Sports Med. Phys. Fitness (in press).

Wright, G.R., Clarke, J., Niinimaa, V., and Shephard, R.J. 1976. Some reactions to a dry-land training programme for sailors. Brit. J. Sports Med. *10*, 4-10.

Wright, G.R., Jewczyk, S., Onrot, J., Tomlinson, P., and Shephard, R.J. 1975. Carbon monoxide in the urban atmosphere. Arch. Env. Health *30*, 123-9.

Wright, G.R., Nicoletti, J., and Shephard, R.J. 1976. The selection, training, and development of youth oarsmen. Proc. VIIth Int. Pediatric Work Physiology Symp. Ed. H. Lavallée and R.J. Shephard. Quebec: Pelican Press.

Wydra, O. 1972. Influence of an anabolic steroid (Dianabol) and muscular training on skeletal muscles of the mouse. Z. Anat. Entwicklungsgesch. *136*, 73-86.

Wyman, A.H. 1913. Thesis, International Y.M.C.A. college. Cited by McCurdy (1928).

Wyndham, C.H., Benade, A.J.S., Williams, C.G., Strydom, N.B., Goldin, A., and Heyns, A.J.A. 1968. Changes in central circulation and body fluid spaces during acclimatization to heat. J. appl. Physiol. *25*, 586-93.

Wyndham, C.H., and Sluis-Cremer, G. 1968a. The capacity for physical work of white miners in South Africa. 1. The effects of age on weight and height of miners. S. Afr. Med. J. *42*, 280-6.

– 1968b. The capacity for physical work of white miners in South Africa. 2. The rates of oxygen consumption during a step test. S. Afr. Med. J. *42*, 841-4.

Wyndham, C.H., Rogers, G.G., Benade, A.J.S., and Strydom, N.B. 1971. Physiological effects of the amphetamines during exercise. S. Afr. Med. J. *45*, 247-52.

Wyndham, C.H., and Strydom, N.B. 1972. Körperliche Arbeit bei höher Temperatur. In: Zentrale Themem der Sportmedizin. Ed. W. Hollmann. Berlin: Springer Verlag.

Wyndham, C.H., Strydom, N.B., Leary, W.P., and Williams, C.G. 1966a. A comparison of methods of assessing the maximum oxygen intake. Int. Z. angew. Physiol. *22*, 285-95.

– 1966b. Studies of the maximum capacity of men for physical effort. Int. Z. angew. Physiol. *22*, 296-303, 304-10.

Wyndham, C.H., Strydom, N.B., Maritz, J.S., Morrison, J.F., Peter, J., and Potgieter, Z.V. 1959. Maximum oxygen intake and maximum heart rate during strenuous work. J. appl. Physiol. *14*, 927-36.

Wyndham, C.H., Strydom, N.B., Morrison, J.F., Williams, J.F., Bredell, C.G., and Heyns, H. 1966. The capacity for endurance effort of Bantu males from different tribes. S. Afr. J. Sci. *62*, 259-63.

Wyndham, C.H., Strydom, N.B., Von Rensburg, A.J., and Rogers, G.G. 1970. Effects on maximal oxygen intake of acute changes in altitude in a deep mine. J. appl. Physiol. *29*, 552–5.

Wyndham, C.H., Watson, M., and Sluis-Cremer, G.K. 1970. The relationship between weight and height of South African males of European descent, between the ages of 20 and 60 years. S. Afr. Med. J. *44*, 406–9.

Yakovlev, N.N. 1958. The importance of vitamins for sportsmen. Theory and Practice of Physical Education, Leningrad.

Yamabayashi, H., Takahashi, T., Tonomura, S., and Takahashi, H. 1970. An analog model of the mechanical properties of lung and airway. In: Airway Dynamics – Physiology and Pharmacology. Ed. A. Bouhuys. Springfield, Ill.: C.C. Thomas.

Yamaji, R. 1951. Studies on protein metabolism during muscular exercise. (i) Nitrogen metabolism in training for heavy muscular exercise. J. Physiol. Soc. Japan *13*, 476–89.

Yarr, A.D. 1968. Prevention of ankle and lower leg problems. Paper presented at First Annual Meeting, Canad. Assoc. Sports Sci., Toronto.

Yeager, S.A., and Bryntson, P. 1970. Effects of varying training periods on the development of cardiovascular efficiency of college women. Res. Quart. *41*, 589–92.

Young, C.M., Blondin, J., Tensuan, R., and Fryer, J.H. 1963. Body composition studies of 'older' women thirty to seventy years of age. Ann. N.Y. Acad. Sci. *110*, 589–607.

Ziegler, E. 1972. A brief chronicle of sport and physical activity for women. Proc. 2nd Canad. Symp. on the History of Sport and Physical Education, Windsor, Ont.

Zimmer, H.G., Steinkopff, G., and Gerlach, E. 1972. Changes of protein synthesis in the hypertrophying rat heart. Pflüg. Arch. *336*, 311–25.

Zitnik, R.S., Ambrosioni, E., and Shepherd, J.T. 1971. Effect of temperature on cutaneous venomotor reflexes in man. J. appl. Physiol. *31*, 507–12.

Zuhlke, V., du Mesuil, de Rochemont, W., Gudbjarnason, S., and Bing, R.J. 1966. Inhibition of protein synthesis in cardiac hypertrophy and its relation to myocardial failure. Circ. Res. *18*, 558–72.

Zuskin, E., Mitchell, C.A., and Bouhuys, A. 1974. Interaction between effects of beta blockade and cigarette smoke on airways. J. appl. Physiol. *36*, 449–52.

Zwiren, L.D., and Bar-Or, O. 1975. Responses to exercise of paraplegics who differ in conditioning level. Med. Sci. Sports 7, 94–8.

Index